Adult and Pediatric Spine Trauma

Editors

DOUGLAS L. BROCKMEYER
ANDREW T. DAILEY

NEUROSURGERY
CLINICS OF NORTH AMERICA

www.neurosurgery.theclinics.com

January 2017 • Volume 28 • Number 1

ELSEVIER

1600 John F. Kennedy Boulevard • Suite 1800 • Philadelphia, Pennsylvania, 19103-2899

http://www.theclinics.com

NEUROSURGERY CLINICS OF NORTH AMERICA Volume 28, Number 1
January 2017 ISSN 1042-3680, ISBN-13: 978-0-323-48264-6

Editor: Stacy Eastman
Developmental Editor: Colleen Viola

Neurosurgery Clinics of North America (ISSN 1042-3680) is published quarterly by Elsevier Inc., 360 Park Avenue South, New York, NY 10010-1710. Months of issue are January, April, July, and October. Business and Editorial Offices: 1600 John F. Kennedy Blvd., Suite 1800, Philadelphia, PA 19103-2899. Customer Service Office: 11830 Westline Industrial Drive, St. Louis, MO 63146. Periodicals postage paid at New York, NY, and additional mailing offices. Subscription prices are $393.00 per year (US individuals), $665.00 per year (US institutions), $423.00 per year (Canadian individuals), $826.00 per year (Canadian institutions), $505.00 per year (international individuals), $826.00 per year (international institutions), $100.00 per year (US students), and $255.00 per year (international and Canadian students). International air speed delivery is included in all *Clinics* subscription prices. All prices are subject to change without notice. **POSTMASTER:** Send address changes to *Neurosurgery Clinics of North America*, Elsevier Periodicals Customer Service, 11830 Westline Industrial Drive, St. Louis, MO 63146. **Customer Service: 1-800-654-2452 (US and Canada). From outside the US and Canada, call: 1-314-453-7041. Fax: 1-314-453-5170. E-mail: JournalsCustomerService-usa@elsevier.com (for print support) and journalsonlinesupport-usa@elsevier.com (for online support).**

Reprints. For copies of 100 or more, of articles in this publication, please contact the Commercial Reprints Department, Elsevier Inc., 360 Park Avenue South, New York, NY 10010-1710. Tel. 212-633-3874; Fax: 212-633-3820; E-mail: reprints@elsevier.com.

Neurosurgery Clinics of North America is covered in *MEDLINE/PubMed (Index Medicus), EMBASE/Excerpta Medica, and Current Contents/Clinical Medicine (CC/CM).*

Contributors

EDITORS

DOUGLAS L. BROCKMEYER, MD
Division of Pediatric Neurosurgery, Professor,
Department of Neurosurgery, Primary
Children's Hospital, University of Utah, Salt
Lake City, Utah

ANDREW T. DAILEY, MD
Professor, Department of Neurosurgery,
Clinical Neurosciences Center, University of
Utah, Salt Lake City, Utah

AUTHORS

TAMIR AILON, MD, MPH, FRCSC
Division of Neurosurgery, Vancouver Spine
Surgery Institute, University of British
Columbia, Vancouver, British Columbia,
Canada

**RICHARD C.E. ANDERSON, MD, FACS,
FAAP**
Department of Neurosurgery, Morgan Stanley
Children's Hospital, Columbia University,
New York, New York

ERICA F. BISSON, MD, MPH
Associate Professor, Department of
Neurosurgery, Clinical Neurosciences
Center, University of Utah, Salt Lake City,
Utah

BARRETT S. BOODY, MD
Resident Physician, Department of
Orthopaedic Surgery, Northwestern University,
Chicago, Illinois

NATHANIEL P. BROOKS, MD, FAANS
Assistant Professor, Department of
Neurosurgery, University of
Wisconsin – Madison, Madison, Wisconsin

STEPHANIE CHEN, MD
Resident, Department of Neurological Surgery,
The Miami Project to Cure Paralysis, University
of Miami Miller School of Medicine, Miami,
Florida

ADAM E. FLANDERS, MD
Regional Spinal Cord Injury Center of the
Delaware Valley (RSCICDV), Professor of
Radiology and Rehabilitation Medicine,
Thomas Jefferson University Hospital,
Philadelphia, Pennsylvania

GEORGE GHOBRIAL, MD
Division of Spine and Peripheral Nerve Surgery,
Department of Neurologic Surgery, Thomas
Jefferson University, Philadelphia,
Pennsylvania

HANNAH E. GOLDSTEIN, MD
Department of Neurosurgery, Morgan Stanley
Children's Hospital, Columbia University,
New York, New York

JIAN GUAN, MD
Resident, Department of Neurosurgery,
Clinical Neurosciences Center, University of
Utah, Salt Lake City, Utah

JAMES S. HARROP, MD, FACS
Director, Division of Spine and Peripheral
Nerve Surgery, Professor, Departments of
Neurologic Surgery and Orthopedic Surgery,
Neurosurgery Director of Delaware Valley SCI
Center, Thomas Jefferson University,
Philadelphia, Pennsylvania

GREGORY HAWRYLUK, MD, PhD, FRCSC
Director of Neurosurgical Critical Care;
Professor, Department of Neurosurgery,
University of Utah, Salt Lake City, Utah

WELLINGTON K. HSU, MD
Director of Research, Clifford C. Raisbeck
Distinguished Professor, Department of
Orthopaedic Surgery, Northwestern University,
Chicago, Illinois

ANDREW JEA, MD
Section of Pediatric Neurosurgery, Department
of Neurosurgery, Goodman Campbell Brain
and Spine, Professor and Chief, Indiana
University School of Medicine, Indianapolis,
Indiana

JAMES M. JOHNSTON Jr, MD
Associate Professor, Division of Pediatric
Neurosurgery, Department of Neurosurgery,
Children's of Alabama, University of Alabama
at Birmingham, Birmingham, Alabama

RICKY RAJ S. KALRA, MD
Chief Resident, Department of Neurosurgery,
Clinical Neurosciences Center, University of
Utah, Salt Lake City, Utah

ADAM S. KANTER, MD, FAANS
Chief, Neurological Surgery Spine Services,
University of Pittsburgh Medical Center, UMPC –
Presbyterian, Pittsburgh, Pennsylvania

MICHAEL KARSY, MD, PhD
Department of Neurosurgery, University of
Utah, Salt Lake City, Utah

NAVID KHEZRI, MD
Division of Neurosurgery, University of British
Columbia, Vancouver, British Columbia,
Canada

BRIAN K. KWON, MD, PhD, FRCSC
Department of Orthopaedic Spine Surgery,
Vancouver Spine Surgery Institute, University
of British Columbia, Vancouver, British
Columbia, Canada

ALLAN D. LEVI, MD, PhD
Professor and Chairman, Department of
Neurological Surgery, The Miami Project to
Cure Paralysis, University of Miami Miller
School of Medicine, Miami, Florida

CASEY J. MADURA, MD, MPH
Fellow, Division of Pediatric Neurosurgery,
Department of Neurosurgery, Children's of
Alabama, University of Alabama at
Birmingham, Birmingham, Alabama

JASON E. McGOWAN, MD
Neurosurgery Resident, Georgetown
University, Washington, DC

MATTHEW PIAZZA, MD
Resident, Department of Neurosurgery,
Hospital of the University of Pennsylvania,
Philadelphia, Pennsylvania

CHRISTIAN B. RICKS, MD
Neurosurgery Resident, University of
Pittsburgh Medical Center, Pittsburgh,
Pennsylvania

BRETT D. ROSENTHAL, MD
Resident Physician, Department of
Orthopaedic Surgery, Northwestern University,
Chicago, Illinois

MEIC H. SCHMIDT, MD, MBA
Professor, Department of Neurosurgery,
Clinical Neuroscience Center, University of
Utah, Salt Lake City, Utah

GREGORY D. SCHROEDER, MD
Department of Orthopaedic Surgery, The
Rothman Institute, Thomas Jefferson
University, Philadelphia, Pennsylvania

JAMES SCHUSTER, MD, PhD
Director of Neurotrauma, Residency Program
Director, Associate Professor, Department of
Neurosurgery, Hospital of the University of
Pennsylvania, Philadelphia, Pennsylvania

LUBDHA M. SHAH, MD
Associate Professor of Radiology, University of
Utah, Salt Lake City, Utah

VISISH SRINIVASAN, MD
Neuro-Spine Program, Division of Pediatric
Neurosurgery, Department of Neurosurgery,
Texas Children's Hospital, Baylor College of
Medicine, Houston, Texas

GEOFFREY STRICSEK, MD
Division of Spine and Peripheral Nerve Surgery,
Department of Neurologic Surgery, Thomas
Jefferson University, Philadelphia,
Pennsylvania

THANA THEOFANIS, MD
Division of Spine and Peripheral Nerve Surgery,
Department of Neurologic Surgery, Thomas
Jefferson University, Philadelphia,
Pennsylvania

ALEXANDER R. VACCARO, MD, PhD, MBA
Department of Orthopaedic Surgery, The Rothman Institute, Thomas Jefferson University, Philadelphia, Pennsylvania

JEFFERSON WILSON, MD
Division of Spine and Peripheral Nerve Surgery, Department of Neurologic Surgery, Thomas Jefferson University, Philadelphia, Pennsylvania

Contents

Preface: Adult and Pediatric Spine Trauma   xiii

Douglas L. Brockmeyer and Andrew T. Dailey

Update on New Imaging Techniques for Trauma   1

Lubdha M. Shah and Adam E. Flanders

> Computed tomography (CT) and MRI are complementary imaging modalities for the evaluation of the traumatic spine. Osseous delineation is best assessed with CT, whereas MRI gives superb soft tissue description. Awareness of the strengths and pitfalls of each modality is critical in the accurate interpretation of images. Advances in MR imaging of the spine, particularly of the spinal cord, provide glimpses into to the pathobiological mechanism of spinal cord injury. Innovative techniques relay microstructural information about the integrity of the axons and myelin sheaths. In addition to clinical status, imaging features may be helpful in prognostication and in monitoring therapeutic interventions.

Thoracolumbar Trauma Classification   23

Gregory D. Schroeder, James S. Harrop, and Alexander R. Vaccaro

> Useful thoracolumbar injury classifications allow for meaningful and concise communication between surgeons, trainees, and researchers. Although many have been proposed, none have been able to obtain universal acceptance. Historically, classifications focused only on the osseous injuries; more recent classifications focused on the injury morphology and other critical determinants of treatment, including the posterior ligamentous complex integrity and the patient's neurologic status. This review details the important historic classifications and reviews more contemporary thoracolumbar injury classifications, such as the Thoracolumbar Injury Classification System and the AOSpine Thoracolumbar Injury Classification System.

Timing of Surgery After Spinal Cord Injury   31

Matthew Piazza and James Schuster

> Although timing for surgical intervention after spinal cord injury remains controversial, there is accumulating evidence suggesting that early surgery may improve neurologic outcomes, particularly with incomplete spinal cord injury, and may reduce non-neurologic complications and health care resource utilization. Moreover, even in patients with complete spinal cord injury, minor improvement in neurologic function can lead to significant changes in quality of life. This article reviews the experimental and clinical data examining surgical timing after spinal cord injury.

Central Cord Syndrome   41

Nathaniel P. Brooks

> Central cord syndrome is a common spinal cord injury. The purpose of this review article is to provide an overview of the anatomy, pathophysiology, prognosis, and management of this disorder.

Pharmacologic Management of Acute Spinal Cord Injury   49

Michael Karsy and Gregory Hawryluk

> Spinal cord injury is a serious global public health problem that often leaves patients with devastating permanent disabilities. Although advances in supportive care have improved outcome in recent decades, there remains great need for a safe and efficacious medical treatment that improves neurologic outcome. This article reviews pharmacologic treatments evaluated or in the process of development in humans. Cellular transplantation strategies are briefly reviewed especially where they have been evaluated with pharmacologic treatments. There is great hope that one or more of these new therapeutics will be successfully translated and improve the neurologic recovery of patients in the near future.

Restorative Treatments for Spinal Cord Injury   63

Stephanie Chen and Allan D. Levi

> Spinal cord injury remains an incurable disease with an enormous impact functionally, financially, and emotionally on affected individuals and their families. Current treatment modalities are focused on minimizing secondary injury and maximizing residual function via rehabilitation. In this article, the authors discuss ambitious advancements under investigation aimed at restoring function. These promising experimental treatments focus on neuroprotection with hypothermia and pharmacologic therapies, regeneration via cell transplantation, and rewiring with electrical stimulation.

Classification and Management of Pediatric Craniocervical Injuries   73

Hannah E. Goldstein and Richard C.E. Anderson

> This article addresses the key features, clinical presentation, patterns of injury, indicated workup, and radiographic findings associated with craniocervical injuries in the pediatric population. It discusses nonsurgical and surgical management of pediatric cervical spine trauma, addressing when each is indicated, and the various techniques available to the pediatric neurosurgeon.

Classification and Management of Pediatric Subaxial Cervical Spine Injuries 91

Casey J. Madura and James M. Johnston Jr

> Appropriate management of subaxial spine injury in children requires an appreciation for the differences in anatomy, biomechanics, injury patterns, and treatment options compared with adult patients. Increased flexibility, weak neck muscles, and cranial disproportion predispose younger children to upper cervical injuries and spinal cord injury without radiographic abnormality. A majority of subaxial cervical spine injuries can be treated nonoperatively. Surgical instrumentation options for children have significantly increased in recent years. Future studies of outcomes for children with subaxial cervical spine injury should focus on injury classification and standardized outcome measures to ensure continued improvement in quality of care for this patient population.

Pediatric Thoracolumbar Spine Trauma   103

Visish Srinivasan and Andrew Jea

> This article reviews thoracolumbar injury patterns that may be seen in children. Although much of the management of these injuries has been extrapolated from

the adult literature, unique surgical and nonsurgical considerations in treating children with thoracolumbar spine fractures are discussed. In conclusion, most children achieve satisfactory outcomes in long-term follow-up after healing.

Treatment of Odontoid Fractures in the Aging Population   115

Jian Guan and Erica F. Bisson

Odontoid fractures are the most common cervical fracture type among the elderly population. Several treatment options exist for these patients, ranging from immobilization with a semirigid orthosis to surgical arthrodesis. This report reviews the key points in the management of odontoid fractures in the aged patient, including diagnosis, the various forms of conservative therapies, and the options for surgical intervention.

Treatment of Facet Injuries in the Cervical Spine   125

Navid Khezri, Tamir Ailon, and Brian K. Kwon

Facet injuries are common in the cervical spine. Many classification systems over the years have characterized the heterogeneity of these injuries. For unilateral facet fractures with minimal displacement and no neurological deficit, there is mounting evidence that better radiographic and clinical outcomes may be achieved with surgical treatment. Anterior and posterior approaches can both be utilized successfully for the surgical management of facet injuries. The anterior approach is well tolerated, allows one to address a disc herniation, and provides a high union rate with good sagittal alignment. The posterior approach allows for easier open reduction and biomechanically superior fixation.

The Role of a Miniopen Thoracoscopic-assisted Approach in the Management of Burst Fractures Involving the Thoracolumbar Junction   139

Ricky Raj S. Kalra and Meic H. Schmidt

Thoracoscopic spinal surgery is a minimally invasive open endoscopic approach to the anterior thoracolumbar spine for decompression and stabilization. It offers an alternative to open thoracotomy for thoracolumbar burst fractures, anterior spinal cord decompression, and spinal reconstruction with interbody and anterolateral plate instrumentation for restoration of biomechanical stability and alignment. Posterior instrumentation may not sufficiently stabilize a significantly disrupted anterior load-bearing spinal column, and the high access morbidity of open procedures is of significant concern. The adoption by spine surgeons of minimally invasive thoracoscopic techniques used by thoracic surgeons has expanded to include treatment of most anterior thoracolumbar disorders.

Complications in the Management of Patients with Spine Trauma   147

Geoffrey Stricsek, George Ghobrial, Jefferson Wilson, Thana Theofanis, and James S. Harrop

More than 50% of patients diagnosed with acute, traumatic spinal cord injury will experience at least 1 complication during their hospitalization. Age, severity of neurological injury, concurrent traumatic brain injury, comorbid illness, and mechanism of injury are all associated with increasing risk of complication. More than 75% of complications will occur within 2 weeks of injury. The complications associated with SCI carry a significant risk of morbidity and mortality; their early identification and management is critical in the care of the SCI patient.

Minimally Invasive Treatment of Spine Trauma   157

Jason E. McGowan, Christian B. Ricks, and Adam S. Kanter

The role for minimally invasive surgery (MIS) continues to expand in the management of spinal pathology. In the setting of trauma, operative techniques that can minimize morbidity without compromising clinical efficacy have significant value. MIS techniques are associated with decreased intraoperative blood loss, operative time, and morbidity, while providing patients with comparable outcomes when compared with conventional open procedures. MIS interventions further enable earlier mobilization, decreased hospital stay, decreased pain, and an earlier return to baseline function when compared with traditional techniques. This article reviews patient selection and select MIS techniques for those who have suffered traumatic spinal injury.

Return to Play for Athletes   163

Brett D. Rosenthal, Barrett S. Boody, and Wellington K. Hsu

Sports-related activities are associated with a variety of spinal injuries. Spine surgeons must be able to determine an athlete's readiness to return to play. Most spine surgeons agree that an athlete should be neurologically intact, be pain free, be at full strength, and have full range of motion before returning to full, unrestricted athletic activity. Certain spine injuries such as stingers may allow for return to play nearly immediately; whereas, other clinical entities such as spear tackler's spine are considered absolute contraindications to return to play.

Index   173

NEUROSURGERY CLINICS OF NORTH AMERICA

FORTHCOMING ISSUES

April 2017
Subdural Hematomas
E. Sander Connolly Jr and Guy M. McKhann II,
Editors

July 2017
Controversies in Spinal and Cranial Surgery
Russell Lonser and Daniel K. Resnick, *Editors*

October 2017
Intraoperative Imaging
J. Bradley Elder and Ganesh Rao, *Editors*

RECENT ISSUES

October 2016
Traumatic Brain Injury
Paul M. Vespa, Daniel Hirt, and
Geoffrey T. Manley, *Editors*

July 2016
Trigeminal Neuralgia
John Y.K. Lee and Michael Lim, *Editors*

April 2016
Memingiomas
Gabriel Zada and Randy L. Jensen, *Editors*

RELATED INTEREST

Emergency Medicine Clinics of North America, November 2016 (Vol. 34, Issue 4)
Neurologic Emergencies
Jonathan A. Edlow and Michael K. Abraham, *Editors*

THE CLINICS ARE AVAILABLE ONLINE!
Access your subscription at:
www.theclinics.com

Preface
Adult and Pediatric Spine Trauma

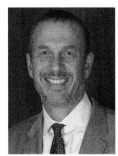
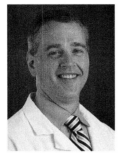

Douglas L. Brockmeyer, MD   Andrew T. Dailey, MD
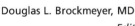
Editors

Almost all neurosurgeons manage spinal trauma in their clinical practice, and most, if not all, are comfortable with their pre-existing knowledge base. Occasionally, however, clinical situations arise in which a neurosurgeon's knowledge is incomplete or insufficient to the task at hand. For instance, questions may arise regarding the management of an odontoid fracture in an elderly patient or the best timing to surgically decompress a spinal cord injury. In those circumstances, a clinician may benefit from an authoritative, up-to-date reference that augments or complements their knowledge. The purpose of this issue of *Neurosurgery Clinics of North America* is to provide such a reference for both adult and pediatric spinal trauma. It is written by leading experts in the field and provides the busy clinician with the latest information about important areas that are either rapidly evolving or controversial in nature.

To accomplish that goal, this issue of *Neurosurgery Clinics of North America* is organized in a stepwise approach to provide maximum learning benefit. It begins with an overview of the latest advances in the imaging of spine trauma, followed by a review of thoracolumbar injury classification schemes. The next four articles discuss spinal cord injury, covering the timing of treatment, pharmacologic aspects, central cord syndrome, and restorative treatment strategies. A comprehensive review of pediatric spinal injury follows, organized into craniocervical, subaxial, and thoracolumbar sections. After that, specific treatment scenarios in adult spine trauma are addressed, including odontoid fractures, facet fractures, and minimally invasive surgery. Finally, the important topics of return to play after spinal injury and complication avoidance in spinal surgery are covered.

The editors and authors hope this issue will prove useful for every neurosurgeon. Each article has been carefully chosen to address important areas in adult and pediatric spinal trauma. We also hope that the patients we serve will benefit from the ideas and information included here.

Douglas L. Brockmeyer, MD
Department of Neurosurgery
Division of Pediatric Neurosurgery
Primary Children's Hospital
100 North Mario Capecchi Drive
Salt Lake City, UT 84113, USA

Andrew T. Dailey, MD
Department of Neurosurgery
Clinical Neurosciences Center
175 North Medical Drive East
Salt Lake City, UT 84132, USA

E-mail addresses:
douglas.brockmeyer@hsc.utah.edu
(D.L. Brockmeyer)
andrew.dailey@hsc.utah.edu (A.T. Dailey)

http://dx.doi.org/10.1016/j.nec.2016.10.001
1042-3680/17/© 2016 Published by Elsevier Inc.

neurosurgery.theclinics.com

Update on New Imaging Techniques for Trauma

Lubdha M. Shah, MD[a],*, Adam E. Flanders, MD[b]

KEYWORDS

- Computed tomography • MRI • Diffusion tensor imaging • Gradient recalled echo
- Susceptibility-weighted imaging

KEY POINTS

- Multidetector computed tomography (CT) is the first-line modality for the rapid evaluation of spinal trauma, with submillimeter axial acquisition and multiplanar reconstructions of the entire spine.
- MRI is complementary to CT in spine trauma evaluation, providing exquisite delineation of soft tissues, that is, ligamentous structures, spinal cord, and vessels.

INTRODUCTION

The first-line imaging evaluation of traumatic spine injury is computed tomography (CT). MRI offers complementary information through direct assessment of soft tissue injury to the disks, ligaments, and spinal cord, thereby obviating the inference of soft tissue damage from the mechanism of injury.[1,2] MRI allows direct examination of the injured soft tissues and provides a unique evaluation of the spinal cord. It is the modality of choice in any patient who has persistent neurologic deficit after spinal trauma. In addition, MRI can provide prognostic information by revealing intramedullary hemorrhage, which portends a poorer prognosis. As the techniques improve, even more microarchitectural and functional information can be attained to guide optimal management and prognosticate. This article focuses on the recent advances in MRI evaluation of spinal trauma.

DISCUSSION

Computed Tomography

CT is used to assess the integrity of the osseous components of the spine. Modern multidetector CT (MDCT) provides rapid assessment with a broad range of coverage in high resolution. Isotropic submillimeter axial datasets are used to create reconstructed images in sagittal and coronal planes of exceptional quality (**Fig. 1**). Different algorithms can be used to assess not only the osseous integrity but also the soft tissues for paraspinal/prevertebral and epidural hematoma (**Fig. 2**) and the lungs for pneumothorax (**Fig. 3**). Most institutions have a polytrauma protocol, which includes MDCT of the chest and abdomen, from which secondary reconstructions of the spine can be performed. The use of image reconstructions reduces radiation exposure to the patient with accurate spinal fracture detection. Roos and colleagues[3] reported 98% sensitivity and 97% specificity of spinal fracture detection with targeted multiplanar reconstructions of the thoracolumbar spine when compared with dedicated spine acquisitions.

The American College of Radiology accepts both the National Emergency X-Radiography Utilization Study and Canadian Cervical Spine Rule criteria in their appropriateness guidelines as a means of screening patients before imaging the cervical spine.[4] Cervical CT is superior to radiographs for the detection of clinically significant cervical spine injury.[5,6] Adams and colleagues[7] found CT to

The authors have no disclosures.

[a] Department of Radiology, University of Utah, 30N 1900E, Room #1A71 Salt Lake City, UT 84132, USA;
[b] Regional Spinal Cord Injury Center of the Delaware Valley, Thomas Jefferson University Hospital, Suite 1080B Main Building, 132 South Tenth Street, Philadelphia, PA 19107, USA
* Corresponding author.
E-mail address: lubdha.shah@hsc.utah.edu

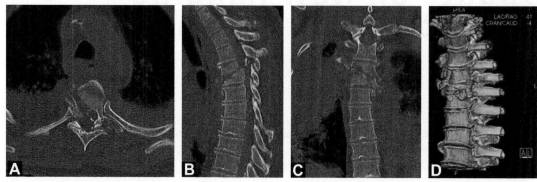

Fig. 1. Axial CT image (*A*) with sagittal (*B*) and coronal (*C*) CT reconstructions demonstrate a complex midthoracic spine fracture with flexion, distraction, and rotational pattern of injury. The T4 and T5 vertebral bodies and posterior elements show comminuted fractures with retropulsion of osseous fragments into the spinal canal. (*D*) The 3-dimensional, surface-rendered image depicts the kyphotic deformity and fracture fragment displacement.

have an overall negative predictive value of 98%, positive predictive value of 78%, and the sensitivity and specificity of 94% and 91%, respectively. A meta-analysis by Holmes and Akkinepalli[8] concluded that CT is the preferred screening method for patients with very high risk of cervical spine injury over radiography and in those patients with a significantly depressed mental status. CT allows for more rapid cervical spine clearance, thereby facilitating expedited clinical management.[9] In this way, cervical CT trauma screening is a more efficient utilization of resources and decreases patient morbidity. Although the pattern of injury on CT and biomechanical principles can suggest the extent of soft tissue injury, and although routine assessment of the CT soft tissue windows can be useful, CT is inadequate as compared with MRI as a screening modality for ligamentous and spinal cord injury. However, the value of a negative MDCT is not without merit. Hogan and colleagues[10] determined the negative predictive value of MDCT for ligament injury as 98.9% and unstable cervical spine injury as 100%. An intervertebral disk angle greater than 2 standard deviations from the average of the remaining disks offers a diagnostic accuracy of 0.972 for the detection of anterior cervical discoligamentous injury.[11] The accuracy of MDCT in detecting acute traumatic features diminishes in the background of severe degenerative disease and osteopenia (**Fig. 4**).

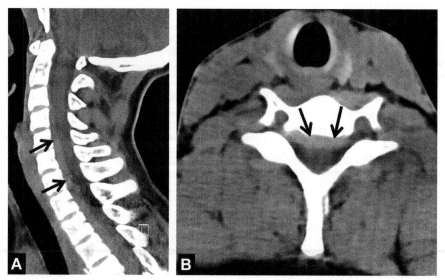

Fig. 2. Sagittal (*A*) and axial (*B*) CT images in soft tissue algorithm reveal a hyperdense epidural hematoma in the ventral thecal sac (*arrows*).

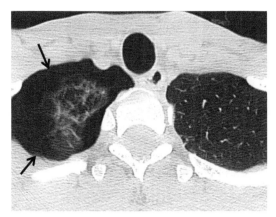

Fig. 3. Axial CT image in lung algorithm demonstrates a pneumothorax on the right (*arrows*).

MRI

MRI has a complementary role in spine trauma evaluation because it routinely depicts ligamentous, intramedullary, and vascular injury in addition to delineating extent of epidural hemorrhage. The pattern of injury on MRI can be used in clinical decision making by precisely determining areas of potential ligamentous instability as well as in characterizing severity of acute spinal cord injury.[12] MRI localizes the level of injury and degree of spinal cord compression. As the force of injury is dissipated at 1 to 2 levels, it is important to assess all tissues (eg, osseous, disk, ligamentous, neural structures) that may be affected. Soft tissue injury evaluation includes assessment of the spinal canal and nerve roots for traumatic pseudomeningocele (**Fig. 5**). MRI findings of intramedullary hemorrhage edema and spinal cord disruption in acute and subacute spinal cord injury (SCI) may contribute to the understanding of severity of injury and potential for recovery. Therefore, the management for SCI entails not only the correction of alignment but also attention to the soft tissue and cord injuries.[13,14] Timing and type of surgery may be affected by identification of MRI findings, such as traumatic disk extrusion or compressive epidural hematoma.[15–17]

Osseous Injury

MRI does not replace MDCT in the evaluation of osseous injury. Spine fractures, particularly nondisplaced types and those involving the posterior elements, can be difficult to identify on MRI.[13,18–20] This decreased sensitivity is greatest in the cervical spine and due to smaller anatomic size with less medullary space. Klein and colleagues[20] found only 11.5% sensitivity of MRI for the diagnosis of posterior element fracture as compared with 36.7% sensitivity for anterior fracture detection. Displaced fractures are easier to detect because of the osseous deformity and associated alteration in thecal sac morphology.[21]

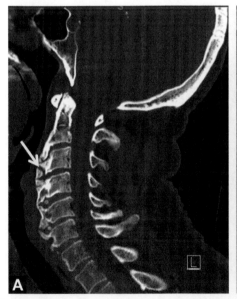
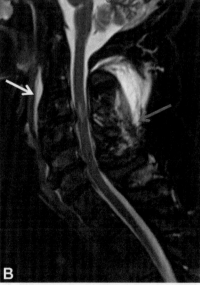

Fig. 4. This 65-year-old man sustained a hyperextension injury in a motor vehicle collision. (*A*) Sagittal CT image shows diffuse idiopathic skeletal hyperostosis. There is a fracture of an osteophyte at the C3-C4 level (*yellow arrow*). Because of upper and lower extremity weakness, an MRI was performed. (*B*) Sagittal STIR image exhibits prevertebral (*white arrow*) and interspinous (*red arrow*) edema. With hyperextension, the underlying disk-osteophyte complex at C3-C4 has caused mechanical injury (contusion) to the cord.

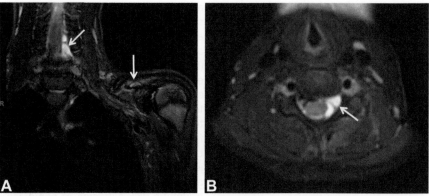

Fig. 5. Coronal STIR image (*A*) and axial T2 image with fat saturation (*B*) show left-sided C4 to C8 ventral and dorsal nerve root avulsions with posttraumatic pseudomeningoceles (*yellow arrows*). Denervation edema of the rotator cuff, superior serratus, and left paraspinal muscles is seen (*white arrow*).

However, one advantage is that MRI is sensitive to acute compressive marrow edema, which can be induced by axial loading alone without associated deformity or cortical break. The microfractures in the medullary bone with compressive injuries result in T1 hypointensity and T2 short tau inversion recovery (STIR) hyperintensity (**Fig. 6**).

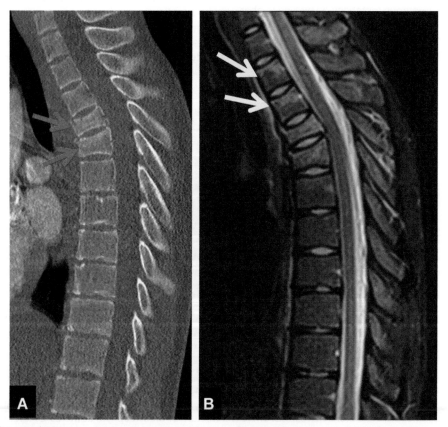

Fig. 6. (*A*) Sagittal CT image demonstrates T4 and T5 burst fractures (*red arrows*). (*B*) Sagittal STIR image also reveals edema in the T1 and T2 vertebral bodies due to acute compressive injury that is not associated with deformity of cortical break (*yellow arrows*).

Ligamentous Injury

MRI is critical for the evaluation of ligamentous integrity. An intervertebral disk angle greater than 18° on CT is concerning for anterior cervical discoligamentous injury and possible additional ligamentous injury and warrants MRI evaluation.[11] Normally, spinal ligaments appear as hypointense with respect to other structures because of their relative avascular, fibroelastic composition. Over-straining or rupture results in focal hyperintense T2/STIR signal in the ligament and in the surrounding tissues due to the increased extracellular fluid and hemorrhage (**Fig. 7**). Ligamentous incompetence may present in several ways on MRI. Overstretching of a ligamentous complex beyond normal capacity may render it incapable to resist against abnormal translation of spinal segments. As ligaments are incomplete normally in a substantial proportion of the population, ligamentous discontinuity alone is not always a reliable measure of injury.[22] Accuracy of detection of ligament injury is reportedly 90% for the supraspinous ligament and up to 97% for the interspinous ligaments.[23,24] Fat-suppressed T2-weighted sagittal sequences are sensitive and T1-weighted sequences provide specificity to ligamentous injury. Subtle damage to the facet joint synovial capsule or cartilaginous surface can be identified with MRI.

Disk Injury

Injury to the discovertebral ligamentous complex, which is a key component of the Subaxial Cervical Spine Injury Classification System,[25] is represented by abnormal T2/STIR signal in these structures (**Fig. 8**). Soft tissue algorithm of MDCT can identify disk herniations, but MRI remains more sensitive to disk abnormality. Posttraumatic disk herniations are more frequently reported in the cervical and thoracic spine.[26–28] In the cervical spine, the incidence of posttraumatic disk herniations is reported as high as 54%[29–31] and occurs more frequently with flexion-distraction and flexion-compression patterns of injury.[32] As spinal cord compression from posttraumatic disk herniation is associated with more severe neurologic injuries,[15,33] surgical management is often advocated. It can be difficult to determine the acuity of a disk herniation on MRI because an acute post-traumatic disk herniation has similar imaging features to a nontraumatic disk herniation (**Fig. 9**). Underlying spondylotic changes further add to the

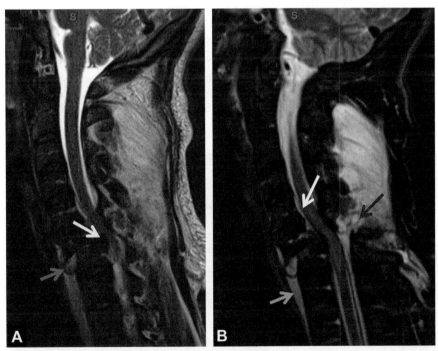

Fig. 7. (A) Sagittal T2 and (B) STIR images demonstrate a flexion-distraction injury at the C6-C7 level. Retropulsion of bone impinges on the spinal canal with cord compression (*yellow arrow*). The anterior subluxation of C6 on C7 results in anterior extrusion of the intervertebral disk material (*red arrow*). The posterior longitudinal ligament (PLL) is stripped off the C5 and C6 vertebral bodies with a small amount of epidural hemorrhage (*white arrow*). The ligamentum flavum and interspinous ligaments are disrupted (*blue arrow*). There is prevertebral edema (*green arrow*).

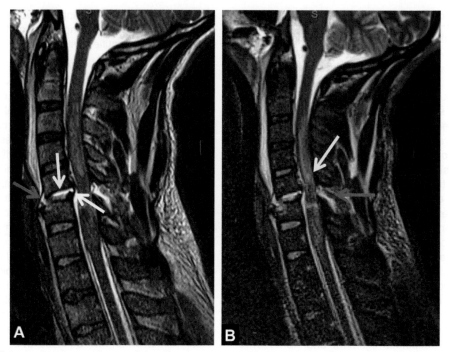

Fig. 8. (*A*) Sagittal T2 image shows a hyperflexion injury at the C6-C7 level. There is extensive injury to the dis-covertebral ligamentous complex with intradiscal T2/STIR hyperintensity (*yellow arrow*), and overstretching of the anterior longitudinal ligament (ALL) (*red arrow*) and PLL (*white arrow*). (*B*) STIR image illustrates disruption of the ligamentum flavum and interspinous ligaments (*red arrow*). There is intramedullary edema and subtle hemorrhage at the site of direct mechanical impact (*yellow arrow*).

challenge of identifying a superimposed acute disk herniation.[26] Some clues to acute disk injury are asymmetric narrowing or widening of an isolated disk space with focal intradiscal T2 hyperintensity and injury of contiguous soft tissues (**Fig. 10**).

Spinal Cord Injury

The primary role of MRI in spinal injury is that it is the only modality that provides an objective assessment of the internal cord architecture. In SCI, the initial MRI spinal cord features correlate

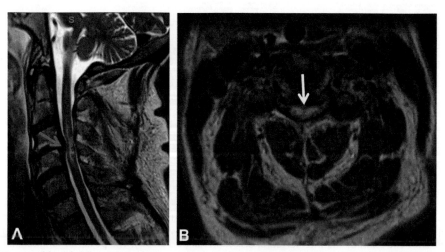

Fig. 9. A 68-year-old with bilateral upper extremity weakness after a fall. (*A*) Sagittal T2 image demonstrates a disk herniation with thickened PLL (*red arrow*) impinging on the cord at the C3-C4 level. (*B*) Axial T2 image illustrates intramedullary hyperintensity, reflecting edema (*yellow arrow*).

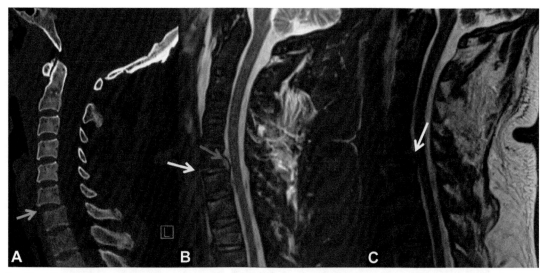

Fig. 10. (*A*) Sagittal CT shows anterior intervertebral disk space widening at C6-C7 (*green arrow*). (*B*) Sagittal STIR and (*C*) T2 images reveal a disk extrusion migrating cephalad at the C6-C7 level (*red arrow*). The ALL (*yellow arrow*) and PLL (*white arrow*) are attenuated and stretched. In addition, there are multiple upper thoracic compression fractures with marrow edema.

with the mechanical and vascular phases of injury. The secondary biochemical cascade results in growth of lesion size and intensity. In experimental studies, the abnormal signal pattern reaches maximum intensity within 3 days after injury and manifests the full MRI correlate of injury. Typically, the injured segment of spinal cord has a spindle-shaped morphology with central hemorrhage and greater surrounding edema. The degree of neurologic deficit is directly related to the severity of these MRI findings.

Spinal cord hemorrhage is commonly in the central gray matter and the point of direct mechanical impact[15,34–36] (**Fig. 11**). In the acute phase of SCI, deoxyhemoglobin predominates and appears hypointense on T2- and T2*-weighted images and isointense to slightly hyperintense on T1-weighted images (**Fig. 12**). Deoxyhemoglobin may evolve into methemoglobin at approximately 8 days, appearing as T1 and T2 hyperintense.[15,34,35] Because current, advanced MRI techniques have increased sensitivity and spatial resolution, miniscule foci of hemorrhage can be detected such that intramedullary hemorrhage is no longer predictive of complete injury and can be seen with incomplete lesions. A sizable hemorrhage (>10 mm in length) is often indicative of complete neurologic injury,[37] particularly if it is located in the cervical region.[15] Boldin and colleagues[38] found that intramedullary hemorrhage less than 4 mm in length and small length of edema were not associated with complete SCI and showed good prognosis. Frank hemorrhage implies a poor prognosis, and the level

of hemorrhage corresponds to the neurologic level of injury.[15,34,35,39,40] Residual cord compression by osseous fragments, disk, or fluid is predictive of intramedullary hemorrhage, and therefore, an important factor in determining poor neurologic recovery and is often an impetus for early surgical decompression in incomplete injuries[33] (**Fig. 13**).

Spinal cord edema is invariably present with hemorrhage but can occur in isolation, as "spinal cord contusion" (**Fig. 14**). It reflects the posttraumatic response with accumulation of intracellular and interstitial fluid.[13,15,34–36,41] There is often associated cord swelling. Spinal cord edema can enlarge the equivalent of one-third of a vertebral body height for every 8 hours due in part to the secondary phase of injury.[42]

Investigators have reported that the length of spinal cord edema is directly proportional to the degree of initial neurologic deficit.[15,30] Without hemorrhage, cord edema alone implies a more favorable prognosis.

MRI findings in SCI show a close correlation with the initial neurologic deficit. The MRI patterns of SCI offer prognostic information regarding neurologic recovery.[34,35,37,39,40,43–45] Negative prognosticators include the presence of intramedullary hemorrhage, length of hemorrhage, length edema, and cord compression.[44,46] Follow-up MRI can also offer prognostic information; those patients with persistent cord signal abnormalities demonstrate little or no clinical improvement as opposed to improvement in those with decreased or resolution of signal abnormalities.[43–45]

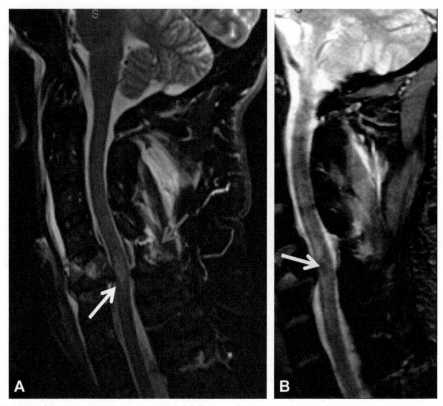

Fig. 11. (*A*) Sagittal STIR image shows a C5 burst fracture with retropulsion of the posterior cortex impinging of the cord (*white arrow*). Interspinous edema and hemorrhage are noted at the C4-C5 level (*red arrow*). (*B*) Sagittal T2* image illustrates intramedullary hemorrhage at the site of direct impact (*yellow arrow*).

The routine use of MRI in the cervical spine clearance (without neurologic injury) remains controversial, and studies suggest that MRI as part of the standard trauma protocol is not warranted.[7,10] Although MRI provides anatomic delineation of ligamentous structures, the lack of a consistent grading scheme and definition of ligamentous injury/disruption makes it a questionable modality for the assessment of ligamentous stability. However, MRI is advocated for cervical spine clearance in the unreliable patient by some investigators. Imaging findings on MRI are objective and highly reproducible, unlike the neurologic examination. In a literature review on blunt trauma patients, Sliker and colleagues[47] found that MRI detected ligamentous injury in 22.7% of population and that 80.8% of these injuries warranted treatment. Of those patients that were obtunded, 19.5% had ligamentous injuries on MRI, 69.2% of which required treatment.[47] Menaker and colleagues[48] found that MRI changed management in 7.9% of 203 CT negative patients, who did not have obvious neurologic deficits but had an unreliable clinical examination. Martinez-Perez and colleagues[49] showed that detection of ligamentous injury (particularly the

ligamentum flavum) correlates with spinal cord lesion length, and hence, may be useful in predicting neurologic outcome. Although their subjects underwent MRI within 96 hours of injury, reasoning that soft tissue injury is static and that acutely unstable patients may not be able to undergo MRI sooner, most studies have recommended that MRI be performed as soon as possible, within 24 to 72 hours of injury[34] due to the dynamic nature of intramedullary edema.[50]

MRI Safety

Imaging patients with MRI, particularly those patients with SCI, requires special considerations. SCI patients, who can be medically and neurologically unstable, require protected transfer to and from the MRI scanner and a myriad of life support, monitoring, and fixation devices. Patient factors can affect the choice of imaging hardware (ie, radiofrequency coils) and sequences. The closer a surface coil is to the area of interest, the better the signal-to-noise ratio, and therefore, the image quality. The risks need to be considered as well as the diagnostic yield of the information to be obtained from the MRI.

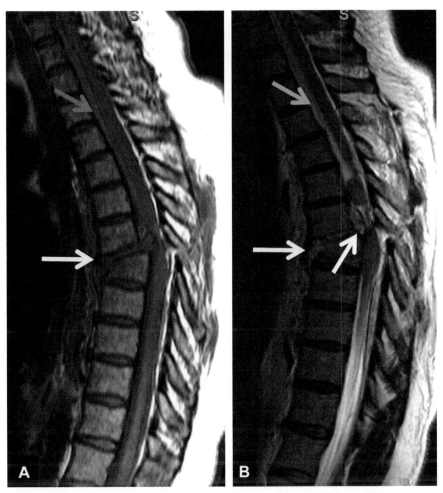

Fig. 12. (*A*) Sagittal T1 and (*B*) T2 images illustrate a T6-T7 fracture dislocation injury with near transection of the cord (*yellow arrows*). The acute epidural hemorrhage appears isointense on T1 (*red arrow*) and hyperintense on T2 (*green arrow*). There is epidural hemorrhage bowing the PLL posteriorly (*white arrow*). Hemorrhage and disk material lies subjacent to the ALL.

Conventional Imaging Sequences

Routine MRI spine protocols include sequences performed in the axial and sagittal planes (**Table 1**). Parallel imaging techniques can be used to reduce imaging time, to decrease blurring with fast spin echo (FSE)/turbo spin echo (TSE) sequences, and to lessen motion artifact.

Fluid-sensitive sequences such as T2-weighted MRI and STIR demonstrate parenchymal contusion and edema (**Fig. 15**). Note that fat-containing structures appear bright on FSE/TSE sequences; therefore, fat-suppression techniques are needed to increase the conspicuity of edema in the marrow and ligamentous structures on long repetition time sequences. FSE sequences exhibit less susceptibility artifact as compared with spin echo and gradient echo sequences. Although intramedullary hemorrhage is visualized on spin echo and FSE T2-weighted MRI,[51] it is made more conspicuous on T2*W MRI sequences, such as gradient recalled echo and susceptibility-weighted imaging (SWI) (**Fig. 16**). The presence and extent of cord edema and hemorrhage are correlated with initial neurologic impairment and predict recovery.[18,26,52,53] The superior and inferior margins of the intramedullary hemorrhage have been shown to have the strongest correlation to the neurologic level of injury,[54] whereas the borders of the cord edema showed weaker correlation. Three-dimensional volumetric acquisitions (such as SPACE, CUBE, VISTA, iso-FSE, 3D MVOX depending on the vendor) enable isotropic acquisitions that can be reformatted with equal resolution in any plane. Such sequences can provide exquisite anatomic delineation (**Fig. 17**).

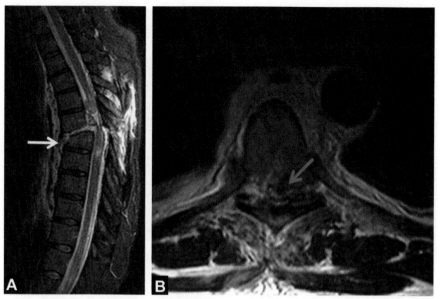

Fig. 13. (*A*) Sagittal STIR image demonstrates a T6-T7 fracture dislocation injury with near transection of the cord (*yellow arrow*). (*B*) Axial T2 image reveals severe thecal sac narrowing due to retropulsed osseous fragments and epidural hemorrhage (*red arrow*).

Vascular Imaging

Because cervical spine trauma,[55,56] particularly craniocervical distraction injury,[57] can be associated with vessel injury, imaging evaluation of the extracranial vasculature is important to assess for posttraumatic dissection of occlusion of the vertebral or carotid arteries. The proportion of patients with clinically symptomatic posttraumatic vascular injury is small, thus not justifying the procedural risks of conventional angiography for all patients with cervical spine trauma. However, evaluation for vascular occlusion, dissection, or significant vasospasm

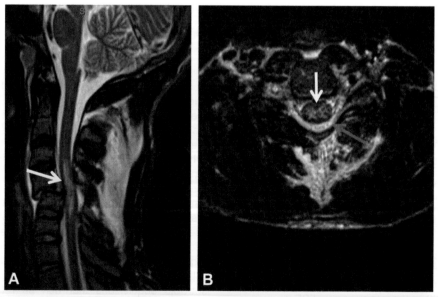

Fig. 14. (*A*) Sagittal T2 image shows a flexion-distraction injury at C4-C5 with cord contusion (*yellow arrow*). The subluxation results in spindle-shaped cord edema and mild swelling. There is ligamentum flavum and interspinous disruption with edema and hemorrhage. (*B*) Axial T2 image reveals hyperintense epidural hemorrhage (*red arrow*) and intramedullary edema (*white arrow*).

Table 1
Standard MRI sequences

MRI Sequence	Information
T1-weighted	Anatomy, hypointense marrow edema in acute fracture, iso-intense to hyperintense epidural hemorrhage
T2-weighted (FSE or TSE)	SCI, ligamentous injury, disk herniation; marrow edema may be masked by unsuppressed fat
Proton density	Ligamentous integrity, epidural collections
STIR	SCI, ligamentous injury, disk herniation, marrow edema
T2*-weighted (gradient echo)	Intramedullary hemorrhage, epidural collections

can be performed with CT angiography or MR angiography. Axial T1 images with fat-saturation or black-blood techniques are helpful to detect subtle subintimal dissection[58,59] (**Fig. 18**).

Advanced Imaging

New MRI techniques such as ultrashort echo time (UTE) imaging can extract signals from structures, such as ligaments, that normally elicit little to no signal using conventional pulse sequences.[60] UTE may be useful to detect subtle ligamentous injury.

Imaging findings on conventional MRI reflect changes in the water content or hemorrhage with SCI. In animal models, lesion length, cord caliber,

and the degree of white matter (WM) preservation on cross-section MRI have a significant relationship not only to pathologic findings but also to functional status.[61–63] However, animal studies also suggest that anatomic MRI techniques do not accurately depict the full extent of injury.[64,65] A significant shortcoming of clinical MRI is its limited capability in demonstrating functionally preserved WM tracts at the level of injury. Newer diffusion-weighted techniques have the ability to assess the integrity of spinal cord WM.

Diffusion-Weighted Imaging and Diffusion-Tensor Imaging

Diffusion-weighted imaging (DWI) exploits free water proton diffusion as a contrast-determining parameter. Diffusion tensor imaging (DTI) solves for proton diffusion in orthogonal directions by measuring diffusion in multiple different directions, which are represented by directional and magnitude vectors. Simple fluid diffuses in equal magnitude in all directions as isotropic diffusion. Cellular structures and membranes inhibit free water diffusion. Myelinated axons preferentially diffuse water along their long axis as relative anisotropy. DTI is able to investigate the 3-dimensional microstructural anatomy of WM and directionality by measuring the anisotropic diffusion of water in the WM. Hydrophobic myelin directs molecular water diffusion preferentially parallel to the long axis of the axon. This diffusion of water along the axis of the axon results in a high longitudinal apparent diffusion coefficient (lADC) and a low transverse apparent diffusion (tADC) coefficient. Several additional DTI metrics can provide

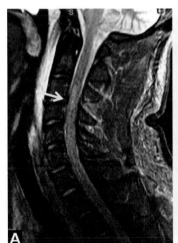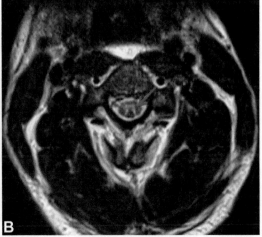

Fig. 15. This 33-year-old man experienced sudden upper and lower extremity weakness after a trampoline accident. (*A*) Sagittal STIR image depicts a traumatic disk protrusion at C3-C4 (*yellow arrow*). There is intramedullary T2 hyperintensity. (*B*) The contusion is more conspicuous on the axial T2 image (*red arrow*).

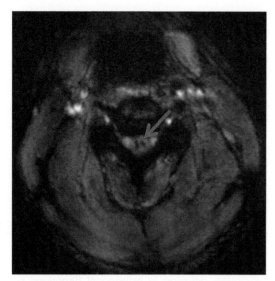

Fig. 16. This 33-year-old man experienced sudden upper and lower extremity weakness after a trampoline accident. Axial T2* image reveals intramedullary hemorrhage (*red arrow*) due to a traumatic disk herniation.

information about WM microstructure. Fractional anisotropy (FA) is a marker of both axonal density[66] and myelin content.[67] It also describes the relative directionality of molecular motion of water, with values ranging between 0 (isotropic) and 1 (anisotropic) (**Fig. 19**). Axial diffusivity (AD) and radial diffusivity (RD) reflect the integrity of axons and myelin, respectively.[68] Morphometric axonal features, such as axon density, spacing, and diameter, significantly correlate with different directional water diffusion values.[69,70]

DTI may provide microstructural information regarding the full extent of SCI in conjunction with features from conventional MRI. Different DWI and DTI parameters can be used to evaluate axonal health quantitatively. SCI shows increased tADC and decreased lADC in not only abnormal-appearing WM but also normal-appearing WM.[65] The preferential anisotropic motion of water along WM in spinal cord is also reduced. In acute SCI, apparent diffusion coefficient (ADC) has been shown to be lower in patients as compared with controls, even in sites remote from the site of injury in normal-appearing spinal cord on conventional MRI[71] (**Fig. 20**). The reduced diffusion values may be due to cellular and axonal swelling.[72] ADC and FA values can be used to quantify SCI and might be useful in assessing efficacy of neuroprotective agents.[73]

Perturbation of linear WM tracts results in isotropic motion. In this way, DTI parameters such as low FA values can serve as surrogate markers of WM integrity. FA values as well as individual directional diffusivities can be used to evaluate endogenous tissue recovery and remyelination.[74] In mouse models of acute SCI, AD value has been shown to correlate with several spared axons and predicts locomotor recovery.[75] In patients with chronic SCI, FA and mean diffusivity (MD) are decreased in comparison to normal subjects. Notably, the FA has been found to be indirectly related to clinical severity, whereas MD is lower throughout the cord.[76,77] DTI parameters (ie, average MD, FA, RD, longitudinal diffusivity) in nonhemorrhagic SCI are strongly correlated with the initial motor scores.[78] Changes of AD and RD not only at the level of injury but also rostral to the lesion suggest there is axonal degeneration and demyelination of descending and ascending central pathways.[78–80]

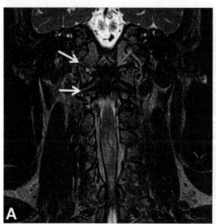
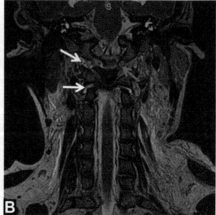

Fig. 17. (*A*) Coronal T2 image (normal) demonstrates intact atlanto-occipital (*yellow arrow*) and atlantoaxial (*white arrow*) articulations. The alar ligaments are homogeneously hypointense (*red arrow*). (*B*) Coronal T2 image (atlanto-occipital dissociation) shows widening of the intact atlanto-occipital (*yellow arrow*) and atlantoaxial (*white arrow*) articulations. There is disruption of bilateral alar ligaments (*red arrow*).

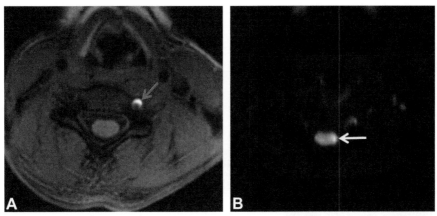

Fig. 18. (*A*) Axial T1 image with fat-saturation image exhibits a hyperintense crescent along the left vertebral artery flow void (*red arrow*). Methemoglobin is along the dissection flap. (*B*) Axial DTI image reveals hyperintensity in the left hemicord due to ischemia (*white arrow*). The cause is likely embolic from a radiculomedullary branch arising from the dissected left vertebral artery.

Fiber tractography is produced when the principal eigenvectors of the tensor, which are aligned with the fiber direction, are mapped to produce a computed visual representation of fiber tracts. Fiber tractography is a graphical representation of DTI data and may be used to evaluate WM integrity and continuity of WM following injury. A "fiber" in tractography is an idealized mathematical representation of a cluster of hundreds or thousands of actual axons that traverse space in a predictable fashion. Both ex vivo[81] and in vivo[70,82] studies have shown that the tractography can illustrate fiber disruption on the transected side.

DTI and tractography are superior at higher magnetic field strengths (ie, 3 T). There are significant technical challenges associated with this type of imaging of the spinal cord, including small cord size, susceptibility artifact of adjacent osseous and ligaments, cerebrospinal fluid and arterial pulsation artifact, and respiratory motion.[83,84] However, advances in MRI techniques (eg, parallel imaging, which enables faster acquisition, thereby reducing the effects of physiologic motion) and hardware development (eg, multiarray coils, which improve the signal-to-noise ratio) have improved image quality and quantifiable metrics.

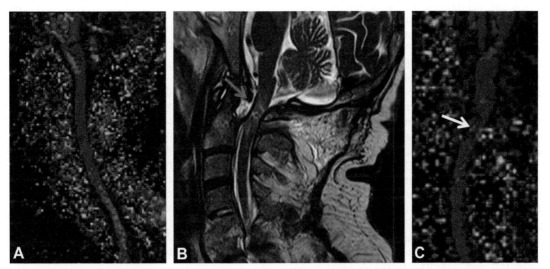

Fig. 19. (*A*) Sagittal color FA map in a normal subject illustrates homogeneous blue color, indicating intact fibers running craniocaudal. (*B*) Sagittal T2 image demonstrates the intramedullary edema and hemorrhage. There is disruption of the tectorial membrane with epidural hemorrhage (*red arrow*). (*C*) Sagittal color FA map shows obscuration of the fibers at the cervicomedullary junction due to cord contusion and hemorrhage (*white arrow*).

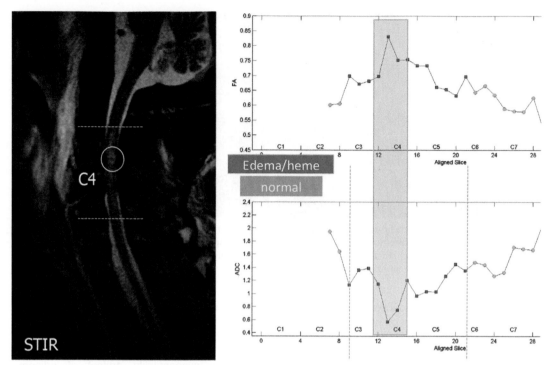

Fig. 20. Sagittal STIR illustrates intramedullary edema and hemorrhage at the C3-C4 level (*yellow circle*) in a patient with complete SCI (C3 ASIA-A). The areas with edema (between the *blue dashed lines*) have corresponding decreased ADC values, with the lowest values in the center of the lesion.

There are several research diffusion techniques, such as diffusion kurtosis imaging (DKI) and Q-space MRI, that supply new information about normal and pathologic tissue. In biological tissues, the presence of barriers (eg, cell membranes) and compartments (eg, intracellular and extracellular) alter water diffusion so that it is non-Gaussian. The degree of non-Gaussianity can be used to characterize tissue microstructure, and this can be quantified by DKI.[85,86] Q-space imaging is also a diffusion-based MRI technique that assesses the diffraction pattern of water molecular spins to provide morphologic information based on water displacement profiles. This detection of diffusion to a few microns can provide indirect measurement to assess the structural integrity of spinal cord at the cellular level resolution. Experimental studies in rat SCI revealed increased mean displacement of water molecules perpendicular to the long axis of the spinal cord with structural damage.[87] High-B radial DWI is a novel type of MRI sequence that can accurately measure relative fractions of intra-axonal water (IAF), extra-axonal water (EAF), and exchange rate between IAF and EAF (D_H) in the cervical spinal cord and add valuable information about the pathologic change, particularly about axonal loss and demyelination[88] (**Fig. 21**).

Susceptibility-Weighted Imaging

SWI is a prolonged echo time gradient echo sequence that combines a magnitude and phase. It is exquisitely sensitive for ferromagnetic substances, such as deoxyhemoglobin, intracellular methemoglobin, hemosiderin, as well as calcium and venous blood (**Fig. 22**). Wang and colleagues[89] have reported the enhanced detection of petechial hemorrhage in SCI with SWI at 3 T.

MR Spectroscopy

MR spectroscopy (MRS) in the spinal cord is technically very challenging. In vivo rat models of SCI demonstrate increased glutamate/glutamine levels in the spinal cord following injury and decreased levels in the brain.[90] Changes in metabolism with SCI are reflected by the early elevations in lactic acid and loss of high-energy metabolites in regions that progressed to necrosis and cavitation in rabbit models of SCI.[91,92] Most human spinal cord MRS studies have focused on the upper cervical cord because it is relatively easier to interrogate with single voxel MRS.

Functional MRI

The blood oxygen level-dependent (BOLD) pulse sequence is the predominant technique for the

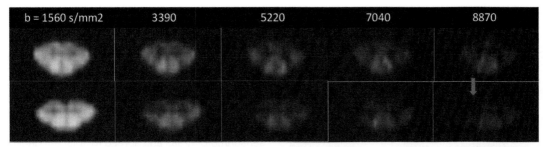

Fig. 21. (*top row*) The normal cord shows expected gradual decay of the signal with increased gradient. The remaining signal is from the intra-axonal compartment. (*bottow row*) An in vivo cord with a lesion in the right hemicord demonstrates that the high-B rDWI (high B gradient, radial diffusion weighted imaging) continues to decay in a focal region at high B values (*red arrow*), thought to be because of leakage from the intra-axonal space due to demyelination. The rate of decay is hypothesized to reflect the degree of demyelination in this region. This high-B rDWI with b = ~3000 and 9000 s/mm^2 may be treated as axonal map and myelin maps, respectively.

evaluation of neuronal activity in functional MRI (fMRI). As with MRS, the method is challenging to perform in the spinal cord because of the small target size, motion, close proximity of large pial vessels, and susceptibility from adjacent osseous structures and ligaments. Several investigators have shown the feasibility of fMRI in the spinal cord with tasks (**Fig. 23**).[93–96] Using the principle that hemodynamic changes with neural activation result in movement of water molecules from the vascular to extravascular spaces, the Signal Enhancement by Extravascular water Protons (SEEP) fMRI has also been used successfully in the spinal cord. When exposed to graded thermal stimuli, the lumbar cord of both SCI patients and controls showed SEEP fMRI activation, although the pattern was altered in the injured patients.[97,98] When patients with varying degrees of SCI were studied with spinal fMRI, there was neuronal activation caudal to the injury site with both active and passive stimulation.[99] The capability of spinal fMRI to show residual motor activity and other studies showing plasticity of sensory neuronal networks in patients with incomplete SCI suggests a potential role of this modality for the assessment of injury and rehabilitation.[100]

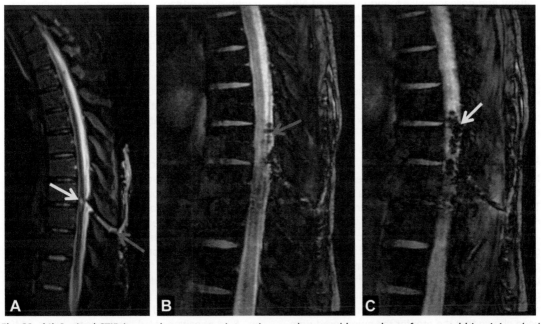

Fig. 22. (*A*) Sagittal STIR image demonstrates interspinous edema and hemorrhage from a stabbing injury (*red arrow*). There is a focal cord laceration, seen as intramedullary hyperintensity (*yellow arrow*). (*B, C*) Sagittal T2* images reveal subarachnoid (*red arrow*) and epidural (*yellow arrow*) hemorrhage.

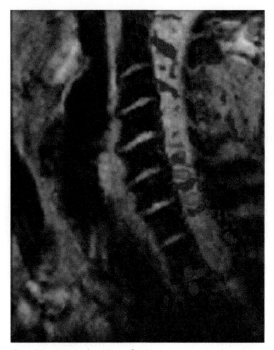

Fig. 23. Cervical spine fMRI in a normal subject showing areas of activation (*red*) and deactivation (*blue*) during isometric forceful contraction of the upper extremity.

Supratentorial Changes with Spinal Cord Injury

SCI can induce changes in the brain. Using MRS, Pattany and colleagues[101] found decreased NAA (a neuronal marker) and increased myo-inositol (a glial marker) in the thalami of paraplegic patients with chronic neuropathic pain. The dysfunction of inhibitory neurons due to deafferentiation is hypothesized to result in the reduced NAA, and the increased myo-inositol may be due to gliosis in the thalami. In patients with incomplete SCI, increased NAA in the motor cortex is suggested to represent neuronal adaptation.[102]

DTI reveals significant differences in the corticospinal tracts including the medullary pyramids, internal capsules, cerebral peduncles, and motor cortex when comparing SCI patients to controls.[103] These microstructural changes are thought to represent trauma-related axonal degeneration and demyelination, which may reflect cortical reorganization. Reduced WM integrity of specific spinal pathways is linked not only to clinical disability[79,80] but also to cortical reorganization.[103] The central pathways show asymmetric changes,[103] which may be due to compensatory overuse.[104] It has been shown that the greater the spinal cord damage, the greater the degree of cortical reorganization, which may be to maximize motor output in

cortical areas that are not normally recruited during a specific movement.[105,106]

BOLD fMRI[107,108] has also used as an imaging surrogate for supratentorial cortical reorganization in paraplegic patients.[109] In patients with complete SCI, cortical activation in the motor regions of the brain are present with attempts to move as well as mental imagery of movement in affected limbs.[110] Task-related increased activation of the sensorimotor areas and spread to adjacent denervated area, such as the leg representation, has been reported in SCI patients. This increased activation in the primary motor cortex (M1) and sensory cortex (S1) is present during movement and/or sensory stimulation of the paralyzed and nonaffected limbs.[106,111–114] These findings suggest that sensorimotor cortical networks not only remain intact but also may recruit adjacent neurons. This finding suggests that treatment strategies in SCI should address these associated cortical changes. For example, a recent pilot investigation of American Spine Injury Association-A subjects with continuous intrathecal baclofen to relieve spasticity demonstrated increased sensorimotor cortex activation, possibly due to functional reorganization.[115]

MRI Limitations

All imaging modalities have their strengths and weakness; therefore, the limitations of MRI should be considered when evaluating spinal trauma. Because of the longer acquisition times and susceptibility to artifact, the percentage of highly diagnostic MRI studies may be lower compared with the CT studies. As stated earlier, fluid-sensitive sequences (eg, STIR, T2-weighted with fat saturation) are helpful in detecting marrow edema of acute fractures. However, the reliability of MRI in determining the acuity of fractures has been increased by recent studies. Lensing and colleagues[116] found that in older patients, the underlying osteopenia and decreased vascularity in the odontoid may yield STIR images unreliable for depicting acute marrows edema. Therefore, the investigators concluded that correlation with CT as well as clinical history is crucial for determining the acuity of an odontoid fracture. Similarly, Brinckman and colleagues[117] found that there is variability in the presence of marrow edema on MRI, which is affected by trauma mechanism. They found that only fractures due to compression reliably produce edema, whereas those from distraction and/or without compression may not exhibit expected hyperintense marrow signal on fluid-sensitive MRI sequences. Also, MRI has high sensitivity for detection of ligamentous injury but has a low specificity for correlative intraoperative findings of disruption.[118,119] Furthermore, there is a lack of consistency in the grading of ligament injury in studies without validation of the methods. Even if there is a paucity of signal abnormality on MRI in the ligamentous complex, this does not predict mechanical stability.

SUMMARY

CT and MRI are complementary imaging modalities for the evaluation of the traumatic spine. CT is best for osseous assessment, whereas MRI gives superb soft tissue delineation. To ensure accurate interpretation of images, it is critical to be cognizant of the strengths and pitfalls of each modality.

Advances in MRI, particularly of the spinal cord, offer clues to the pathobiological mechanism of spinal cord injury. Innovative techniques, such as DTI, provide microstructural information about the axonal and myelin integrity. As such, imaging features may serve as biomarkers for prognostication and for monitoring therapeutic interventions.

REFERENCES

1. Denis F. The three column spine and its significance in the classification of acute thoracolumbar spinal injuries. Spine 1983;8(8):817–31.
2. Holdsworth F. Fractures, dislocations, and fracture-dislocations of the spine. J bone Jt Surg Am 1970; 52(8):1534–51.
3. Roos JE, Hilfiker P, Platz A, et al. MDCT in emergency radiology: is a standardized chest or abdominal protocol sufficient for evaluation of thoracic and lumbar spine trauma? AJR Am J Roentgenol 2004;183(4):959–68.
4. Stiell IG, Wells GA, Vandemheen KL, et al. The Canadian C-spine rule for radiography in alert and stable trauma patients. JAMA 2001;286(15): 1841–8.
5. Bailitz J, Starr F, Beecroft M, et al. CT should replace three-view radiographs as the initial screening test in patients at high, moderate, and low risk for blunt cervical spine injury: a prospective comparison. J Trauma 2009;66(6):1605–9.
6. Nunez DB Jr. Helical CT for the evaluation of cervical vertebral injuries. Semin Musculoskelet Radiol 1998;2(1):19–26.
7. Adams JM, Cockburn MI, Difazio LT, et al. Spinal clearance in the difficult trauma patient: a role for screening MRI of the spine. Am Surg 2006;72(1): 101–5.
8. Holmes JF, Akkinepalli R. Computed tomography versus plain radiography to screen for cervical spine injury: a meta-analysis. J Trauma 2005; 58(5):902–5.
9. Blackmore CC, Mann FA, Wilson AJ. Helical CT in the primary trauma evaluation of the cervical spine: an evidence-based approach. Skeletal Radiol 2000;29(11):632–9.
10. Hogan GJ, Mirvis SE, Shanmuganathan K, et al. Exclusion of unstable cervical spine injury in obtunded patients with blunt trauma: is MR imaging needed when multi-detector row CT findings are normal? Radiology 2005;237(1):106–13.
11. Alhilali LM, Fakhran S. Evaluation of the intervertebral disk angle for the assessment of anterior cervical diskoligamentous injury. AJNR Am J Neuroradiol 2013;34(12):2399–404.
12. Bozzo A, Marcoux J, Radhakrishna M, et al. The role of magnetic resonance imaging in the management of acute spinal cord injury. J Neurotrauma 2011;28(8):1401–11.
13. Chakeres DW, Flickinger F, Bresnahan JC, et al. MR imaging of acute spinal cord trauma. AJNR Am J Neuroradiol 1987;8(1):5–10.
14. Robertson PA, Ryan MD. Neurological deterioration after reduction of cervical subluxation. Mechanical compression by disc tissue. J Bone Joint Surg Br 1992;74(2):224–7.
15. Flanders AE, Schaefer DM, Doan HT, et al. Acute cervical spine trauma: correlation of MR imaging findings with degree of neurologic deficit. Radiology 1990;177(1):25–33.
16. Beers GJ, Raque GH, Wagner GG, et al. MR imaging in acute cervical spine trauma. J Comput Assist Tomogr 1988;12(5):755–61.
17. Hayashi K, Yone K, Ito H, et al. MRI findings in patients with a cervical spinal cord injury who do not show radiographic evidence of a fracture or dislocation. Paraplegia 1995;33(4):212–5.
18. Kerslake RW, Jaspan T, Worthington BS. Magnetic resonance imaging of spinal trauma. Br J Radiol 1991;64(761):386–402.
19. Goldberg AL, Rothfus WE, Deeb ZL, et al. Hyperextension injuries of the cervical spine. Magnetic resonance findings. Skeletal Radiol 1989;18(4):283–8.
20. Klein GR, Vaccaro AR, Albert TJ, et al. Efficacy of magnetic resonance imaging in the evaluation of posterior cervical spine fractures. Spine 1999; 24(8):771–4.
21. Meoded A, Singhi S, Poretti A, et al. Tectorial membrane injury: frequently overlooked in pediatric traumatic head injury. AJNR Am J Neuroradiol 2011;32(10):1806–11.
22. Saifuddin A, Green R, White J. Magnetic resonance imaging of the cervical ligaments in the absence of trauma. Spine 2003;28(15):1686–91 [discussion: 91–2].
23. Lee HM, Kim HS, Kim DJ, et al. Reliability of magnetic resonance imaging in detecting posterior ligament complex injury in thoracolumbar spinal fractures. Spine 2000;25(16):2079–84.

24. Haba H, Taneichi H, Kotani Y, et al. Diagnostic accuracy of magnetic resonance imaging for detecting posterior ligamentous complex injury associated with thoracic and lumbar fractures. J Neurosurg 2003;99(1 Suppl):20–6.

25. Vaccaro AR, Hulbert RJ, Patel AA, et al, Spine Trauma Study Group. The subaxial cervical spine injury classification system: a novel approach to recognize the importance of morphology, neurology, and integrity of the disco-ligamentous complex. Spine 2007;32(21):2365–74.

26. Goldberg AL, Rothfus WE, Deeb ZL, et al. The impact of magnetic resonance on the diagnostic evaluation of acute cervicothoracic spinal trauma. Skeletal Radiol 1988;17(2):89–95.

27. Davis SJ, Teresi LM, Bradley WG Jr, et al. Cervical spine hyperextension injuries: MR findings. Radiology 1991;180(1):245–51.

28. Pratt ES, Green DA, Spengler DM. Herniated intervertebral discs associated with unstable spinal injuries. Spine 1990;15(7):662–6.

29. Dai L, Jia L. Central cord injury complicating acute cervical disc herniation in trauma. Spine 2000;25(3):331–5 [discussion: 336].

30. Schaefer DM, Flanders A, Northrup BE, et al. Magnetic resonance imaging of acute cervical spine trauma. Correlation with severity of neurologic injury. Spine 1989;14(10):1090–5.

31. Rizzolo SJ, Piazza MR, Cotler JM, et al. Intervertebral disc injury complicating cervical spine trauma. Spine 1991;16(6 Suppl):S187–9.

32. Harrington JF, Likavec MJ, Smith AS. Disc herniation in cervical fracture subluxation. Neurosurgery 1991;29(3):374–9.

33. Silberstein M, Tress BM, Hennessy O. Prediction of neurologic outcome in acute spinal cord injury: the role of CT and MR. AJNR Am J Neuroradiol 1992;13(6):1597–608.

34. Bondurant FJ, Cotler HB, Kulkarni MV, et al. Acute spinal cord injury. A study using physical examination and magnetic resonance imaging. Spine 1990;15(3):161–8.

35. Kulkarni MV, McArdle CB, Kopanicky D, et al. Acute spinal cord injury: MR imaging at 1.5 T. Radiology 1987;164(3):837–43.

36. Weirich SD, Cotler HB, Narayana PA, et al. Histopathologic correlation of magnetic resonance imaging signal patterns in a spinal cord injury model. Spine 1990;15(7):630–8.

37. Ramon S, Dominguez R, Ramirez L, et al. Clinical and magnetic resonance imaging correlation in acute spinal cord injury. Spinal Cord 1997;35(10):664–73.

38. Boldin C, Raith J, Fankhauser F, et al. Predicting neurologic recovery in cervical spinal cord injury with postoperative MR imaging. Spine 2006;31(5):554–9.

39. Sato T, Kokubun S, Rijal KP, et al. Prognosis of cervical spinal cord injury in correlation with magnetic resonance imaging. Paraplegia 1994;32(2):81–5.

40. Marciello MA, Flanders AE, Herbison GJ, et al. Magnetic resonance imaging related to neurologic outcome in cervical spinal cord injury. Arch Phys Med Rehabil 1993;74(9):940–6.

41. Mirvis SE, Geisler FH, Jelinek JJ, et al. Acute cervical spine trauma: evaluation with 1.5-T MR imaging. Radiology 1988;166(3):807–16.

42. Leypold B, Flanders AE, Sharma D, et al. Dynamic characteristics of acute spinal cord injury: is absolute lesion length affected by delay in MR imaging?. Radiological Society of North America Scientific Assembly and Annual Meeting. Chicago, November 27–December 2, 2005.

43. Yamashita Y, Takahashi M, Matsuno Y, et al. Acute spinal cord injury: magnetic resonance imaging correlated with myelopathy. Br J Radiol 1991;64(759):201–9.

44. Selden NR, Quint DJ, Patel N, et al. Emergency magnetic resonance imaging of cervical spinal cord injuries: clinical correlation and prognosis. Neurosurgery 1999;44(4):785–92 [discussion: 92–3].

45. Shimada K, Tokioka T. Sequential MR studies of cervical cord injury: correlation with neurological damage and clinical outcome. Spinal Cord 1999;37(6):410–5.

46. Flanders AE, Spettell CM, Tartaglino LM, et al. Forecasting motor recovery after cervical spinal cord injury: value of MR imaging. Radiology 1996;201(3):649–55.

47. Sliker CW, Mirvis SE, Shanmuganathan K. Assessing cervical spine stability in obtunded blunt trauma patients: review of medical literature. Radiology 2005;234(3):733–9.

48. Menaker J, Philp A, Boswell S, et al. Computed tomography alone for cervical spine clearance in the unreliable patient—are we there yet? J Trauma 2008;64(4):898–903 [discussion: 903–4].

49. Martinez-Perez R, Paredes I, Cepeda S, et al. Spinal cord injury after blunt cervical spine trauma: correlation of soft-tissue damage and extension of lesion. AJNR Am J Neuroradiol 2014;35(5):1029–34.

50. Leypold BG, Flanders AE, Burns AS. The early evolution of spinal cord lesions on MR imaging following traumatic spinal cord injury. AJNR Am J Neuroradiol 2008;29(5):1012–6.

51. Flanders AE, Tartaglino LM, Friedman DP, et al. Magnetic resonance imaging in acute spinal injury. Semin Roentgenol 1992;27(4):271–98.

52. Parashari UC, Khanduri S, Bhadury S, et al. Diagnostic and prognostic role of MRI in spinal trauma, its comparison and correlation with clinical profile and neurological outcome, according to ASIA

impairment scale. J Craniovertebr Junction Spine 2011;2(1):17–26.

53. Talbott JF, Whetstone WD, Readdy WJ, et al. The brain and spinal injury center score: a novel, simple, and reproducible method for assessing the severity of acute cervical spinal cord injury with axial T2-weighted MRI findings. J Neurosurg Spine 2015;23(4):495–504.

54. Zohrabian VM, Parker L, Harrop JS, et al. Can anatomic level of injury on MRI predict neurological level in acute cervical spinal cord injury? Br J Neurosurg 2016;30(2):204–10.

55. Desouza RM, Crocker MJ, Haliasos N, et al. Blunt traumatic vertebral artery injury: a clinical review. Eur Spine J 2011;20(9):1405–16.

56. Jacobson LE, Ziemba-Davis M, Herrera AJ. The limitations of using risk factors to screen for blunt cerebrovascular injuries: the harder you look, the more you find. World J Emerg Surg 2015;10:46.

57. Vilela MD, Kim LJ, Bellabarba C, et al. Blunt cerebrovascular injuries in association with craniocervical distraction injuries: a retrospective review of consecutive cases. Spine J 2015;15(3):499–505.

58. Takano K, Yamashita S, Takemoto K, et al. MRI of intracranial vertebral artery dissection: evaluation of intramural haematoma using a black blood, variable-flip-angle 3D turbo spin-echo sequence. Neuroradiology 2013;55(7):845–51.

59. Edjlali M, Roca P, Rabrait C, et al. 3D fast spin-echo T1 black-blood imaging for the diagnosis of cervical artery dissection. AJNR Am J Neuroradiol 2013;34(9):E103–6.

60. Gatehouse PD, He T, Hughes SP, et al. MR imaging of degenerative disc disease in the lumbar spine with ultrashort TE pulse sequences. MAGMA 2004;16(4):160–6.

61. Hackney DB, Finkelstein SD, Hand CM, et al. Post-mortem magnetic resonance imaging of experimental spinal cord injury: magnetic resonance findings versus in vivo functional deficit. Neurosurgery 1994;35(6):1104–11.

62. Hackney DB, Ford JC, Markowitz RS, et al. Experimental spinal cord injury: MR correlation to intensity of injury. J Comput Assist Tomogr 1994;18(3):357–62.

63. Metz GA, Curt A, van de Meent H, et al. Validation of the weight-drop contusion model in rats: a comparative study of human spinal cord injury. J Neurotrauma 2000;17(1):1–17.

64. Falconer JC, Narayana PA, Bhattacharjee MB, et al. Quantitative MRI of spinal cord injury in a rat model. Magn Reson Med 1994;32(4):484–91.

65. Ford JC, Hackney DB, Alsop DC, et al. MRI characterization of diffusion coefficients in a rat spinal cord injury model. Magn Reson Med 1994;31(5):488–94.

66. Gouw AA, Seewann A, Vrenken H, et al. Heterogeneity of white matter hyperintensities in Alzheimer's disease: post-mortem quantitative MRI and neuropathology. Brain 2008;131(Pt 12):3286–98.

67. Schmierer K, Wheeler-Kingshott CA, Boulby PA, et al. Diffusion tensor imaging of post mortem multiple sclerosis brain. Neuroimage 2007;35(2):467–77.

68. Zhang J, Jones M, DeBoy CA, et al. Diffusion tensor magnetic resonance imaging of Wallerian degeneration in rat spinal cord after dorsal root axotomy. J Neurosci 2009;29(10):3160–71.

69. Schwartz ED, Cooper ET, Fan Y, et al. MRI diffusion coefficients in spinal cord correlate with axon morphometry. Neuroreport 2005;16(1):73–6.

70. Schwartz ED. Experimental techniques of spinal imaging. In: Flanders ED, editor. Spinal trauma: imaging, diagnosis, and management. Philadelphia: Lipincott Williams & Wilkins; 2007. p. 373–407.

71. Shanmuganathan K, Gullapalli RP, Zhuo J, et al. Diffusion tensor MR imaging in cervical spine trauma. AJNR Am J Neuroradiol 2008;29(4):655–9.

72. Sagiuchi T, Tachibana S, Endo M, et al. Diffusion-weighted MRI of the cervical cord in acute spinal cord injury with type II odontoid fracture. J Comput Assist Tomogr 2002;26(4):654–6.

73. Hauben E, Nevo U, Yoles E, et al. Autoimmune T cells as potential neuroprotective therapy for spinal cord injury. Lancet 2000;355(9200):286–7.

74. Deo AA, Grill RJ, Hasan KM, et al. In vivo serial diffusion tensor imaging of experimental spinal cord injury. J Neurosci Res 2006;83(5):801–10.

75. Kim JH, Loy DN, Wang Q, et al. Diffusion tensor imaging at 3 hours after traumatic spinal cord injury predicts long-term locomotor recovery. J Neurotrauma 2010;27(3):587–98.

76. Ellingson BM, Kurpad SN, Schmit BD. Functional correlates of diffusion tensor imaging in spinal cord injury. Biomed Sci Instrum 2008;44:28–33.

77. Ellingson BM, Ulmer JL, Schmit BD. A new technique for imaging the human spinal cord in vivo. Biomed Sci Instrum 2006;42:255–60.

78. Cheran S, Shanmuganathan K, Zhuo J, et al. Correlation of MR diffusion tensor imaging parameters with ASIA motor scores in hemorrhagic and nonhemorrhagic acute spinal cord injury. J Neurotrauma 2011;28(9):1881–92.

79. Cohen-Adad J, Leblond H, Delivet-Mongrain H, et al. Wallerian degeneration after spinal cord lesions in cats detected with diffusion tensor imaging. Neuroimage 2011;57(3):1068–76.

80. Petersen JA, Wilm BJ, von Meyenburg J, et al. Chronic cervical spinal cord injury: DTI correlates with clinical and electrophysiological measures. J Neurotrauma 2012;29(8):1556–66.

81. Schwartz ED, Duda J, Shumsky JS, et al. Spinal cord diffusion tensor imaging and fiber tracking can identify white matter tract disruption and glial scar orientation following lateral funiculotomy. J Neurotrauma 2005;22(12):1388–98.

82. Schwartz ED. In vivo diffusion tensor imaging (DTI) and fiber tractography in the normal and injured rat spinal cord Radiological Society of North America (RSNA) Annual Meeting. Chicago, 2006.

83. Ries M, Jones RA, Dousset V, et al. Diffusion tensor MRI of the spinal cord. Magn Reson Med 2000; 44(6):884–92.

84. Quencer RM, Pattany PM. Diffusion-weighted imaging of the spinal cord: is there a future? AJNR Am J Neuroradiol 2000;21(7):1181–2.

85. Rangwala NA, Hackney DB, Dai W, et al. Diffusion restriction in the human spinal cord characterized in vivo with high b-value STEAM diffusion imaging. Neuroimage 2013;82:416–25.

86. Hori M, Fukunaga I, Masutani Y, et al. New diffusion metrics for spondylotic myelopathy at an early clinical stage. Eur Radiol 2012;22(8):1797–802.

87. Nossin-Manor R, Duvdevani R, Cohen Y. q-Space high b value diffusion MRI of hemi-crush in rat spinal cord: evidence for spontaneous regeneration. Magn Reson Imaging 2002;20(3):231–41.

88. Sapkota N, Yoon S, Thapa B, et al. Characterization of Spinal Cord White Matter by Suppressing Signal from Hindered Space: a Monte Carlo Simulation and an Ex Vivo Ultrahigh-b Diffusion-Weighted Imaging Study. The Journal of Magnetic Resonance, in press.

89. Wang M, Dai Y, Han Y, et al. Susceptibility weighted imaging in detecting hemorrhage in acute cervical spinal cord injury. Magn Reson Imaging 2011; 29(3):365–73.

90. Erschbamer M, Oberg J, Westman E, et al. 1H-MRS in spinal cord injury: acute and chronic metabolite alterations in rat brain and lumbar spinal cord. Eur J Neurosci 2011;33(4):678–88.

91. Vink R, Knoblach SM, Faden AI. 31P magnetic resonance spectroscopy of traumatic spinal cord injury. Magn Reson Med 1987;5(4):390–4.

92. Vink R, Noble LJ, Knoblach SM, et al. Metabolic changes in rabbit spinal cord after trauma: magnetic resonance spectroscopy studies. Ann Neurol 1989;25(1):26–31.

93. Yoshizawa T, Nose T, Moore GJ, et al. Functional magnetic resonance imaging of motor activation in the human cervical spinal cord. Neuroimage 1996;4(3 Pt 1):174–82.

94. Backes WH, Mess WH, Wilmink JT. Functional MR imaging of the cervical spinal cord by use of median nerve stimulation and fist clenching. AJNR Am J Neuroradiol 2001;22(10):1854–9.

95. Stroman PW, Nance PW, Ryner LN. BOLD MRI of the human cervical spinal cord at 3 tesla. Magn Reson Med 1999;42(3):571–6.

96. Madi S, Flanders AE, Vinitski S, et al. Functional MR imaging of the human cervical spinal cord. AJNR Am J Neuroradiol 2001;22(9):1768–74.

97. Stroman PW, Kornelsen J, Bergman A, et al. Noninvasive assessment of the injured human spinal cord by means of functional magnetic resonance imaging. Spinal Cord 2004;42(2):59–66.

98. Stroman PW, Tomanek B, Krause V, et al. Mapping of neuronal function in the healthy and injured human spinal cord with spinal fMRI. Neuroimage 2002;17(4):1854–60.

99. Kornelsen J, Stroman PW. Detection of the neuronal activity occurring caudal to the site of spinal cord injury that is elicited during lower limb movement tasks. Spinal Cord 2007;45(7):485–90.

100. Cadotte DW, Bosma R, Mikulis D, et al. Plasticity of the injured human spinal cord: insights revealed by spinal cord functional MRI. PLoS One 2012;7(9): e45560.

101. Pattany PM, Yezierski RP, Widerstrom-Noga EG, et al. Proton magnetic resonance spectroscopy of the thalamus in patients with chronic neuropathic pain after spinal cord injury. AJNR Am J Neuroradiol 2002;23(6):901–5.

102. Puri BK, Smith HC, Cox IJ, et al. The human motor cortex after incomplete spinal cord injury: an investigation using proton magnetic resonance spectroscopy. J Neurol Neurosurg Psychiatry 1998; 65(5):748–54.

103. Freund P, Wheeler-Kingshott CA, Nagy Z, et al. Axonal integrity predicts cortical reorganisation following cervical injury. J Neurol Neurosurg Psychiatry 2012;83(6):629–37.

104. Elbert T, Flor H, Birbaumer N, et al. Extensive reorganization of the somatosensory cortex in adult humans after nervous system injury. Neuroreport 1994;5(18):2593–7.

105. Freund P, Weiskopf N, Ward NS, et al. Disability, atrophy and cortical reorganization following spinal cord injury. Brain 2011;134(Pt 6):1610–22.

106. Lundell H, Christensen MS, Barthelemy D, et al. Cerebral activation is correlated to regional atrophy of the spinal cord and functional motor disability in spinal cord injured individuals. Neuroimage 2011; 54(2):1254–61.

107. Friston KJ, Josephs O, Rees G, et al. Nonlinear event-related responses in fMRI. Magn Reson Med 1998;39(1):41–52.

108. Turner R, Howseman A, Rees GE, et al. Functional magnetic resonance imaging of the human brain: data acquisition and analysis. Exp Brain Res 1998;123(1–2):5–12.

109. Kokotilo KJ, Eng JJ, Curt A. Reorganization and preservation of motor control of the brain in spinal cord injury: a systematic review. J Neurotrauma 2009;26(11):2113–26.

110. Sabbah P, de SS, Leveque C, et al. Sensorimotor cortical activity in patients with complete spinal cord injury: a functional magnetic resonance imaging study. J Neurotrauma 2002;19(1):53–60.

111. Curt A, Alkadhi H, Crelier GR, et al. Changes of non-affected upper limb cortical representation in

paraplegic patients as assessed by fMRI. Brain 2002;125(Pt 11):2567–78.

112. Freund P, Rothwell J, Craggs M, et al. Corticomotor representation to a human forearm muscle changes following cervical spinal cord injury. Eur J Neurosci 2011;34(11):1839–46.

113. Jurkiewicz MT, Mikulis DJ, McIlroy WE, et al. Sensorimotor cortical plasticity during recovery following spinal cord injury: a longitudinal fMRI study. Neurorehabil Neural Repair 2007;21(6): 527–38.

114. Jurkiewicz MT, Mikulis DJ, Fehlings MG, et al. Sensorimotor cortical activation in patients with cervical spinal cord injury with persisting paralysis. Neurorehabil Neural Repair 2010;24(2):136–40.

115. Keller J, Robert J, Ivana S. Longitudinal fMRI assessment in chronic spinal cord injury treated by intrathecal baclofen—pilot data. Clin Neurophysiol 2015;126(3):e36–7.

116. Lensing FD, Bisson EF, Wiggins RH 3rd, et al. Reliability of the STIR sequence for acute type II odontoid fractures. AJNR Am J Neuroradiol 2014;35(8): 1642–6.

117. Brinckman MA, Chau C, Ross JS. Marrow edema variability in acute spine fractures. Spine J 2015; 15(3):454–60.

118. Goradia D, Linnau KF, Cohen WA, et al. Correlation of MR imaging findings with intraoperative findings after cervical spine trauma. AJNR Am J Neuroradiol 2007;28(2):209–15.

119. Rihn JA, Fisher C, Harrop J, et al. Assessment of the posterior ligamentous complex following acute cervical spine trauma. J bone Jt Surg Am 2010; 92(3):583–9.

Thoracolumbar Trauma Classification

Gregory D. Schroeder, MD[a], James S. Harrop, MD[b], Alexander R. Vaccaro, MD, PhD, MBA[a],*

KEYWORDS

- Spine trauma • Thoracolumbar trauma • Thoracolumbar injury • Spine injury classification
- AOSpine thoracolumbar spine injury classification system
- The thoracolumbar injury classification system (TLICS)

KEY POINTS

- Useful thoracolumbar injury classifications allow meaningful and concise communication between surgeons, trainees and researchers; although many have been proposed, none have obtained universal acceptance.
- Regional treatment algorithms for spine trauma are often similar in regions that use the same classification systems.
- The AOSpine Thoracolumbar Spine Injury Classification System was developed recently.
- Given the unique and globally inclusive development process used in the design of the AOSpine classification, there is cautious optimism for global acceptance.

INTRODUCTION

An ideal spine injury classification permits clear, easy, accurate, and reproducible communication between surgeons, residents, fellows, researchers, and other health care professionals. Many historical classifications were either mechanistic or based solely on the radiographic morphology of the injury. In an effort to more accurately guide treatment and possibly predict long-term outcomes, multiple recent classifications have been developed that consider the patient's entire clinical picture. Although many thoracolumbar injury classifications have been proposed, currently there is no single, globally accepted classification. In North America, many surgeons use the Thoracolumbar Injury Classification System (TLICS)[1,2]; in contrast, many European surgeons commonly use the Magerl system.[3–7] Most recently the AOSpine Thoracolumbar Injury Classification system was published and validated;[8–14] however, it remains unclear if this classification will be able to achieve global acceptance. The failure of surgeons to agree on a unified classification system for these injuries may initially seem unimportant, but the lack of a universal classification system has resulted in dramatically different treatment algorithms for similar fractures throughout the world; furthermore, the regional treatment algorithms tend to be similar in areas that use the same classification system.[2,5,6,10,15–17]

HISTORICAL CLASSIFICATIONS

The first published thoracolumbar injury classification in the English literature was by Watson-Jones in 1938. He identified 3 distinct fracture types—the simple wedge fracture, the comminuted fracture, and the fracture dislocation—and he recommended different treatments for these fracture types.[18] Additionally in the middle of the 20th century, many unique thoracolumbar fractures were identified, and a different treatment algorithm was proposed for the individual fractures. One such injury is the Chance fracture, which was originally described in 1948 by G.Q. Chance as a flexion injury resulting in a wedge deformity of the vertebral body that may result in the disruption of the

a Department of Orthopaedic Surgery, The Rothman Institute, Thomas Jefferson University, 925 Chestnut St, 5th floor, Philadelphia, PA 19107, USA; b Department of Neurosurgery, Thomas Jefferson University, 909 Walnut St, Philadelphia, PA 19107, USA
* Corresponding author.
E-mail address: alexvaccaro3@aol.com

Neurosurg Clin N Am 28 (2017) 23–29
http://dx.doi.org/10.1016/j.nec.2016.07.007
1042-3680/17/© 2016 Elsevier Inc. All rights reserved.

posterior elements.[19] Another classic thoracolumbar fracture is the burst fracture. The term burst fracture was coined by Holdsworth in 1970 in a series of more than 1000 spinal injuries, and he defined a burst fracture as any vertebral body compression fracture that disrupted the posterior vertebral wall.[20] In the same publication, Holdsworth proposed the first mechanistic classification. He divided fractures into 6 basic types (simple wedge, dislocation, rotational fracture–dislocation, extension, burst, and shear injuries). Perhaps the most important and controversial finding in this publication was that Holdsworth reported that all fractures with an intact posterior ligamentous complex (PLC) were stable. Although this classification offered basic treatment guidelines, the classification has never been validated independently, and so although the term burst fracture has persisted, the remainder of the classification is no longer used.[20–22]

TWO- AND THREE-COLUMN CLASSIFICATIONS

Kelly and Whiteside[23] proposed the next major classification in 1968 when they divided the spine into 2 columns. The anterior column, which they considered the entire vertebral body and intervertebral disc, and the posterior column, which comprised the neural arch and ligamentous complex. They postulated that any injury that involved only one of the columns was stable, but any injury resulting in disruption of both columns was unstable.[23] This classification was never validated independently, and it was challenged in 1983 when Denis published a comprehensive classification for thoracolumbar fractures based off of 412 patients with a thoracolumbar injury. The Denis classification is commonly thought of as dividing each spinal segment into 3 columns: the anterior column—from the anterior longitudinal ligament through the anterior two-thirds of the vertebral body; the middle column—from the posterior third of the vertebral body/intervertebral disc to the posterior longitudinal ligament; and the posterior column—everything posterior to the posterior longitudinal ligament. However, the classification actually divides fractures into 4 major types (compression fractures, burst fractures, seatbelt-type injuries, and fracture–dislocations), and then subdivides each fracture into 1 of 16 total subtypes (**Table 1**). The 3-column theory was described in the same publication as an alteration to the 2-column theory of stability proposed by Kelly and Whiteside[23,24]; Denis reported that the individual fracture pattern should not dictate treatment, but rather the treatment was determined by

Table 1 The Denis classification	
Compression (may be anterior or lateral)	
Type A	Coronal split of the anterior column
Type B	Fracture of the superior endplate of the anterior column
Type C	Fracture of the inferior endplate of the anterior column
Type D	Anterior cortex fracture with intact endplates
Burst	
Type A	Fracture involving both endplates and the posterior wall
Type B	Fracture involving the superior endplate and the posterior wall
Type C	Fracture involving the inferior endplate and the posterior wall
Type D	Burst fracture associated with significant rotation
Type E	Lateral Burst fracture which involves the both endplates and the posterior wall, but only involves the left or right side
Seatbelt type	
Type A	Single-level osseous injury
Type B	Single-level ligamentous injury
Type C	Two-level injury with osseous involvement of the middle column
Type D	Two-level injury with ligamentous involvement of the middle column
Fracture–dislocations	
Type A	Flexion with rotation
Type B	Shear injury
Type C	Flexion distraction injury

From Denis F. The three column spine and its significance in the classification of acute thoracolumbar spinal injuries. Spine (Phila Pa 1976) 1983;8:817–31; with permission.

the integrity of the middle column. Denis proposed that isolated anterior or poster column injuries were stable, but if the injury resulted in concomitant disruption of the middle column, the fracture was unstable.[24] This 3-column concept of stability achieved widespread acceptance, and to this day is responsible for many surgeons recommending operative treatment of thoracolumbar burst fractures in a neurologically intact patient[14,24]; despite its widespread use and moderate to substantial interobserver reliability of identifying the 4 main types of fractures,[25] when attempting to classify the fractures into these subtypes, the reliability is poor.[26] Furthermore, the importance of the middle column as the critical piece in spinal stability continues to be debated in the scientific community today.

Building on the work of Denis,[24] McAfee and colleagues[27] published a classification that was both a morphologic and mechanistic classification. Fractures were initially classified into 1 of 6 fracture types: wedge compression, stable burst, unstable burst, flexion distraction, Chance, and translation injuries. Similar to the Denis classification, the spine was divided into 3 columns, and any fractures that involved the middle column were considered unstable; however, McAfee and colleagues[27] proposed that the mechanism of failure of the middle column was critical to determining the appropriate treatment. Injuries of the middle column that occurred from either a compressive (burst fractures) or a distractive (Chance and flexion distraction injuries) could be treated posteriorly with distraction or compression instrumentation. Conversely, translational injuries were a contraindication to posterior distraction and required segmental instrumentation of each level.[27]

Following the Denis classification, the Ferguson and Allen[28] classification was published in 1984; importantly, this is a mechanistic classification that did not challenge Denis' 3-column biomechanical concept of stability. Because of this, although the classification contributed significantly to the nomenclature of thoracolumbar injuries, it failed to alter the treatment paradigm for any fractures. This classification identified 7 injury types with 5 additional injury subtypes (**Box 1**), and presented treatment recommendations based on the type of injury.[28] Likely because this classification did not alter the treatment paradigm and is derived from an inferred injury mechanism rather than verifiable imaging characteristics, it has never been validated independently.[22]

The next substantial contribution to thoracolumbar fracture classification came in 1994 when Magerl and colleagues[3] published a hierarchical classification. The Magerl system divides fractures into 3 types based on mechanism (compression/A-type fractures, distraction/B-type fractures and rotational/C-type fractures) and then it further incrementally subdivides the fractures into a total of 53 subtypes based on specific morphologic characteristics of the fracture. Although this classification was designed such that there was an incremental increase in severity of the injury when increasing the overall fracture type (A → B → C) and fracture subtype, the classification is still designed around the 3-column concept of spinal stability. Because of this, it had little impact on

---

Box 1
The Ferguson and Allen classification
Vertical compression
Burst fracture with diffuse retropulsion
Burst fracture with retropulsion at the superior and inferior endplates
Compression flexion
Anterior wedge
Anterior wedge with associated posterior tension band disruption
Burst fracture with associated posterior tension band disruption
Distraction flexion
Lateral flexion
Translation
Torsional flexion
Distractive extension
From Ferguson RL, Allen BL Jr. A mechanistic classification of thoracolumbar spine fractures. Clin Orthop Relat Res 1984;(189):77–88; with permission.

---

the treatment algorithm of controversial fractures. Furthermore, owing to the complexity of the classification, multiple authors have demonstrated either poor or fair interobserver reliability,[25,29] so a clinically validated treatment algorithm based off of this classification has not been possible. Additionally, although the Magerl system is criticized for being overly complex with its 53 unique injury types, it still fails to formally consider to critical factors in determining the treatment algorithm, the integrity of the PLC, and the neurologic status of the patient.[3]

THE THORACOLUMBAR INJURY CLASSIFICATION SYSTEM

In 2005, Vaccaro and colleagues[1] published the TLICS, the first major thoracolumbar classification system to repudiate the notion that all injuries involving the middle column are unstable (**Table 2**). Additionally, the TLICS is the first classification to incorporate the integrity of the PLC and the neurologic status of the patient into the system. Initially fractures are separated into 1 of 3 major morphologic categories: compression injuries, translational/rotational injuries, and distraction injuries. Next, the integrity of the PLC is graded as either intact, disrupted, or indeterminate. Finally, the neurology is graded as either neurologically intact, a nerve root deficit, a complete spinal cord injury,

Table 2	
The Thoracolumbar Injury Classification System	
Injury Variables	**Score**
Morphology	
Compression fracture	1
Burst fracture	2
Rotational or translation injury	3
Distraction injury	4
Posterior ligamentous complex	
Intact	0
Unclear	2
Disrupted	3
Neurology	
Neurologically intact	0
Nerve root injury	2
Complete spinal cord injury	2
Incomplete spinal cord injury/ cauda equina syndrome	3

From Vaccaro AR, Lehman RA Jr, Hurlbert RJ, et al. A new classification of thoracolumbar injuries: the importance of injury morphology, the integrity of the posterior ligamentous complex, and neurologic status. Spine (Phila Pa 1976) 2005;30:2325–33; with permission.

or an incomplete spinal cord injury/cauda equine syndrome. In addition to classifying the injury, the TLICS was supplemented with an associated injury severity score that assigned an integer value to each category to determine an injury score[30]; in this way, the TLICS is able to both classify the fracture as well as make a treatment recommendation based on the injury score. The TLICS recommends nonoperative treatment for all injuries that result in a score of less than 4, and operative intervention for all injuries with a score of more than 4; if the injury score is 4, either operative on nonoperative treatment may be appropriate depending on patient and surgeon variables.

The TLICS is also the first thoracolumbar injury classification to be validated externally. Vaccaro and colleagues[30] reported that 96.2% of surgeons agree on the final treatment recommendation of the TLICS, and Joaquim and colleagues[31] reported that the TLICS recommendation accurately predicted the treatment of 96% of thoracolumbar injuries. Furthermore, the TLICS has even been validated in pediatric patients, with Savage and colleagues[32] reporting good validity (0.84 sensitivity, 0.79 specificity, 0.68 positive predictive value, and 0.90 negative predictive value) for the TLICS when 20 pediatric thoracolumbar injuries were reviewed prospectively by 20 surgeons of differing experience levels.

Although there is significant literature demonstrating the validity of the TLICS,[30–32] it has failed to gain universal acceptance, in large part owing to its recommended management of thoracolumbar burst fractures in neurologically intact patients. In a neurologically intact patient with a burst fracture, the recommended treatment is based on the integrity of the PLC. If the PLC is intact, nonoperative treatment is recommended (injury score of 2), and if the PLC is disrupted, surgical treatment is recommended (injury score of 5). Finally, if the status of the PLC is unclear, TLICS does not make a firm recommendation for or against surgery (injury score of 4).[1] However, using the imaging modalities available today, surgeons cannot agree on the integrity of the PLC in these fractures. Schroeder and colleagues[11] reported a poor reliability ($\kappa = 0.11$) when more than 500 surgeons worldwide were asked to determine the integrity of the PLC in 10 cases of compression-type injuries. Similarly, Harrop and colleagues[2,4–7,33] reported only slightly better reliability ($\kappa = 0.34$) when 48 surgeons reviewed 56 thoracolumbar injuries. Furthermore, even when the integrity of the PLC is not in question, the need for surgical stabilization in a burst fracture is still debated in the literature, and this ambiguity is responsible for the majority of deviations from the TLICS treatment recommendations. In a review of 458 consecutive patients with thoracolumbar injuries, Joaquim and colleagues[34] reported that of the 310 patients initially treated nonoperatively, 307 had a TLICS score of 3 or less; however, of the 148 patients treated surgically, 53.4% (79 patients) had a score of less than 4, and all 79 patients with a score of less than 4 that were treated surgically had a burst fractures without neurologic involvement (TLICS score of 2).

THE AOSPINE THORACOLUMBAR SPINE INJURY CLASSIFICATION SYSTEM

Recognizing the failure of these classifications to achieve global acceptance, Vaccaro and colleagues incorporated aspects of the Magerl system and the TLICS when they designed the new AOSpine Thoracolumbar Spine Injury Classification System in 2013. Furthermore, in an effort to gain universal acceptance, this is the first thoracolumbar injury classification system that used a modified Delphi method to determine the treatment algorithm. To do this, the authors first published the initial classification, and then performed multiple follow-up studies before publishing the accompanying surgical algorithm.[8–14,35,36]

The morphologic classification is a simplified version of the Magerl system with a total of 9 injury patterns. Injuries are first separated into 3 major types: A—compression injuries; B—tension band injuries; and C—translation injures. Then, type A and B injuries are subclassified into 5 and 3 subtypes, respectively (**Table 3**). Similar to the TLICS, evaluation of the neurologic status of the patient, as well as 2 patient-specific modifiers are also formally considered in the AOSpine classification (**Table 4**).

After publication of the classification, Kepler and colleagues[8] performed a reliability analysis of 100 worldwide surgeons, and they found substantial ($\kappa = 0.74$) overall interobserver reliability for the 3 main types, and excellent ($\kappa = 0.81$) intraobserver reliability. Additionally, they reported moderate interobserver ($\kappa = 0.56$) and intraobserver ($\kappa = 0.43–0.57$) reliability of the fracture subtypes. These results have since been validated independently by multiple authors; Urrutia and colleagues[37] found substantial interobserver reliability of the 3 main types ($\kappa = 0.62$) and moderate reliability of the subtypes ($\kappa = 0.55$), and Azimi and colleagues[38] reported excellent interobserver reliability of the 3 main types of injures ($\kappa = 0.83–0.89$). After establishing the reliability of the classification, the hierarchical nature of the classification system was verified by

Schroeder and colleagues[12] in a survey of 74 surgeons, and these results were used to develop the Thoracolumbar AOSpine Injury Score (TL AOSIS; see **Tables 3** and **4**).[9] Similar to the TLICS score, the TL AOSIS has an integer assigned to each possible variable in the AOSpine Thoracolumbar Injury Classification System. The values of all variables are then summed to determine the total TL AOSIS.

In an attempt to prevent regional rejection of the classification, the treatment algorithm was developed with the input of more than 500 surgeons from all regions of the world. If fewer than 30% of the respondents recommended surgical intervention, nonoperative treatment was recommended for the injury, and if more than 70% of respondents recommended surgical intervention, surgical management was recommended for the injury. Using these results and the TL AOSIS, a simple and easy to use surgical algorithm was proposed. Patients with a total TL AOSIS of less than 4 should undergo a trial of nonoperative treatment, and early operative intervention is appropriate for patients with a TL AOSIS of greater than 5. Treatment of patients with a TL AOSIS of 4 or 5 should be individualized based on surgeon and patient variables, because

Table 3
The TL AOSIS types

Subgroup	Description	TL AOSIS
Type A—compression fractures		
A0	An injury that has no possibility of affecting the structural integrity of the spine (ie, fracture spinous or transverse process fracture)	0
A1	A fracture through a single endplate that does not extend into the posterior wall	1
A2	A fracture through a both endplate that does not extend into the posterior wall	2
A3	A fracture through a single endplate that does extend into the posterior wall (incomplete burst)	3
A4	A fracture through both endplates that does extend into the posterior wall (complete burst)	5
Type B—tension band injuries		
B1	A completely osseous tension band injury (ie, a bony chance fracture)	5
B2	An injury that disrupts the posterior tension bade	6
B3	An injury that disrupts the anterior tension band	7
Type C—translational injuries		
C	Any injury that results in translation of the vertebral body	8

The TL AOSIS divides fractures into 3 main types, and 8 subtypes. Each injury type is accompanied by the TL AOSIS.
Abbreviation: TL AOSIS, Thoracolumbar AOSpine Injury Score.
From Kepler CK, Vaccaro AR, Schroeder GD, et al. The Thoracolumbar AOSpine Injury Score (TL AOSIS). Global Spine J 2016;6(4):329–34; and Vaccaro AR, Oner C, Kepler CK, et al. AOSpine thoracolumbar spine injury classification system: fracture description, neurological status, and key modifiers. Spine (Phila Pa 1976) 2013;38:2028–37; with permission.

Table 4
The TL AOSIS status and modifiers

Subgroup	Description	TL AOSIS
Neurologic status		
N0	No neurologic injury	0
N1	Resolved temporary neurologic injury	1
N2	Injury to a nerve root	2
N3	Incomplete spinal cord injury or cauda equina syndrome	4
N4	Complete spinal cord injury	4
Nx	A reliable neurologic examination cannot be obtained	3
Patient-specific modifiers		
M1	Ambiguity in the integrity of the PLC	1
M2	Patient specific concerns that will affect the treatment algorithm (ie, ankylosing spondylitis, severe burns etc.)	0

The TL AOSIS has 6 possible grades for the patient's neurologic status and 2 patient-specific modifiers. Each variable is accompanied by the TL AOSIS.

Abbreviation: TL AOSIS, Thoracolumbar AOSpine Injury Score.

From Schroeder GD, Kepler CK, Koerner JD, et al. A worldwide analysis of the reliability and perceived importance of an injury to the posterior ligamentous complex in AO Type A Fractures. Global Spine J 2015;5:378–82; and Savage JW, Moore TA, Arnold PM, et al. The reliability and validity of the thoracolumbar injury classification system in pediatric spine trauma. Spine (Phila Pa 1976) 2015;40:E1014–8; with permission.

either operative or nonoperative care may be appropriate.[14]

SUMMARY

Currently, there is significant regional variability in the treatment of thoracolumbar trauma, and one of the possible causes for this is the lack of a globally accepted classification system. Historic classifications often separated each spinal segment into 2 or 3 columns, and then classified the injury based on either specific osseous injuries or an inferred injury mechanism. Contemporary classifications have focused not only on the morphology of the injury, but also other critical determinants of treatment, such as the integrity of the PLC and the neurology. Most recently, the

AOSpine Thoracolumbar Spine Injury Classification System and its accompanying treatment algorithm were developed, and given the unique and globally inclusive development process used in the design of the system, there is cautious optimism for global acceptance.

REFERENCES

1. Vaccaro AR, Lehman RA Jr, Hurlbert RJ, et al. A new classification of thoracolumbar injuries: the importance of injury morphology, the integrity of the posterior ligamentous complex, and neurologic status. Spine (Phila Pa 1976) 2005;30:2325–33.
2. Bailey CS, Urquhart JC, Dvorak MF, et al. Orthosis versus no orthosis for the treatment of thoracolumbar burst fractures without neurologic injury: a multicenter prospective randomized equivalence trial. Spine J 2014;14(11):2557–64.
3. Magerl F, Aebi M, Gertzbein SD, et al. A comprehensive classification of thoracic and lumbar injuries. Eur Spine J 1994;3:184–201.
4. Schnake KJ. Expert's comment concerning Grand Rounds case entitled "progressive kyphotic deformity in comminuted burst fractures treated non-operatively: the Achilles tendon of the Thoracolumbar Injury Classification and Severity Score (TLICS)" (T.A. Mattei, J. Hanovnikian, D. Dinh). Eur Spine J 2014;23:2263–4.
5. Reinhold M, Knop C, Beisse R, et al. Operative treatment of 733 patients with acute thoracolumbar spinal injuries: comprehensive results from the second, prospective, Internet-based multicenter study of the Spine Study Group of the German Association of Trauma Surgery. Eur Spine J 2010;19:1657–76.
6. Schnake KJ, Stavridis SI, Kandziora F. Five-year clinical and radiological results of combined anteroposterior stabilization of thoracolumbar fractures. J Neurosurg Spine 2014;20:497–504.
7. Schnake KJ, Stavridis SI, Krampe S, et al. Additional anterior plating enhances fusion in anteroposteriorly stabilized thoracolumbar fractures. Injury 2014;45:792–8.
8. Kepler C, Vaccaro A, Koerner J, et al. Reliability analysis of the AOSpine thoracolumbar spine injury classification system by a worldwide group of naïve spinal surgeons. Eur Spine J 2016;25(4):1082–6.
9. Kepler CK, Vaccaro AR, Schroeder GD, et al. The Thoracolumbar AOSpine Injury Score (TL AOSIS). Global Spine J 2016;6(4):329–34.
10. Schroeder GD, Kepler CK, Koerner JD, et al. Is there a regional difference in morphology interpretation of A3 and A4 fractures among different cultures? J Neurosurg Spine 2015;1–8.
11. Schroeder GD, Kepler CK, Koerner JD, et al. A worldwide analysis of the reliability and perceived

importance of an injury to the posterior ligamentous complex in AO Type A Fractures. Global Spine J 2015;5:378–82.

12. Schroeder GD, Vaccaro AR, Kepler CK, et al. Establishing the injury severity of thoracolumbar trauma: confirmation of the hierarchical structure of the AO-Spine thoracolumbar spine injury classification system. Spine (Phila Pa 1976) 2015;40:E498–503.

13. Vaccaro AR, Oner C, Kepler CK, et al. AOSpine thoracolumbar spine injury classification system: fracture description, neurological status, and key modifiers. Spine (Phila Pa 1976) 2013;38:2028–37.

14. Vaccaro AR, Schroeder GD, Kepler CK, et al. The surgical algorithm for the AOSpine thoracolumbar spine injury classification system. Eur Spine J 2016;25(4):1087–94.

15. Gertzbein SD. Scoliosis Research Society. Multicenter spine fracture study. Spine (Phila Pa 1976) 1992;17:528–40.

16. Weinstein JN, Collalto P, Lehmann TR. Thoracolumbar "burst" fractures treated conservatively: a long-term follow-up. Spine (Phila Pa 1976) 1988;13:33–8.

17. Wood K, Buttermann G, Mehbod A, et al. Operative compared with nonoperative treatment of a thoracolumbar burst fracture without neurological deficit. A prospective, randomized study. J Bone Joint Surg Am 2003;85-A:773–81.

18. Watson-Jones R. The results of postural reduction of fractures of the spine. J Bone Joint Surg Am 1938; 20:567–86.

19. Chance GQ. Note on a type of flexion fracture of the spine. Br J Radiol 1948;21:452.

20. Holdsworth F. Fractures, dislocations, and fracture-dislocations of the spine. J Bone Joint Surg Am 1970;52:1534–51.

21. Mirza SK, Mirza AJ, Chapman JR, et al. Classifications of thoracic and lumbar fractures: rationale and supporting data. J Am Acad Orthop Surg 2002;10:364–77.

22. Patel AA, Vaccaro AR. Thoracolumbar spine trauma classification. J Am Acad Orthop Surg 2010;18:63–71.

23. Kelly RP, Whitesides TE Jr. Treatment of lumbodorsal fracture-dislocations. Ann Surg 1968;167:705–17.

24. Denis F. The three column spine and its significance in the classification of acute thoracolumbar spinal injuries. Spine (Phila Pa 1976) 1983;8:817–31.

25. Oner FC, Ramos LM, Simmermacher RK, et al. Classification of thoracic and lumbar spine fractures: problems of reproducibility. A study of 53 patients using CT and MRI. Eur Spine J 2002;11:235–45.

26. Wood KB, Khanna G, Vaccaro AR, et al. Assessment of two thoracolumbar fracture classification systems as used by multiple surgeons. J Bone Joint Surg Am 2005;87:1423–9.

27. McAfee PC, Yuan HA, Fredrickson BE, et al. The value of computed tomography in thoracolumbar fractures. An analysis of one hundred consecutive cases and a new classification. J Bone Joint Surg Am 1983;65:461–73.

28. Ferguson RL, Allen BL Jr. A mechanistic classification of thoracolumbar spine fractures. Clin Orthop Relat Res 1984;(189):77–88.

29. Aebi M. Classification of thoracolumbar fractures and dislocations. Eur Spine J 2010;19(Suppl 1): S2–7.

30. Vaccaro AR, Baron EM, Sanfilippo J, et al. Reliability of a novel classification system for thoracolumbar injuries: the thoracolumbar injury severity score. Spine (Phila Pa 1976) 2006;31:S62–9 [discussion: S104].

31. Joaquim AF, Fernandes YB, Cavalcante RA, et al. Evaluation of the thoracolumbar injury classification system in thoracic and lumbar spinal trauma. Spine (Phila Pa 1976) 2011;36:33–6.

32. Savage JW, Moore TA, Arnold PM, et al. The reliability and validity of the thoracolumbar injury classification system in pediatric spine trauma. Spine (Phila Pa 1976) 2015;40:E1014–8.

33. Wood KB, Buttermann GR, Phukan R, et al. Operative compared with nonoperative treatment of a thoracolumbar burst fracture without neurological deficit: a prospective randomized study with follow-up at sixteen to twenty-two years. J Bone Joint Surg Am 2015;97:3–9.

34. Joaquim AF, Daubs MD, Lawrence BD, et al. Retrospective evaluation of the validity of the thoracolumbar injury classification system in 458 consecutively treated patients. Spine J 2013;13:1760–5.

35. Sadiqi S, Oner FC, Dvorak MF, et al. The influence of spine surgeons' experience on the classification and intraobserver reliability of the novel AOSpine thoracolumbar spine injury classification system - an international study. Spine (Phila Pa 1976) 2015; 40(23):E1250–6.

36. Schroeder GD, Kepler CK, Koerner JD, et al. Can a thoracolumbar injury severity score be uniformly applied from T1 to L5 or are modifications necessary? Global Spine J 2015;5:339–45.

37. Urrutia J, Zamora T, Yurac R, et al. An independent interobserver reliability and intraobserver reproducibility evaluation of the new AOSpine thoracolumbar spine injury classification system. Spine (Phila Pa 1976) 2015;40:E54–8.

38. Azimi P, Mohammadi HR, Azhari S, et al. The AO-Spine thoracolumbar spine injury classification system: a reliability and agreement study. Asian J Neurosurg 2015;10:282–5.

Timing of Surgery After Spinal Cord Injury

Matthew Piazza, MD, James Schuster, MD, PhD*

KEYWORDS

- Spinal cord injury • Spine trauma • Surgical timing • Surgical decompression

KEY POINTS

- Early surgical decompression of spinal cord injury, in particular incomplete injury, may lead to improved neurologic recovery.
- Although the data for early surgery are less clear in patients with complete injury, even small gains in neurologic function can have significant impact on quality of life.
- Sacral sparing has a significant impact on prognosis, and patients with an unreliable assessment should undergo early intervention if stable for surgery.
- Early surgery after spinal cord injury may also reduce the rate of non-neurologic complications and health care resource utilization.

INTRODUCTION

Spinal cord injury, affecting approximately 54 per 1 million people annually in the United States, can be a devastating injury for the trauma patient and is associated with a significant morbidity and high mortality rate, particularly among the elderly.[1] Approximately 71.7% of patients with spinal injury suffer polytrauma and the incidence of spinal cord injury among the elderly is rising, making this patient population particularly challenging to manage.[2,3] Moreover, the socioeconomic burden of spinal cord injury in the United States is substantial.[4] There is a need to optimize treatment paradigms for this patient population. Once patients are resuscitated and stabilized, the cornerstones of management of spinal cord injury include rapid clinical assessment and characterization of injury and, if indicated, definitive surgical decompression and/or stabilization. The surgical approach for decompression and fusion depends on the injury pattern. A critical question faced by the neurosurgeon is the optimal timing for decompression and stabilization. Despite having been studied extensively in the literature, there remains considerable controversy regarding the safety and efficacy of early decompressive surgery. This article examines the evidence for early surgery in patients presenting with spinal cord injury.

PATHOPHYSIOLOGIC BASIS FOR SPINAL CORD INJURY AND EXPERIMENTAL EVIDENCE FOR TIMELY DECOMPRESSIVE SURGERY

Blunt traumatic spinal cord injuries, distinct from penetrating injuries, begin with a mechanical insult that results in biomechanical failure of the spinal column leading to bony fractures and/or discoligamentous disruption. Resultant osteoligamentous instability and/or displaced bone fragments can exert compressive, sheer, or distractive forces on the spinal cord itself and can lead to immediate disruption of neural tissue or vasculature. This initial mechanical event constitutes the primary phase of spinal cord injury and the degree of primary injury is correlated with the magnitude of the force of insult.[5] After this inciting event, the secondary phase of injury ensues propagated by

Disclosures: The authors have nothing to disclose.
Department of Neurosurgery, Hospital of the University of Pennsylvania, 3400 Spruce Street, 3rd Floor Silverstein, Philadelphia, PA 19104, USA
* Corresponding author.
E-mail address: James.schuster@uphs.upenn.edu

Neurosurg Clin N Am 28 (2017) 31–39
http://dx.doi.org/10.1016/j.nec.2016.08.005
1042-3680/17/© 2016 Elsevier Inc. All rights reserved.

neurosurgery.theclinics.com

vascular ischemia, inflammation, neuronal hyper-excitability, and free radical generation, ultimately leading to further neuronal cell death.[6] Treatment of spinal cord injury focuses on curtailing the extent of secondary injury. Emerging novel therapies target these pathophysiologic processes on a molecular level. Although targeting these secondary processes is appealing and is the focus of intense research, preserving any residual viable neural tissue, even in those patients with complete injury, may optimize the chances of neurologic recovery with these newer treatment modalities.

Persistent compression or forces imparted on the spinal cord through motion from instability are the primary immediate concerns with regard to protecting a patient from further spinal cord injury. Experimental evidence in animal models suggests that the extent of spinal cord injury is correlated both with the degree of cord compression and timing to decompression.[7–9] Animal studies have demonstrated that a cerebrospinal fluid pressure differential is generated at the level of the compression; this higher pressure cephalad to compression may impair perfusion of viable tissue, leading to ischemia and further secondary injury.[10] Early decompression (<8 hours compared with >72 hours) has been associated with decreased levels of tumor necrosis factor α and fewer apoptotic cells in injured spinal cord tissue, and these factors were associated with improved neurologic recovery.[8] Timely decompression and/or stabilization of spine injuries may preserve remaining viable tissue and reduce the risk of secondary injury.

INITIAL NEUROLOGIC ASSESSMENT AFTER SPINAL CORD INJURY

Given the neurologic examination may influence the timing of surgical decision making, the initial assessment and management of spinal cord injury are reviewed briefly here.[11] Once a patient with suspected spinal cord injury is identified, a critical first step in management is a thorough neurologic assessment. This allows the neurosurgeon to determine the severity of spinal cord injury and to establish the baseline neurologic status, both of which are important for guiding further management and surgical decision making. Using well-established and validated injury severity grading scales is important because they provide a standardized way to classify spinal cord injury and facilitate communication among practitioners. The American Spinal Injury Association Classifications Standards/International Standards for Neurological Classification of Spinal Cord Injury (ASIA/ISNCSCI) is a widely used and validated clinical grading scale both for the initial evaluation of patients with spinal cord injury and for the assessment of postinjury recovery long term.[12,13] The ASIA Impairment Scale (AIS) integrates the detailed neurologic assessment captured by the ASIA/ISNCSCI into a simple grading scale of neurologic injury severity (**Table 1**).[14] The presence of sacral sparing distinguishes a complete injury (ASIA grade A) from incomplete injuries (ASIA grade B–E). A complete spinal cord injury is classified by no evidence of neurologic function,

---

Table 1
American Spinal Injury Association Impairment Scale grade and relationship with long-term functional ambulation

American Spinal Injury Association Impairment Scale Grade	Definition[14]	Percent Ambulation at 6 mo to 12 mo[58] (%)
A	No preservation of neurologic function at the S4-5 segments	3.7
B	Preservation of some sensory but no motor function no more than 3 levels below the level of injury, including S4-5 segments	24
C	Preservation of motor function below level with <50% of muscle groups with power rating of 3 or greater	58
D	Preservation of motor function below level with >50% of muscle groups with power rating of 3 or greater	100

Adapted from Kirshblum SC, Burns SP, Biering-Sorensen F, et al. International standards for neurological classification of spinal cord injury (revised 2011). J Spinal Cord Med 2011;34(6):535–46; and van Middendorp JJ, Hosman AJF, Pouw MH; EM-SCI Study Group. ASIA impairment scale conversion in traumatic SCI: is it related with the ability to walk? A descriptive comparison with functional ambulation outcome measures in 273 patients. Spinal Cord 2009;47(7):555–60.

either sensory or motor, at the level of the lower sacral roots (S4-5), indicating the probability of a complete conduction block at the level of injury. On the other hand, the most severe grading of incomplete spinal cord injury, classified as ASIA grade B, requires preservation of some sensory function but no motor function below the level of injury, including the sacral segments. According to the definitions proposed by the International Standards Committee of ASIA, patients with no neurologic function in sacral segments but some retained motor or sensory function elsewhere below the level of injury are still classified as ASIA grade A.[14] Zariffa and colleagues[15] investigated the incidence of this somewhat paradoxic classification in patients with spinal cord injury and found that approximately 3.4% and 34.3% of patients diagnosed as ASIA grade A 1 week from injury would otherwise be designated ASIA grade D and ASIA grade C, respectively, if graded by motor scores alone. Accurate assessment of the lower sacral segments is paramount, because there is clear evidence within the literature of spontaneous recovery of neurologic function in the presence of spared lower sacral nerve root function.[16] In patients in whom lower sacral nerve root function via the anorectal examination is equivocal or unreliable, assessment of sensory function within the high sacral segments is closely correlated and may serve as an adjunct.[17]

Numerous studies have used the ASIA score to categorize injury severity, and there is ample evidence within the literature that more severe spinal cord injury is associated with poor outcome; outcomes are especially poor among those patients with complete injury.[18–20] There is a clear relationship with AIS grade and functional ambulation, with few patients who are initially ASIA A recovering functional ambulation (see **Table 1**).[21] There is less urgency to definitively treat patients with complete spinal cord injury[11] and well-established surgical grading scales, such as the thoracolumbar injury classification and severity scale[22] and the subaxial cervical spine injury classification system,[23] place less emphasis on operative intervention on patients with complete injury. Hence, distinguishing between an ASIA grade A and ASIA grade B injury may significantly surgical decision making. Although there is ample evidence in the literature for high inter-rater reliability of the ASIA/ISNCSCI among trained professionals,[24] given the reliance on injury severity for operative decision making, it is imperative that an accurate reliable assessment is performed in patients without confounding factors if a neurosurgeon is to use the neurologic examination in the decision making regarding surgery and its timing. Burns and

colleagues[25] identified a small but not negligible fraction of patients who were initially diagnosed as ASIA grade A injuries convert to ASIA grade B on follow-up assessment. This is especially important given that 16% to 35% of patients with spinal cord injury have concomitant moderate to severe traumatic brain injury, a confounding factor when attempting a detailed neurologic assessment of spinal cord function.[26,27] Although the initial neurologic assessment is an important component of surgical decision making, this should not be the sole factor in determining timing of surgery, especially in the setting of confounding factors.

TIMING OF DECOMPRESSION AND NEUROLOGIC RECOVERY

There is growing evidence within the clinical literature supporting early surgical intervention after traumatic spinal cord injury. The Surgical Timing in Acute Spinal Cord Injury Study (STASCIS) was a multicenter, prospective study of 313 patients with cervical spinal cord injury undergoing surgical decompression and instrumentation.[28] In this study, early surgery was defined as less than 24 hours after the initial injury. The investigators found that even after adjusting for preoperative neurologic status and steroid administration, patients undergoing early surgery were 2.8 times more likely to have at least a 2-grade improvement in AIS score. Patients undergoing early surgery were significantly more likely to be motor complete (ASIA grade A/B; 57.7% vs 38.2%). In another prospective study, Wilson and colleagues[29] examined 55 patients with traumatic spinal cord injury undergoing either early or late decompressive surgery (<24 hours vs >24 hours); after adjusting for presence of complete injury and level of injury, early surgery was predictive of improved neurologic outcomes at discharge from rehabilitation as assessed by the ASIA motor score. Dvorak and colleagues[30] examined changes in ASIA motor score in patients with incomplete spinal cord injury and found significantly greater degree of neurologic recovery in patients undergoing early surgery (a 6-point motor difference). Although a 6-point motor score difference may not seem substantial, such an improvement may lead to functional recovery of 1 or 2 neurologic levels that may translate into greater independence and quality of life.[31] For example, patients who convert to a C7 from a C6 neurologic level regain the arm extension and the ability to perform independent transfers. Dvorak and colleagues[30] did not observe improvement with early surgery in patients with complete spinal cord injury.

As suggested previously, in the subgroup of patients with complete spinal cord injury, the timing of decompressive surgery is even more controversial. In general, outcomes within this subgroup of patients are poor, although few studies have closely examined patients with complete spinal cord injury. Recently, Bourassa-Moreau and colleagues[32] specifically studied patients with complete spinal cord injury, defined as AIS grade A on initial assessment who underwent surgery either in an early or delayed fashion (less than or greater than 24 hours after injury, respectively). Although the observed frequency of neurologic improvement with early surgery did not reach statistical significance overall, the investigators noted that among patients with cervical injuries, AIS grade A patients had significantly greater rate of neurologic improvement in the early surgery group when compared with the delayed surgery group (64% vs 0%, respectively). There are several studies that contradict this finding, showing no benefit in neurologic recovery in patients with early versus later surgery.[18,30,33]

Not all studies support early surgical intervention. Vaccaro and colleagues[34] conducted a prospective study of 62 patients examining surgery performed within 72 hours or greater than 5 days after cervical spinal cord injury. In this early clinical study, the investigators did not find any difference in neurologic outcomes at follow-up. In a retrospective study of 595 patients with cervical spinal cord injury, patients who underwent surgery either 72 hours before or after the initial injury were assessed for neurologic improvement.[35] In this study, neurologic improvement was not significantly different between the surgical groups; patients undergoing early surgery experienced greater degrees of postoperative neurologic decline and perioperative mortality.[35] In another retrospective review, Pollard and colleagues[36] studied 412 patients with incomplete cervical spinal cord injury and found no relationship between early surgery (<24 hours postinjury) and late surgery.

Given the inconsistent findings in the literature, several meta-analyses have been published to address the issue of timing of surgical decompression. A recent meta-analysis of published studies by Liu and colleagues[37] found that patients undergoing surgery within 24 hours of injury had greater degrees of neurologic improvement and overall motor function. In another meta-analysis, van Middendorp and colleagues[38] found a similar benefit in the early surgery group; the investigators, however, found significant evidence of publication bias secondary to study heterogeneity and advised readers to interpret their results with caution.

More recently, the impact of even earlier decompressive surgery within 8 hours of injury has been investigated. Grassner and colleagues[39] performed a retrospective analysis of patients undergoing decompressive surgery within 8 hours or after 8 hours of injury; in addition to baseline neurologic status and age, timing of surgery independently predicted neurologic improvement at follow-up as assed by change in Spinal Cord Independence Measure. In another study, Jug and colleagues[40] examined patients who underwent early decompressive surgery dichotomized by intervention less than 8 hours from injury and between 8 hours and 24 hours from injury; even within this group of patients undergoing early surgery, decompression less than 8 hours from injury was associated with a significantly increased odds of a 2-grade improvement in AIS score even after controlling for baseline neurologic function and amount of canal compromise. There was no difference in perioperative complications or mortality in these 2 groups, suggesting that surgical intervention can be performed very early after injury without added perioperative risk.

In summary, there is accumulating evidence within the literature regarding the neurologic benefit of early surgery after spinal cord injury. In particular, there seems to be a more robust impact on neurologic recovery with early surgery in patients with incomplete injury, and there are data that the earlier the surgery, the greater the neurologic benefit. Moreover, there is emerging evidence that even in patients with complete spinal cord injury, early intervention may yield neurologic improvement. This topic remains controversial given the overall small sample, the heterogeneity of published studies, and lack of level I data. Randomized clinical trials examining timing of surgery are unfeasible due to obvious ethical issues. Moreover, definitions of early surgery within published studies are varied. Larger, multicenter studies that are adequately powered are needed to (1) identify the optimal definition of early surgery, (2) elucidate the true role of decompression after neurologically complete injuries, and (3) delineate patient factors (ie, specific level of injury) that are predictive of improved neurologic recovery and functional outcome with early surgery.

SURGICAL TIMING IN PATIENTS WITH CENTRAL CORD SYNDROME

Traumatic central cord syndrome is a clinical entity that is typically seen after a hyperextension injury in which there is preferential involvement of the medial anterior and posterior columns of the spinal cord, resulting in predominant upper extremity symptoms, although the presentation can be fairly heterogeneous. Cervical spondylosis is commonly seen with this syndrome, can occur in the absence of frank osteoligamentous injury, and can result from mild trauma. The evidence for early surgery, or surgery at all, in this patient population is even more controversial than in patients without spinal fractures or instability. Lenehan and colleagues[41] analyzed a prospective cohort of 73 patients with central cord syndrome with cervical spondylosis without instability; the investigators found that patients undergoing early surgery (<24 hours) had a significant increase in motor recovery scores and Functional Independence Measure total scores with late surgery group at 12-month follow-up. Yamakazi and colleagues,[42] in their retrospective study of 47 patients with traumatic central cord syndrome, found that time to surgery was the only predictor of improved postoperative neurologic function. Guest and colleagues[43] divided their cohort of patients with central cord syndrome into those with fracture and/or acute disc herniation and those with purely cervical stenosis. In the former group, there was a significant difference in neurologic improvement with early surgery defined as less than 24 hours after injury; however, there was no relationship between degree of neurologic recovery and surgical timing in the subgroup with isolated cervical stenosis. In a prospective study, Kepler and colleagues[44] studied 68 patients undergoing either surgery within or after 24 hours from injury and did not observe any significant difference in neurologic improvement although, again, there was a significant fraction of patients with cervical fractures and only short-term outcomes were available (1 week from injury). Stevens and colleagues[45] examined 3 different time points for surgical intervention in their retrospective study of 67 patients: surgery within 24 hours of injury, surgery 24 hours after injury but prior to discharge, and surgery performed after discharge after the initial admission. Although there was no difference with regard to neurologic outcome among the different time points, there was a nonsignificant trend toward decreased length in stay and fewer complications in patients receiving surgery during the first admission. In another respective study of 49 patients with central cord syndrome, Chen and colleagues[46] examined the impact of several clinical factors on neurologic, including surgical, intervention with or after 4 days from injury. The investigators found no significant difference in neurologic improvement as assessed by the AIS; the study population was heterogeneous, however, regarding the presence of associated fracture. Delaying surgery may provide some clinical benefit. In a large national database-based study of 1060 patients with acute central cord syndrome, Samuel and colleagues[47] found that with each 24-hour delay of surgery there was a 19% reduction in mortality; the investigators also found an association between early surgery and more frequent minor, but not major,

complications. In a systematic review of studies examining timing of surgery after traumatic central cord syndrome, Anderson and colleagues[48] concluded that although surgery within 24 hours seemed safe, there was insufficient evidence to recommend routine early surgical decompression. Given the lack of consistent data within the literature regarding surgical timing for central cord syndrome, there is understandably disagreement within the surgical community regarding when to operate. In a survey study of 971 spine surgeons conducted by AOSpine regarding timing of surgery for spinal cord injury, there was little consensus among the spine surgeons surveyed regarding the optimal timing of surgery for central cord syndrome; in particular, central cord syndrome was the only pathology examined in which a majority of surgeons did not prefer to operate within 24 hours.[11]

THE IMPACT OF TIMING OF SURGERY ON NON-NEUROLOGIC OUTCOMES

Early surgery may have potential benefits in reducing non-neurologic–related complications and clinical outcomes. Bliemel and colleagues,[49] in their large series of patients with spinal cord injury, demonstrated that patients undergoing late surgery (>72 hours postinjury) experienced greater rates of sepsis, duration of ventilation, and ICU and hospital length of stay. Bourassa-Moreau and colleagues[50] identified early surgery defined as less than 24 hours from injury as predictive of fewer overall complications, pneumonia, and pressure ulcers; a more severe ASIA score was also significantly predictive of complications. In another study, the same group examined patients with complete spinal cord injury and found that early surgery, again defined as less than 24 hours from injury, was predictive of fewer total complications, pneumonia, and urinary tract infections.[51] Several meta-analyses and systematic reviews have strengthened these findings. Liu and colleagues[37] demonstrated that patients undergoing surgery within 24 hours had lower complication rates and shorter hospital length of stay in their meta-analysis. In a systematic review, Dimar and colleagues[52] found that early surgery in patients with spinal cord injury, especially those patients with more severe injury, is associated with fewer complications, days of ventilation, and ICU and hospital length of stays. The length of hospitalization is especially important for spinal cord injury patients because longer hospital stays result in delays to rehabilitation; in a recent study by Herzer and colleagues,[53] time to rehabilitation was associated with lower functional independence at 1 year postinjury.

Given the potential reduction in in-hospital complications and length of stay, several studies have evaluated the impact of timing of surgery on associated cost of hospitalization. In the previously cited study examining non-neurologic complications in patients undergoing early decompression for complete spinal cord injury, Bourassa-Moreau and colleagues[51] also found that early surgery led to lower cost of hospitalization. This latter finding may reflect the increased cost of care associated with complication management as well as length of stay with delay in definitive surgical management, which was not assessed in this study. Furlan and colleagues,[54] in a cost-utility analysis of patients undergoing early versus late decompression for spinal cord injury using the data from STASCIS study, found that patients with both complete and incomplete motor injuries undergoing early decompression experienced substantial savings with an associated $58,368,024.12 and $536,217.33 per quality-adjusted life year gained, respectively. Similarly, in their study examining 477 patients undergoing either early or late surgery dichotomized at 24 hours, Mac-Thiong and colleagues[55] demonstrated that surgical timing was significantly associated cost of hospitalization ($20,525 $\pm$ $13,791 vs $25,036 $\pm$ $17,886, respectively). Together, these findings are highly suggestive that not only does early surgery reduce non-neurologic–related complications but also leads to a decrease in health care resource utilization and health care costs.

FACTORS THAT INFLUENCE TIMING OF SURGERY

Several studies have attempted to identify the impact of other patient-related and health system–related variables on timing to surgery. Bliemel and colleagues[49] examined factors that influenced timing of surgery in trauma patients with spinal cord injury and found that patients with polytrauma, in particular chest, abdominal, extremity, or head injury, were more likely to undergo delayed surgical intervention. Similarly, patients with severe head injury, those requiring hemodynamic support with catecholamines, and those intubated or receiving chest tubes, underwent delayed surgery as well. Patients admitted prior to surgery, either as a transfer or primarily, did not experience differences in surgical timing. Use of closed reduction prior to definitive surgical treatment reduced the delay to the operating room. Furlan and colleagues[56] assessed extrinsic factors and intrinsic factors potentially related to delay of surgical decompression using data from the STASCIS study. The investigators found that extrinsic factors (ie, those related to health systems issues)

but not intrinsic factors (ie, those that are patient related) were significantly different among early versus delayed surgical groups. In particular, patients undergoing late surgery had a significantly longer wait at the first general hospital prior to transfer to a spine center, longer time to assessment by a spine surgeon, and longer time for decision to operate. Similarly, Battistuzzo and colleagues,[57] in their series of 192 patients with spinal cord injury undergoing surgical decompression, found a significant difference in time to the operating room for patients initially transferred to nonsurgical hospital versus surgical hospital directly (26 hours vs 12 hours, respectively). Together, these studies suggest that certain modifiable non–patient-related factors may have a potential impact on surgical timing and can inform the development of streamlined spinal cord injury acute care paradigms.

SUMMARY

The evidence presented in this article suggests that early surgical decompression of spinal cord injury may lead not only to improved neurologic recovery but also to reduction in non-neurologic complications, health care resource utilization, and spinal cord injury–associated hospitalization costs. In particular, there is significant support within the literature that early decompression in patients with incomplete spinal cord injury is associated with improved neurologic outcomes; the data are less clear regarding complete spinal cord injuries. That said, small gains in neurologic function, even with complete injury, can lead to substantial improvements in quality of life. Sacral sparing has significant impact on prognosis; when using the clinical examination to drive decision making for timing of surgery, if there is any question about the reliability of the examination, especially with the assessment of the lower sacral segments, the surgeon should lean toward earlier, more aggressive intervention. Moreover, early intervention seems to correlate with shorter length of stay and hence shorter time to rehabilitation, which may have an impact on long-term functional outcome. Further large, multicenter, adequately powered prospective studies, however, especially within the subgroup of patients with complete injury and central cord syndrome, are needed to confirm these findings and identify the optimal definition of early decompression. Moreover, efforts at the health care system level should be implemented to streamline initial care of spinal cord injury patients to further reduce the time between the injury and surgical decompression.

REFERENCES

1. Jain NB, Ayers GD, Peterson EN, et al. Traumatic spinal cord injury in the United States, 1993-2012. JAMA 2015;313(22):2236–43.

2. Hebert JS, Burnham RS. The effect of polytrauma in persons with traumatic spine injury. A prospective database of spine fractures. Spine (Phila Pa 1976) 2000;25(1):55–60.

3. Selvarajah S, Hammond ER, Haider AH, et al. The burden of acute traumatic spinal cord injury among adults in the united states: an update. J Neurotrauma 2014;31(3):228–38.

4. Mahabaleshwarkar R, Khanna R. National hospitalization burden associated with spinal cord injuries in the United States. Spinal Cord 2014;52(2):139–44.

5. Blight AR, Decrescito V. Morphometric analysis of experimental spinal cord injury in the cat: the relation of injury intensity to survival of myelinated axons. Neuroscience 1986;19(1):321–41.

6. Kwon BK, Tetzlaff W, Grauer JN, et al. Pathophysiology and pharmacologic treatment of acute spinal cord injury. Spine J 2004;4(4):451–64.

7. Dimar JR, Glassman SD, Raque GH, et al. The influence of spinal canal narrowing and timing of decompression on neurologic recovery after spinal cord contusion in a rat model. Spine (Phila Pa 1976) 1999;24(16):1623–33.

8. Xie J-B, Zhang X, Li Q-H, et al. Inhibition of inflammatory cytokines after early decompression may mediate recovery of neurological function in rats with spinal cord injury. Neural Regen Res 2015; 10(2):219–24.

9. Batchelor PE, Wills TE, Skeers P, et al. Meta-analysis of pre-clinical studies of early decompression in acute spinal cord injury: a battle of time and pressure. PLoS One 2013;8(8):e72659.

10. Jones CF, Newell RS, Lee JHT, et al. The pressure distribution of cerebrospinal fluid responds to residual compression and decompression in an animal model of acute spinal cord injury. Spine (Phila Pa 1976) 2012;37(23):E1422–31.

11. Fehlings MG, Rabin D, Sears W, et al. Current practice in the timing of surgical intervention in spinal cord injury. Spine (Phila Pa 1976) 2010;35(Suppl 21):S166–73.

12. Marino RJ, Barros T, Biering-Sorensen F, et al. International standards for neurological classification of spinal cord injury. J Spinal Cord Med 2003; 26(Suppl 1):S50–6.

13. Hadley MN, Walters BC, Aarabi B, et al. Clinical assessment following acute cervical spinal cord injury. Neurosurgery 2013;72(Suppl 2):40–53.

14. Kirshblum SC, Burns SP, Biering-Sorensen F, et al. International standards for neurological classification of spinal cord injury (revised 2011). J Spinal Cord Med 2011;34(6):535–46.

15. Zariffa J, Curt A, Steeves JD. Functional motor preservation below the level of injury in subjects with American spinal injury association impairment scale grade a spinal cord injuries. Arch Phys Med Rehabil 2012;93(5):905–7.

16. Kirshblum S, Botticello A, Lammertse DP, et al. The impact of sacral sensory sparing in motor complete spinal cord injury. Arch Phys Med Rehabil 2011; 92(3):376–83.

17. Zariffa J, Kramer JLK, Jones LAT, et al. Sacral sparing in SCI: beyond the S4-S5 and anorectal examination. Spine J 2012;12(5):389–400.e3.

18. Petitjean ME, Mousselard H, Pointillart V, et al. Thoracic spinal trauma and associated injuries: should early spinal decompression be considered? J Trauma 1995;39(2):368–72.

19. McCarthy MJH, Gatehouse S, Steel M, et al. The influence of the energy of trauma, the timing of decompression, and the impact of grade of SCI on outcome. Evid Based Spine Care J 2011; 2(2):11–7.

20. Marino RJ, Burns S, Graves DE, et al. Upper- and lower-extremity motor recovery after traumatic cervical spinal cord injury: an update from the national spinal cord injury database. Arch Phys Med Rehabil 2011;92(3):369–75.

21. Spiess MR, Müller RM, Rupp R, et al, EM-SCI Study Group. Conversion in ASIA impairment scale during the first year after traumatic spinal cord injury. J Neurotrauma 2009;26(11):2027–36.

22. Vaccaro AR, Lehman RA, Hurlbert RJ, et al. A new classification of thoracolumbar injuries: the importance of injury morphology, the integrity of the posterior ligamentous complex, and neurologic status. Spine (Phila Pa 1976) 2005;30(20):2325–33.

23. Vaccaro AR, Hulbert RJ, Patel AA, et al. The subaxial cervical spine injury classification system: a novel approach to recognize the importance of morphology, neurology, and integrity of the disco-ligamentous complex. Spine (Phila Pa 1976) 2007; 32(21):2365–74.

24. Marino RJ, Jones L, Kirshblum S, et al. Reliability and repeatability of the motor and sensory examination of the international standards for neurological classification of spinal cord injury. J Spinal Cord Med 2008;31(2):166–70.

25. Burns AS, Lee BS, Ditunno JF, et al. Patient selection for clinical trials: the reliability of the early spinal cord injury examination. J Neurotrauma 2003;20(5): 477–82.

26. Iida H, Tachibana S, Kitahara T, et al. Association of head trauma with cervical spine injury, spinal cord injury, or both. J Trauma 1999;46(3):450–2.

27. Macciocchi S, Seel RT, Thompson N, et al. Spinal cord injury and co-occurring traumatic brain injury: assessment and incidence. Arch Phys Med Rehabil 2008;89(7):1350–7.

28. Fehlings MG, Vaccaro A, Wilson JR, et al. Early versus delayed decompression for traumatic cervical spinal cord injury: results of the surgical timing in acute spinal cord injury study (STASCIS). PLoS One 2012;7(2):e32037.

29. Wilson JR, Singh A, Craven C, et al. Early versus late surgery for traumatic spinal cord injury: the results of a prospective Canadian cohort study. Spinal Cord 2012;50(11):840–3.

30. Dvorak MF, Noonan VK, Fallah N, et al. The influence of time from injury to surgery on motor recovery and length of hospital stay in acute traumatic spinal cord injury: an observational Canadian cohort study. J Neurotrauma 2015;32(9):645–54.

31. Kramer JLK, Lammertse DP, Schubert M, et al. Relationship between motor recovery and independence after sensorimotor-complete cervical spinal cord injury. Neurorehabil Neural Repair 2013;26(9):1064–71.

32. Bourassa-Moreau É, Mac-Thiong J-M, Li A, et al. Do Patients with complete spinal cord injury benefit from early surgical decompression? analysis of neurological improvement in a prospective cohort study. J Neurotrauma 2016;33(3):301–6.

33. Rahimi-Movaghar V. Efficacy of surgical decompression in the setting of complete thoracic spinal cord injury. J Spinal Cord Med 2005;28(5):415–20.

34. Vaccaro AR, Daugherty RJ, Sheehan TP, et al. Neurologic outcome of early versus late surgery for cervical spinal cord injury. Spine (Phila Pa 1976) 1997;22(22):2609–13.

35. Liu Y, Shi CG, Wang XW, et al. Timing of surgical decompression for traumatic cervical spinal cord injury. Int Orthop 2015;39(12):2457–63.

36. Pollard ME, Apple DF. Factors associated with improved neurologic outcomes in patients with incomplete tetraplegia. Spine (Phila Pa 1976) 2003;28(1):33–9.

37. Liu J-M, Long X-H, Zhou Y, et al. Is urgent decompression superior to delayed surgery for traumatic spinal cord injury? A Meta-Analysis. World Neurosurg 2016;87:124–31.

38. van Middendorp JJ, Hosman AJF, Doi SA. The effects of the timing of spinal surgery after traumatic spinal cord injury: a systematic review and meta-analysis. J Neurotrauma 2013;30(21):1781–94.

39. Grassner L, Wutte C, Klein B, et al. "Early decompression (<8 h) after traumatic cervical spinal cord injury improves functional outcome as assessed by spinal cord independence measure (SCIM) after 1 year". J Neurotrauma 2016;33(18):1658–66.

40. Jug M, Kejžar N, Vesel M, et al. Neurological recovery after traumatic cervical spinal cord injury is superior if surgical decompression and instrumented fusion are performed within 8 hours versus 8 to 24 hours after injury: a single center experience. J Neurotrauma 2015;32(18):1385–92.

41. Lenehan B, Fisher CG, Vaccaro A, et al. The urgency of surgical decompression in acute central cord injuries with spondylosis and without instability. Spine (Phila Pa 1976) 2010;35(Suppl 21):S180–6.

42. Yamazaki T, Yanaka K, Fujita K, et al. Traumatic central cord syndrome: analysis of factors affecting the outcome. Surg Neurol 2005;63(2):95–9 [discussion: 99–100].

43. Guest J, Eleraky MA, Apostolides PJ, et al. Traumatic central cord syndrome: results of surgical management. J Neurosurg 2002;97(Suppl 1):25–32.

44. Kepler CK, Kong C, Schroeder GD, et al. Early outcome and predictors of early outcome in patients treated surgically for central cord syndrome. J Neurosurg Spine 2015;23(4):490–4.

45. Stevens EA, Marsh R, Wilson JA, et al. A review of surgical intervention in the setting of traumatic central cord syndrome. Spine J 2010;10(10):874–80.

46. Chen L, Yang H, Yang T, et al. Effectiveness of surgical treatment for traumatic central cord syndrome. J Neurosurg Spine 2009;10(1):3–8.

47. Samuel AM, Grant RA, Bohl DD, et al. Delayed surgery after acute traumatic central cord syndrome is associated with reduced mortality. Spine (Phila Pa 1976) 2015;40(5):349–56.

48. Anderson KK, Tetreault L, Shamji MF, et al. Optimal timing of surgical decompression for acute traumatic central cord syndrome: a systematic review of the literature. Neurosurgery 2015;77(Suppl 4):S15–32.

49. Bliemel C, Lefering R, Buecking B, et al. Early or delayed stabilization in severely injured patients with spinal fractures? Current surgical objectivity according to the trauma registry of DGU: treatment of spine injuries in polytrauma patients. J Trauma Acute Care Surg 2014;76(2):366–73.

50. Bourassa-Moreau É, Mac-Thiong J-M, Ehrmann Feldman D, et al. Complications in acute phase hospitalization of traumatic spinal cord injury: does surgical timing matter? J Trauma Acute Care Surg 2013;74(3):849–54.

51. Bourassa-Moreau E, Mac-Thiong J-M, Feldman DE, et al. Non-neurological outcomes after complete traumatic spinal cord injury: the impact of surgical timing. J Neurotrauma 2013;30(18):1596–601.

52. Dimar JR, Carreon LY, Riina J, et al. Early versus late stabilization of the spine in the polytrauma patient. Spine (Phila Pa 1976) 2010;35(Suppl 21):S187–92.

53. Herzer KR, Chen Y, Heinemann AW, et al. Association between time-to-rehabilitation and outcomes following traumatic spinal cord injury. Arch Phys Med Rehabil 2016;97(10):1620–7.

54. Furlan JC, Craven BC, Massicotte EM, et al. Early versus delayed surgical decompression of spinal cord after traumatic cervical spinal cord injury: a cost-utility analysis. World Neurosurg 2016;88:166–74.

55. Mac-Thiong J-M, Feldman DE, Thompson C, et al. Does timing of surgery affect hospitalization costs and length of stay for acute care following a traumatic spinal cord injury? J Neurotrauma 2012; 29(18):2816–22.

56. Furlan JC, Tung K, Fehlings MG. Process benchmarking appraisal of surgical decompression of spinal cord following traumatic cervical spinal cord injury: opportunities to reduce delays in surgical management. J Neurotrauma 2013;30(6): 487–91.

57. Battistuzzo CR, Armstrong A, Clark J, et al. Early decompression following cervical spinal cord injury: examining the process of care from accident scene to surgery. J Neurotrauma 2016; 33(12):1161–9.

58. van Middendorp JJ, Hosman AJF, Pouw MH, EM-SCI Study Group. ASIA impairment scale conversion in traumatic SCI: is it related with the ability to walk? A descriptive comparison with functional ambulation outcome measures in 273 patients. Spinal Cord 2009;47(7):555–60.

Central Cord Syndrome

Nathaniel P. Brooks, MD, FAANS

KEYWORDS

- Central cord syndrome • Spinal cord injury • Management • Pathophysiology

KEY POINTS

- Central cord syndrome (CCS) is an injury to the cervical spinal cord that causes arm greater than leg weakness, mixed modalities of sensory impairment, and bladder dysfunction.
- CCS has a good prognosis, although factors, such as older age and more severe neurologic injury at presentation, are associated with lower likelihood for neurologic recovery.
- Conservative treatment remains the most common treatment of CCS. The role and timing of surgical treatment of CCS remains controversial because there is limited evidence to support any particular treatment. Patients who have had a high-energy mechanism, evidence of spinal instability, or ongoing spinal cord compression should be considered for early surgery.

INTRODUCTION

Central cord syndrome (CCS) is most commonly caused by blunt trauma. Schneider and colleagues[1] initially described this syndrome in the 1950s, and its clinical description has changed very little since that time. CCS results in weakness of the arms with relative preservation of leg strength. Thus, CCS has been given the colloquial name of man in a barrel syndrome.[2] Mixed modalities of sensory impairment below the level of the lesion can occur. Bladder dysfunction in the form of urinary retention can also be seen in this syndrome. CCS often occurs in patients with underlying cervical stenosis and is prevalent in the elderly.[3] However, CCS occurs more frequently in younger patient populations and is more likely to be associated with cervical spine fractures or traumatic disc herniation in this group.[4–6] The management of patients with CCS is variable as there is no high-level evidence to guide treatment recommendations.[7]

The goal of this review is to provide the reader with a broad understanding of CCS from pathophysiology to management. Care must be taken to use the surgeon's training, experience, and clinical results to help select the appropriate treatments for each patient.

INCIDENCE/PREVALENCE

CCS represents about 9.0% of adult spinal cord injuries and 6.6% of pediatric spinal cord injuries.[3] The distribution of affected ages tends to be bimodal, with a young group of patients and an older group of patients that develop CCS.[5] Patients with CCS have similar neurologic presentations; but the underlying traumatic cause is heterogeneous and seems to be age related, with an age cutoff around 45 to 50 years old (depending on the study). In patients less than about 45 to 50 years old, the cause of CCS includes high-energy events: high-speed motor vehicle crashes (MVC), falls, athletic injuries/diving, gunshot wounds, and assault. In patients greater than 45 to 50 years old, the cause of CCS is more likely to be low-energy events: low-speed MVC and falls.[5] The variation in injury patterns is probably not secondary to age but due to morphologic and biomechanical differences between young versus old patients in the degree of

Disclosures: None.
Department of Neurosurgery, University of Wisconsin – Madison, 600 Highland Avenue, K4/860, Madison, WI 53792, USA
E-mail address: n.brooks@neurosurgery.wisc.edu

Neurosurg Clin N Am 28 (2017) 41–47
http://dx.doi.org/10.1016/j.nec.2016.08.002
1042-3680/17/© 2016 Elsevier Inc. All rights reserved.

neurosurgery.theclinics.com

cervical spondylosis, baseline cervical stenosis, and spinal flexibility.

ANATOMY AND PATHOPHYSIOLOGY

CCS was originally described as a clinical syndrome. Schneider originally proposed that mechanical compression of the spinal cord caused injury to the central region of the spinal cord, causing central cord edema and occasionally hematoma formation, leading to the eventual dysfunction of the medial portion of the lateral corticospinal tract.[1] However, more recent autopsy studies by Quencer and colleagues[8] suggest that the injury and axonal breakdown is localized to the white matter of the lateral corticospinal tracts with sparing of the central gray matter. Although previously reported as a classic component of CCS, hemorrhage is a rare finding in subsequent imaging and autopsy studies. Further pathologic findings demonstrate that the axons are diffusely injured in the lateral corticospinal tract.[8] The pathophysiologic mechanism of weakness remains poorly understood, although recent study of cadaveric specimens revealed that there does not seem to be axon loss at the level of injury but rather Wallerian degeneration of the axons adjacent to the epicenter of the injury that is the likely cause of persistent neurologic findings.[9]

MECHANISM OF INJURY

The mechanism of injury is secondary to trauma in most cases, but the subsequent injury morphologies are heterogeneous. Schneider and colleagues[10] initially described this in 1958 and subsequently has been supported by more recent studies.[5,10–26] The original proposed mechanism is secondary to cervical degenerative disease with subsequent hyperextension, which causes buckling of the ligamentum flavum (**Fig. 1**).[1] This mechanism was initially demonstrated in cadavers

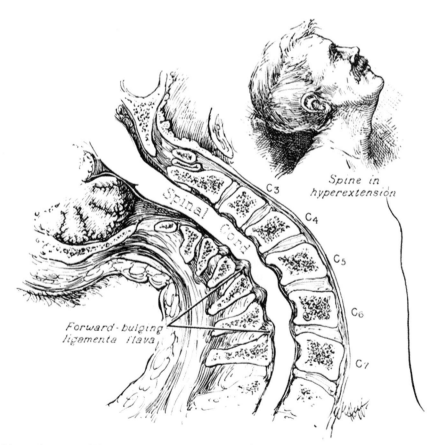

Fig. 1. In older patients, aged 45 years or greater, CCS is most often caused by low-energy cervical hyperextension in the setting of chronic cervical spondylosis and stenosis. Younger patients tend to have CCS secondary to high-energy fracture dislocation or acute disc herniations. (*From* Schneider RC, Cherry G, Pantek H. The syndrome of acute central cervical spinal cord injury; with special reference to the mechanisms involved in hyperextension injuries of cervical spine. J Neurosurg 1954;11(6):552; with permission.)

using myelography.[27] Further studies have demonstrated that the mechanism is often associated with age. Young patients (less than about 45–50 years old) are more likely to have fracture dislocations or disc herniation secondary to a flexion-compression mechanism, and older patients (greater than about 45–50 years old) are more likely to have hyperextension injuries in the setting of chronic spinal stenosis.[5,11] Few studies have shown CCS to occur because of hyperextension injuries without underlying stenosis or other radiographic abnormality.[19,26,28] In fact, cadaveric studies have demonstrated that whiplash-type injures are unlikely to cause spinal cord injury if patients have a normal canal diameter.[29]

DIAGNOSIS
Clinical

The primary diagnostic criteria for CCS was proposed by Schneider and colleagues[1] in 1954: "It is characterized by disproportionately more motor impairment of the upper than of the lower extremities, bladder dysfunction, usually urinary retention, and varying degrees of sensory loss below the level of the lesion." The practical application of these diagnostic criteria is variable based on results of a global surgeon survey.[30] A proposal has been made to include a criterion of a positive difference of 10 points in the lower extremity motor score compared with the upper extremity motor score on the American Spinal Injury Association (ASIA) spinal cord injury scale.[31] However, there are even differences of opinion regarding the severity of motor deficit that is necessary to diagnose CCS. As an example, the phenomena of burning hands syndrome is thought to be a variant of CCS that preferentially affects the lateral spinothalamic tracts.[32]

Radiographic

Plain radiographs and/or computed tomography scans should be performed to evaluate for fracture or dislocation because of the traumatic nature of these injuries. Subsequently, an MRI scan of the cervical spine without contrast is the best imaging modality to assess injury to the spinal cord.[33] The most consistent finding on MRI is hyperintense signal on gradient T2 echo MRI within the cervical spinal cord and evidence of cord compression. In cases of spine fracture or dislocation, it is possible that no ongoing compression will be identified and care must be taken to screen for instability if T2 signal change is identified. Miranda and colleagues[24] demonstrated that the length of the T2 signal (cord edema) correlates with the initial motor score.

NATURAL HISTORY/PROGNOSIS

The natural history of CCS is reasonably well understood. Some degree of motor and sensory recovery is common. Recovery generally plateaus between 1 to 2 years. Prognostic factors most commonly associated with improvement after CCS are age, severity of initial neurologic presentation, and MRI findings. Although most patients will achieve some recovery, there is still a risk of persistent weakness, difficulties with ambulation, spasticity, bladder dysfunction, sensory dysfunction, and neuropathic pain.

Overall Recovery

Generally, patients will double their ASIA motor scores at the 1-year follow-up.[34] Bosch and colleagues[12] reviewed 60 patients and found that 75% of patients improved in the postinjury period, but a functional ambulatory level was seen in only 59% of cases. Ishida and colleagues[6] studied 22 conservatively treated patients prospectively and noted a nearly full neurologic recovery in 6 weeks. Aito and colleagues[22] studied 87 patients over a 2-year follow-up and noted that approximately 86% of patients will recover the ability to ambulate and 80% of patients will have recovered functional independence. Persistent neuropathic pain was seen in 47% of patients. Spontaneous voiding and bladder emptying was seen in 68% of patients. Shavelle and colleagues[35] evaluated long-term mortality in a retrospective study of patients with ASIA D injury. Patients who are ambulatory and/or do not require bladder catheterization have a lower mortality than wheelchair-bound patients or those requiring bladder catheterization.[35]

Severity of Neurologic Injury on Presentation

Multiple studies have demonstrated that patients who present with mild to moderate motor impairment are likely to have a good recovery.[11,17] This finding was initially noted by Shosbree[11] in 1977 and has been reproduced in multiple subsequent studies.[14,17,21,26,36]

Youth Is an Advantage in Recovery

Multiple studies demonstrate a recovery advantage for patients less than 40 to 50 years old. Roth and colleagues[5] performed a retrospective review of 81 patients with CCS. The study found that factors associated with a good prognosis were: younger patients, preinjury employment, absence of lower extremity neurologic weakness on admission and documentation of upper and lower extremity strength improvement during rehabilitation. Penrod and colleagues[4] reviewed a matched cohort of patients selecting for a young group and an old group. Patients younger than 50 years had more improvement in neurologic function (walking, independence in activities of daily living, and control of bowel or bladder) than patients older than 50 years. Generally younger patients had minimal sensory complaints at 3 months. Chen and colleagues[33] performed a retrospective study of 28 patients with CCS. Clinical recovery to walk with assistance was 5 days in 90% of patients. Ninety percent of young patients (aged <40 years) recover walking in 3.4 days versus 4.9 days in older patients (aged >40 years). Additionally, partial recovery of hand activities of daily living was obtained in 3 days for young patients and 12 days for older patients.

Lenehan and colleagues[25] noted that patients younger than 50 years had better neurologic improvement. Aito and colleagues[22] showed similar age-associated improvements in patients younger than 65 years. These findings have been reproduced in other studies demonstrating that older patients had worse neurologic outcomes.[16,18]

Imaging Findings

MRI imaging characteristics have also been studied to attempt to predict recovery. Schroeder and colleagues[37] note that the presence of T2 signal increase on MRI is associated with a worse neurologic examination on presentation, but this group of patients tends to recover some of their function initially. Conversely, the cohort of patients who do not have T2 signal have better neurologic presentation but have a higher risk of a declining neurologic examination over time. Hohl and colleagues[36] developed a classification system that seeks to predict recovery. The findings of the investigators were that ASIA motor score and degree of edema seen on T2 MRI represented predictors of motor improvement at 1 year.

TREATMENT INTERVENTIONS

The treatment of CCS remains controversial, although there has been an evolution regarding treatment since the initial description of the disease process. The data regarding this evolution are summarized in **Table 1**. This evolution represents a dramatic change from Schneider's era when he advocated against surgical intervention in CCS because the natural history (or conservative treatment) seemed to be better than the surgical treatment at the time.[1] Granted at that time the surgical approach was quite extensive, involving a posterior approach, opening the dura, sectioning the dentate ligament, and performing a transdural discectomy.[10] In the modern era research from Brodkey, Bosch and colleagues,[12] and Bose and colleagues[13] revisited Schneider's recommendation and demonstrated that in patients with ongoing compression there seemed to be a benefit to surgical decompression.[12,13] The use of surgery to treat patients with CCS still does not represent the most common treatment modality, but surgical intervention has become more common in the treatment of CCS over the last decade, increasing from 15% to 30%.[39] Treatment should depend on the mechanism and morphology of the spinal injury. Patients with

Table 1
Evidentiary table of studies evaluating treatment options (surgery or conservative) for central cord syndrome

Reference	Study Description	Recommendation
Schneider et al,[1] 1954	Case series, 14 cases (mixed morphology of injury)	Conservative treatment
Schneider et al,[10] 1958	Retrospective 12 patients (11 conservative, 1 surgery)	Conservative treatment
Bosch et al,[12] 1971	Retrospective 42 patients (all conservative)	Chronic CCS may benefit from surgery
Brodkey,[38] 1980	Retrospective 7 surgical patients	Surgery (all patients improved rapidly with surgery)
Bose et al,[13] 1984	Retrospective 28 patients (14 conservative, 14 surgery)	Surgery (surgical patients did better than treated group)
Chen et al,[33] 1997	Retrospective study of 37 patients (16 surgical)	Surgery (patients improved more rapidly)

It is worth noting that the use of surgery became more common in the 1970s and 1980s. However, surgery is still not the most common treatment option based on survey data.
Data from Refs.[1,10,12,13,33,38]

high-energy fracture dislocations or disc herniation mechanisms should be considered for surgery. Patients with low-energy hyperextension injuries in the setting of cervical spondylosis and stenosis could benefit from surgery or conservative treatment based on the available data.

Guideline Recommendations

Aarabi and colleagues[7] published an evidence-based guideline for the management of acute traumatic CCS in 2013. The guidelines did not find any high-level evidence to produce treatment standards. The recommendations from the guideline are provided as treatment options and are as follows: Patients with severe neurologic deficits should be initially managed in an intensive care unit. Patients should have a mean arterial pressure goal of 85 to 90 mm Hg, although no recommendation is provided for duration. Patients with fracture dislocation should undergo early reduction. Surgical decompression should be considered particularly if the compression is focal and anterior.

Timing of Surgery

The timing of surgery is a contentious subject. There are multiple studies that have attempted to answer the question of timing that are summarized in **Table 2**. Fehlings and colleagues[40] surveyed 971 spine surgeons regarding the timing of surgical decompression for a 65-year-old man with CCS secondary to hyperextension and underlying stenosis. The responses were quite variable and inconclusive. Thirteen percent of surgeons would operate within 24 hours, but 16% would operate at 6 weeks. Management did seem to have a training bias as orthopedic surgeons were more likely to operate earlier than neurosurgeons. Conversely, Samuel and colleagues[41] reviewed 1060 patients in the National Trauma Data Bank Research Set and found that delayed surgery is associated with decrease mortality. The study demonstrated that the odds of mortality decrease by 19% per day of delay from the initial injury.

Broadly it seems that treating younger patient groups that are likely to have CCS secondary to a high-energy mechanism with ongoing compression or fracture dislocation is reasonable. The exact timing of surgery could be within 24 to 48 hours based on available data. Older patients with underlying cervical spondylosis who develop central cord symptoms after a low-energy hyperextension injury could have early (24–48 hours) or delayed surgery. A systematic review performed by Anderson and colleagues[42] recommends that patients be operated on within 2 weeks based on low levels of evidence showing improved neurologic outcomes and decreased complications. Additionally, a consensus statement from the writing group recommends operating within 24 hours.

Table 2
Evidentiary table of studies evaluating surgical timing in central cord syndrome

Reference	Description of Study	Conclusion
Aarabi et al,[26] 2011	Retrospective review of 42 patients	Timing of surgery before 48 h or after did not effect outcome.
Lenehan et al,[25] 2010	Ambispective review of 73 patients, follow-up at 6 and 12 mo	Patients decompressed within 24 h did better than after 24 h.
Stevens et al,[43] 2010	Retrospective review, 50 patients, 16 <24 h, 34 >24 h	There was no difference in outcome.
Chen et al,[23] 2009	Retrospective, 49 patients, surgical decompression <4 d and >4 d	Timing of 4 d did not effect outcome.
Aito et al,[22] 2006	Retrospective review of 82 patients	Surgical decompression did not affect outcome. Timing was not evaluated.
Song et al,[20] 2005	Retrospective review of 22 patients who had surgery with no comparison group	Surgical decompression improved recovery and prevented deterioration.
Guest et al,[19] 2002	Retrospective 50 patients	Surgery <24 h improved motor recovery in fracture dislocation but not in patients with chronic spinal stenosis.

There is no study that provides consensus on how rapidly central cord patients should be decompressed. However, the opinion of this author is that patients who present with high-energy mechanisms of injury and acute compressive morphology (fracture dislocation or disc herniation) should be decompressed early.
Data from Refs.[19,20,23,25,26,33,43]

Surgical Approach

There is no evidence providing guidance of approach for surgical intervention. The surgeon should select the surgical approach based on injury morphology and sound biomechanical principles. The surgeon should select the techniques that they are most comfortable and that have provided good results in the past. Typically, if the compressive lesion is anterior then an anterior approach should be considered. If the compressive pathology extends over multiple levels and is circumferential, then a posterior decompressive approach should be considered. Fracture dislocations should be reduced and stabilized, which can necessitate a combined anterior and posterior surgical approach.

FUTURE DIRECTIONS/RESEARCH

Further study of CCS remains necessary. It is clear that there are subgroups of patients who benefit from surgical intervention, but there is a lack of diagnostic tools to help identify those patients. A multicenter prospective cohort study could provide further evidence to guide treatment options. Although a multicenter randomized trial would provide high-level evidence, the heterogeneity of this patient population would make the development of useful inclusion and exclusion criteria quite onerous.

SUMMARY

CCS is a common type of spinal cord injury. Most patients will recover with conservative management, but surgery has also been shown to be beneficial in some patients with ongoing compression. There is no high-level evidence to guide treatment decisions. Therefore, surgeons must draw on their training and experience to determine the best treatment options.

REFERENCES

1. Schneider RC, Cherry G, Pantek H. The syndrome of acute central cervical spinal cord injury; with special reference to the mechanisms involved in hyperextension injuries of cervical spine. J Neurosurg 1954;11(6):546–77.
2. Butterfield MC, DeBlieux P, Palacios E. Man in a barrel: acute central cord syndrome after minor injury. J Emerg Med 2015;48(3):333–4.
3. McKinley W, Santos K, Meade M, et al. Incidence and outcomes of spinal cord injury clinical syndromes. J Spinal Cord Med 2007;30(3):215–24.
4. Penrod LE, Hegde SK, Ditunno JF. Age effect on prognosis for functional recovery in acute, traumatic central cord syndrome. Arch Phys Med Rehabil 1990;71(12):963–8.
5. Roth EJ, Lawler MH, Yarkony GM. Traumatic central cord syndrome - clinical-features and functional outcomes. Arch Phys Med Rehabil 1990; 71(1):18–23.
6. Ishida Y, Tominaga T. Predictors of neurologic recovery in acute central cervical cord injury with only upper extremity impairment. Spine (Phila Pa 1976) 2002;27(15):1652–8.
7. Aarabi B, Hadley MN, Dhall SS, et al. Management of acute traumatic central cord syndrome (ATCCS). Neurosurgery 2013;72:195–204.
8. Quencer RM, Bunge RP, Egnor M, et al. Acute traumatic central cord syndrome: MRI-pathological correlations. Neuroradiology 1992;34(2):85–94.
9. Jimenez O, Marcillo A, Levi ADO. A histopathological analysis of the human cervical spinal cord in patients with acute traumatic central cord syndrome. Spinal Cord 2000;38(9):532–7.
10. Schneider RC, Thompson JM, Bebin J. The syndrome of acute central cervical spinal cord injury. J Neurol Neurosurg Psychiatry 1958;21(3):216–27.
11. Shrosbree RD. Acute central cervical spinal cord syndrome–aetiology, age incidence and relationship to the orthopaedic injury. Spinal Cord 1977;14(4): 251–8.
12. Bosch A, Stauffer ES, Nickel VL. Incomplete traumatic quadriplegia. A ten-year review. JAMA 1971; 216(3):473–8.
13. Bose B, Northrup BE, Osterholm JL, et al. Reanalysis of central cervical cord injury management. Neurosurgery 1984;15(3):367–72.
14. Merriam WF, Taylor TK, Ruff SJ, et al. A reappraisal of acute traumatic central cord syndrome. J Bone Joint Surg Br 1986;68(5):708–13.
15. Cheng JS, Lee MJ, Massicotte E, et al. Clinical guidelines and payer policies on fusion for the treatment of chronic low back pain. Spine (Phila Pa 1976) 2011;36:S144–63.
16. Newey ML, Sen PK, Fraser RD. The long-term outcome after central cord syndrome: a study of the natural history. J Bone Joint Surg Br 2000; 82(6):851–5.
17. Tow AM, Kong KH. Central cord syndrome: functional outcome after rehabilitation. Spinal Cord 1998;36(3):156–60.
18. Dai L, Jia L. Central cord injury complicating acute cervical disc herniation in trauma. Spine (Phila Pa 1976) 2000;25(3):331–5 [discussion: 336].
19. Guest J, Eleraky MA, Apostolides PJ, et al. Traumatic central cord syndrome: results of surgical management. J Neurosurg 2002;97(1 Suppl):25–32.
20. Song J, Mizuno J, Nakagawa H, et al. Surgery for acute subaxial traumatic central cord syndrome without fracture or dislocation. J Clin Neurosci 2005;12(4):438–43.

21. Dvorak MF, Fisher CG, Hoekema J, et al. Factors predicting motor recovery and functional outcome after traumatic central cord syndrome: a long-term follow-up. Spine (Phila Pa 1976) 2005;30(20): 2303–11.

22. Aito S, D'Andrea M, Werhagen L, et al. Neurological and functional outcome in traumatic central cord syndrome. Spinal Cord 2006;45(4):292–7.

23. Chen L, Yang H, Yang T, et al. Effectiveness of surgical treatment for traumatic central cord syndrome clinical article. J Neurosurg Spine 2009;10(1):3–8.

24. Miranda P, Gomez O, Alday R. Acute traumatic central cord syndrome: analysis of clinical and radiological correlations. J Neurosurg Sci 2008;52(4): 107–12.

25. Lenehan B, Fisher CG, Vaccaro A, et al. The urgency of surgical decompression in acute central cord injuries with spondylosis and without instability. Spine (Phila Pa 1976) 2010;35(21 Suppl):S180–6.

26. Aarabi B, Alexander M, Mirvis SE, et al. Predictors of outcome in acute traumatic central cord syndrome due to spinal stenosis. J Neurosurg Spine 2011; 14(1):122–30.

27. Taylor AR. The mechanism of injury to the spinal cord in the neck without damage to vertebral column. J Bone Joint Surg Br 1951;33-B(4):543–7.

28. Yamazaki T, Yanaka K, Fujita K, et al. Traumatic central cord syndrome: analysis of factors affecting the outcome. Surg Neurol 2005;63(2):95–100.

29. Ito S, Panjabi MM, Ivancic PC, et al. Spinal canal narrowing during simulated whiplash. Spine (Phila Pa 1976) 2004;29(12):1330–9.

30. van Middendorp JJ, Pouw MH, Hayes KC, et al. Diagnostic criteria of traumatic central cord syndrome. Part 2: a questionnaire survey among spine specialists. Spinal Cord 2010;48(9):657–63.

31. Pouw MH, van Middendorp JJ, van Kampen A, et al. Diagnostic criteria of traumatic central cord syndrome. Part 1: a systematic review of clinical descriptors and scores. Spinal Cord 2010;48(9):652–6.

32. Wilberger JE, Abla A, Maroon JC. Burning hands syndrome revisited. Neurosurgery 1986;19(6): 1038–40.

33. Chen TY, Lee ST, Lui TN, et al. Efficacy of surgical treatment in traumatic central cord syndrome. Surg Neurol 1997;48(5):435–40.

34. Waters RL, Adkins RH, Sie IH, et al. Motor recovery following spinal cord injury associated with cervical spondylosis: a collaborative study. Spinal Cord 1996;34(12):711–5.

35. Shavelle RM, Paculdo DR, Tran LM, et al. Mobility, continence, and life expectancy in persons with ASIA impairment scale grade D spinal cord injuries. Am J Phys Med Rehabil 2015;94(3):180–91.

36. Hohl JB, Lee JY, Horton JA, et al. A novel classification system for traumatic central cord syndrome: the Central Cord Injury Scale (CCIS). Spine (Phila Pa 1976) 2010;35(7):E238–43.

37. Schroeder GD, Hjelm N, Vaccaro AR, et al. The effect of increased T2 signal intensity in the spinal cord on the injury severity and early neurological recovery in patients with central cord syndrome. J Neurosurg Spine 2016;24(5):792–6.

38. Brodkey JS, Miller CF, Harmody RM. The syndrome of acute central cervical spinal cord injury revisited. Surgical Neurology 1980;14(4):251–7.

39. Yoshihara H, Yoneoka D. Trends in the treatment for traumatic central cord syndrome without bone injury in the United States from 2000 to 2009. J Trauma Acute Care Surg 2013;75(3):453–8.

40. Fehlings MG, Rabin D, Sears W, et al. Current practice in the timing of surgical intervention in spinal cord injury. Spine (Phila Pa 1976) 2010;35(21): S166–73.

41. Samuel AM, Grant RA, Bohl DD, et al. Delayed surgery after acute traumatic central cord syndrome is associated with reduced mortality. Spine (Phila Pa 1976) 2015;40(5):349–56.

42. Anderson KK, Tetreault L, Shamji MF, et al. Optimal timing of surgical decompression for acute traumatic central cord syndrome. Neurosurgery 2015; 77:S15–32.

43. Andrew SE, Robert M, John AW, et al. A review of surgical intervention in the setting of traumatic central cord syndrome. The Spine Journal 2010; 10(10):874–80.

Pharmacologic Management of Acute Spinal Cord Injury

Michael Karsy, MD, PhD, Gregory Hawryluk, MD, PhD, FRCSC*

KEYWORDS

- Spinal cord injury • Secondary injury • Neuroprotective agent • Neuroregenerative agent
- Methylprednisolone • Central nervous system

KEY POINTS

- The recognition of delayed, progressive damage to the spinal cord after injury, termed secondary injury, provides a rationale for therapeutic intervention.
- Methylprednisolone is the most extensively studied therapeutic agent for acute spinal cord injury, and it remains a treatment option despite controversy.
- Numerous neuroprotective or regeneration-stimulating agents are in human trials and hold great promise for improving neurologic recovery after acute spinal cord injury.

INTRODUCTION

Spinal cord injury (SCI) has a global incidence of 10.4 to 83.0 cases per million per year, with most cases resulting in incomplete injury and permanent disability.[1,2] After the initial SCI, a complex pathophysiological process involving multiple molecular mechanisms ensues, which causes further damage for months and even years after the initial injury. The notion of inhibiting this secondary injury provides the possibility of neuroprotection and, to this end, numerous therapeutic targets have been identified. Moreover, we have learned of various inhibitors of central nervous system (CNS) regeneration that might be targeted therapeutically to improve recovery from SCI. This review discusses various historical and contemporary medical treatments investigated in humans for the treatment of acute SCI.

MECHANISMS OF SPINAL CORD INJURY

Two stages of SCI first conceptualized by Allen[3] in 1911 are now recognized, although this paradigm was not generally accepted by the scientific community until recently. *Primary injury* refers to the initial traumatic impact to the spinal cord resulting in neuronal damage (**Table 1**).[4,5] Injury to neurons can involve shear, laceration, contusion, and compression, and there can be acute stretch of neurons, glia, and spinal cord vasculature. Full anatomic disruption (or transection) rarely occurs in SCI; approximately 50% of patient cases show complete injury and 50% show incomplete injury, although the ratio can greatly vary depending on the study evaluated.[2,6] Trauma to the spinal cord can occur from the force of the trauma along with disruption of bone, muscle, or ligaments with associated cord contusion. *Secondary injury* involves the delayed progression of injury occurring weeks to months after initial trauma and is defined by complex and highly interrelated molecular processes that progressively damage CNS tissue.[1,7,8] *Secondary insults* are distinct from secondary injury and represent systemic events resulting in insufficient nutrient supply to the spinal cord.[9] These events

Department of Neurosurgery, University of Utah, Salt Lake City, UT, USA
* Corresponding author. Department of Neurosurgery, Clinical Neurosciences Center, University of Utah, 175 North Medical Drive East, Salt Lake City, UT 84132.
E-mail address: gregory.hawryluk@hsc.utah.edu

Neurosurg Clin N Am 28 (2017) 49–62
http://dx.doi.org/10.1016/j.nec.2016.07.002
1042-3680/17/© 2016 Elsevier Inc. All rights reserved.

Table 1
Summary of injury mechanisms in spinal cord injury

Category	Timing	Mechanism
Primary injury	Seconds	Compression, laceration, distraction, shearing, contusion, transection, stretching
Secondary injury	Seconds-minutes	Hemorrhage, decreased adenosine triphosphate, increased lactate
	Hours	Vasogenic and cytotoxic edema, microvessel vasospasm, thrombosis, ionic excitotoxicity, loss of Na/K gradient, release of neurotoxic opioids, inflammatory cascade, lipid peroxidation, glutamatergic excitotoxicity, oxidative stress
	Days/weeks	Microglial stimulation, gliosis, macrophage activation, apoptosis

most commonly include hypotension and hypoxia.

Secondary injury involves a complex interrelated signaling cascade and tissue changes causing continued damage long after the primary injury has ceased. These injurious cascades can theoretically be targeted by pharmacologic therapies, but there has been little success with this to date.[1,2] The timing of the various types of secondary injury after SCI can vary (see **Table 1**). Cellular insults involve vasospasm, localized ischemia, oxidative stress, reperfusion injury, and ischemia during compromise of spinal cord vasculature.[10] Ischemia involves insufficient oxygen supply to meet metabolic demands. Diminished production of adenosine triphosphate (ATP) causes dysfunction of energy-dependent sodium-potassium channels resulting in cytotoxic intracellular edema and ion-mediated cell damage. Intracellular acidosis also results in cellular enzymatic dysfunction, including diminished DNA repair. Elevation of intracellular calcium levels can cause myelin dysfunction,[11] as well as the inactivation of beneficial antioxidant enzymes and activation of those that are injurious to the cell, such as calpain, caspases, and nitric oxide synthase. This can ultimately lead to cell death through apoptosis.[12] Mitochondrial dysfunction also can be triggered by elevated intracellular calcium, and this causes increased mitochondrial permeability through mitochondrial permeability transition pores. This generates free radicals, which cause oxidative stress, and it impairs the ability of mitochondria to generate ATP.[13] Neuroinflammatory cascades and immune dysregulation also follow SCI.[14] Upregulation of inflammatory cytokines, such as tumor necrosis factor alpha (TNF-α), interleukins, and interferons, can induce aberrant cell signaling. Immune cells, such as microglia, T cells, neutrophils, and monocytes, can invade the injured area following SCI. Spinal cord inflammation is a challenging therapeutic target, as it can both improve and inhibit recovery. For instance, the inflammatory response can clear myelin debris, which inhibits axonal regrowth, but it can also produce injurious free radicals.

A large body of recent research has improved understanding of the mechanisms governing impediments to SCI recovery and regeneration.[1,2] Targeting these inhibitors to regrowth following SCI is a promising therapeutic approach for SCI. Cells from the CNS have long been known to show diminished capacity for regeneration compared with those of the peripheral nerves. In a landmark study, however, axons from the CNS demonstrated the ability to grow through peripheral nerve grafts. This demonstrates that the CNS has greater capacity for regeneration than previously believed.[15–19] As CNS axons have demonstrated an ability to regenerate, this implies that the CNS environment inhibits this inherent regenerative capacity. This premise inspired work from Schwab and others, which led to the identification of molecules inhibiting regeneration in the CNS, including Nogo,[19] myelin-associated glycoprotein (MAG),[20] oligodendrocyte myelin glycoprotein (OMgp),[21] semaphorin 4D,[22] ephrin B3,[23] repulsive guidance molecule,[24] chondroitin sulfate proteoglycans (CSPGs),[24] and Netrin-1.[25] The family of myelin-associated inhibitor (MAI) proteins includes 3 classic members, including Nogo-A, MAG,[20] and OMgp.[21,26] These bind to shared receptors, namely Nogo-66 receptor-1 (NgR1) and paired immunoglobulin-like receptor B (PirB), to regulate cytoskeletal dynamics and inhibit growth.[27] Downstream molecules inhibiting axonal growth, including RhoA and its effector kinase, ROCK, also have been discovered to impact nerve regeneration.[28] In addition, glial scarring after injury can serve as a physical barrier to regeneration. Growth inhibitory molecules can be secreted by astrocytes within a glial scar, including neurocan, versican, aggrecan, brevican, phosphacan, and neural/glial antigen 2 (NG2).[28] The barriers to axonal regeneration are thus numerous and complex.

THERAPEUTICS FOR ACUTE SPINAL CORD INJURY

Ongoing research efforts seek to prevent or reduce the effects of secondary insults as well as secondary injury. Broadly, these treatments can be classified as either neuroprotective aiming to prevent further cord damage, or neuroregenerative, with the goal of improving neuronal regrowth or myelination. Here we will discuss vasoactive medications that can play an important role in maintaining spinal perfusion, especially during neurogenic shock with loss of sympathetic tone. We discuss neuroprotective agents, such as methylprednisolone (MPSS), tirilazad mesylate, naloxone, thyrotropin-releasing hormone (TRH), minocycline, glyburide, magnesium, granulocyte colony-stimulating factor (G-CSF), riluzole, and gacyclidine. We also discuss treatments that aim to augment neural regeneration, such as myelin associated inhibitors (MAI) (eg, anti-Nogo antibodies [ATI-355]), Rho inhibitor VX-210/Cethrin, gangliosides (GM-1), and fibroblast growth factor (FGF). Regeneration is also a major goal of cell transplantation therapies for SCI, and we discuss strategies that have been used to date.

LESSONS LEARNED FROM HISTORIC CLINICAL TRIALS IN SPINAL CORD INJURY

A variety of agents were evaluated in early clinical trials with the goal of identifying neuroprotective and neuroregenerative treatments after SCI (**Table 2**). Although these studies led to little benefit for patients with acute SCI, much has been learned from them. These lessons are now being applied to a new generation of trials.

TRH was evaluated in a phase I randomized controlled trial. It was thought to inhibit secondary mediators of excitotoxicity, such as excitotoxic amino acids, peptidoleukotrienes, endogenous opioids, and platelet-activating factor.[29] The trial results suggested neurologic benefit in patients with initially incomplete injuries, but loss to follow-up and small sample size ultimately detracted from the findings.[30]

Gacyclidine/GK-11 (Beaufour-Ipsen Pharma, Basking Ridge, NJ) is a noncompetitive N-methyl-D-aspartate receptor antagonist designed to reduce excitotoxicity by reducing glutamate-mediated calcium influx after SCI.[31] A phase II trial of gacyclidine reported evaluation in 280 patients with incomplete SCI but did not show a long-term therapeutic benefit.[32,33] These results were, however, reported only in abstract form and were not published in a peer-reviewed journal.

Ganglioside (GM-1) is a glycosphingolipid located in neuronal cell membranes that can anchor secondary proteins that regulate signaling pathways involved in differentiation, regeneration, apoptosis, and neuroplasticity, among other roles.[34] A landmark trial of ganglioside performed in 37 patients showed significant improvement in American Spinal Injury Association (ASIA) motor score and Frankel grade.[35] Improvement predominantly on lower extremity function was seen as soon as 48 hours after treatment, and it was thought the compound had an effect on traversing neurons. These findings led to a large phase III trial of more than 750 patients in 28 institutions, but the results of this study failed to reach their ambitious primary outcome (a 2-point improvement on the modified Benzel walking scale).[36] The study did show that patients had improvements in bowel/bladder recovery and sacral function, and patients in both groups achieved significant improvement of Functional Independence Measure and Modified Barthel Index.[37] In this study, intensive physical therapy was also combined with the pharmacologic treatment to achieve improved patient outcomes. A major criticism of the study was the delay in time to GM-1 treatment, as most patients first received MPSS as part of their clinical treatment. Several meta-analyses evaluating the efficacy of GM-1 treatment in SCI have failed to support its widespread use.[38,39]

Despite the many clinical trials evaluating treatments in SCI, a safe and markedly effective therapeutic has been elusive (see **Table 2**). Nevertheless, the lessons learned from these historic clinical trials have aided later studies and drug development.[40] The results of these trials have helped formulate multiple guidelines and consensus statements informing how experimental trials for acute SCI should be conducted.[41,42] These recommendations encourage the evaluation of treatments early after SCI even though this will require larger numbers of patients and multicenter approaches. In addition, large numbers of patients are required to account for the variation in disease severity (eg, ASIA categories) to ensure adequate representation of patients and clinical translation of the research. A standardized metric of injury severity and objective assessment of neurologic improvement have been shown to be important in comparing studies. Adequate duration for follow-up after trials (eg,

Table 2
Summary of clinical trials and experimental therapies with potential benefit in humans

Treatment	Highest Level of Evidence	Mechanism	Findings
Neuroprotective treatments			
Vasopressors	Cohort studies	Augmentation of heart rate and blood pressure to improve spinal cord perfusion	• Improved recovery in patients with higher mean arterial blood pressures for 5–7 d post-injury in some studies[43,44,103] • Independent risk factor of worsened cardio-vascular effects with dopamine and phenylephrine[16]
NASCIS I (MPSS)	Phase III (low-dose vs high-dose MPSS)	Reduces antioxidant stress, calcium influx, excitotoxicity, and immune-mediated phagocytosis during hypoperfusion of the spinal cord	NASCIS I: No difference in neurologic improvement but increased morbidity and mortality with high dose[47] • No difference in outcome[104]
NASCIS II (MPSS)	Phase III (MPSS vs placebo/naloxone within 24 h injury)		NASCIS II: Improved motor scores but not functional recovery in patients treated <8 h after injury[46] • No difference in outcome[51,55,105]
NASCIS III (MPSS)	Phase III (MPSS/tirilazad mesylate within 8 h of injury for 24 vs 48 h)		NASCIS III: Improved neurologic function in patients <8 h from injury and treated for 48 h[48,52]
Minocycline	Phase II	Synthetic tetracycline class antibiotic that regulates inflammatory and apoptotic signaling pathways	• No improvement in outcome for lumbar SCI[57] • Subgroup analysis showed potential improve-ment for cervical injury[57]
Glyburide/glibenclamide	Pre-clinical	Sulfonylurea receptor 1 (SUR1)–regulated, Trpm4 channel, a Ca^{2+}-activated nonspecific cation channel blocker that acts on microvessels to reduce progressive hemorrhagic necrosis, edema, and inflammation in SCI	• Reduced hemorrhage at 24 h postinjury and diminished lesion size at 1 and 6 wk in vivo[61,63] • Improved functional outcome in animals[60]
Magnesium	Pre-clinical	Blocks N-methyl-D-aspartate receptors to prevent glutamatergic excitotoxicity	Improved white matter preservation, reduced apoptosis, improved vascular permeability, reduced inflammation, and improved functional outcome in vivo[67]
Riluzole	Phase I	Blocks voltage-sensitive calcium channels to prevent glutamatergic excitotoxicity	• Increase in cervical injury improvement at 3 mo compared with matched registry control patients[69,71,72] • Improved motor scores not seen at 6 mo[73]

Gacyclidine/GK-11	Phase II	Noncompetitive N-methyl-D-aspartate receptor antagonist designed to reduce glutamatergic excitotoxicity	No improvement in outcome[32,33]
Thyrotropin-releasing hormone (TRH)	Phase I	Inhibit secondary mediators of excitotoxicity (excitotoxic amino acids, peptidoleukotrienes, endogenous opioids, and platelet-activating factor)	Improved outcome in a limited series[30]
Naloxone	Phase II	Opioid receptor antagonist	Limited therapeutic efficacy[46,49,50]
Granulocyte colony-stimulating factor (G-CSF)	Phase II	Mitogen of leukocyte proliferation and differentiation along granulocyte lineages, possible effects on neuroprotection and immune regulation	Induces bone marrow stromal cells to SCI sites and functional improvement in vivo[76,78]
Neuroregenerative treatments			
IN-1, ATI355	Phase I	Anti-Nogo targeting molecule that improves axonal sprouting, long-distance axonal regeneration, and functional recovery	Safe delivery of drug by infusion pump[19,79–81]
Cethrin, BA-210		Clostridium botulinum toxin, C3 transferase–derived targeting molecule of guanosine triphosphatase Rho that affects axonal growth, functional recovery, and neuroprotection	Improvement in motor function (27.3 points) at 12 mo in cervical-injured patients[82,83]
Gangliosides (GM-1)/Syngen	Phase III	Glycosphingolipid involved in neuronal physiology, neuroplasticity, and cellular signaling	• Improvement in ASIA grade, Frankel score, Functional Independence Measure, and Modified Barthel Index[35] • Synergistically combined with intensive physical therapy[37] • Improvement in bladder/bowel and sacral function[36] • No improvement in Benzel walking scale outcome[39] • No therapeutic benefit in meta-analyses[38]
Fibroblast growth factor	Experimental	Mitogen inducing cellular proliferation and stem cell properties	Neuroprotective and angiogenic features in vivo[87–89]

Abbreviations: ASIA, American Spinal Injury Association; MPSS, methylprednisolone sodium succinate; SCI, spinal cord injury.

6–12 months for neuroprotection trials, 12–24 months for regenerative therapies) has also been suggested to properly evaluate potential treatments. The use of SCI clinical treatment guidelines for other management strategies and uniform application during trials is also important to ensure that evaluated treatments are biased by other factors.[41,42]

ESTABLISHED AND EMERGING PHARMACOLOGIC TREATMENTS
Neuroprotective Treatments for Acute Spinal Cord Injury

Vasoactive agents
Initial supportive care of acute SCI involves the maintenance of spinal cord perfusion and oxygenation. Injuries above T6 can result in sympathetic disruption and neurogenic shock, characterized by low cardiac output, low inotropic activity, bradycardia, hypotension, and hypothermia. Meticulous attention to such secondary insults is believed to reduce the secondary injury after SCI. Fluid administration and vasoactive agents are used for treatment.

After appropriate volume resuscitation, vasopressor medications can be used to augment blood pressure in the hopes of improving spinal cord perfusion. Guidelines recommend prevention of hypotension, defined as a systolic blood pressure less than 90 mm Hg, as well as augmenting mean arterial pressure (MAP) values to 85 to 90 mm Hg for a week after injury. This practice requires the administration of vasopressors in most patients. Moreover, patients with acute SCI have limited tolerance for intravascular volume expansion in the context of impaired sympathetic outflow. Here pharmacologic options include dopamine (1–10 μg/kg per minute), dobutamine (5–15 μg/kg per minute), epinephrine (1–8 μg/min), norepinephrine (1–20 μg/min), and phenylephrine (10–100 μg/min). Norepinephrine and dopamine are favored over other agents because of their α-agonist and β-agonist activity resulting in vasoconstriction and increased cardiac activity, respectively. In a study by Inoue and colleagues[16] of 131 patients with SCI, dopamine was the most commonly used vasoactive medication, followed by phenylephrine, norepinephrine, epinephrine, and vasopressin. Importantly, this study showed dopamine and phenylephrine were independently associated with increased cardiovascular complications suggesting that norepinephrine may be a better agent. A recent "big data" study involving nearly a million blood pressure measurements from 100 patients with acute SCI confirmed that patients with average MAP values of greater than 85 mm Hg had improved recovery in ASIA score.[43,44] Furthermore, the correlation between MAP values declined over time, suggesting that this therapy has greatest effect early after injury.

Corticosteroids
The National Acute Spinal Cord Injury Studies (NASCIS) were large randomized clinical trials in SCI that evaluated the role of corticosteroids in SCI and generated high-quality data. Corticosteroids were believed to reduce oxidative stress associated with hypoperfusion of the spinal cord, to reduce calcium influx and excitotoxicity, and to reduce immune-mediated neuronal phagocytosis.[45] All NASCIS trials failed to show benefit as assessed by the primary outcome measure; however, various secondary analyses have shown an important potential role for corticosteroids.[46–48]

NASCIS I, published in 1984, compared low-dose and high-dose MPSS (100-mg bolus and 100 mg/daily vs 1000-mg bolus and 1000 mg/daily). This study did not detect a difference in neurologic improvement, but high-dose MPSS administration was associated with greater risk of wound infection, gastrointestinal hemorrhage, sepsis, pulmonary embolism, and death.[47] Interestingly, no placebo was used in this study, as corticosteroids were assumed to be efficacious and withholding them was considered unethical.

NASCIS II evaluated high-dose MPSS in comparison to the opioid antagonist naloxone, as well as a placebo within 24 hours of SCI.[46] Several previous studies had evaluated naloxone independently in SCI but had found limited efficacy.[49,50] The results showed no difference in neurologic benefit between the groups; however, subgroup analysis planned a priori showed that patients treated within 8 hours of injury with MPSS had significantly improved motor recovery. Increased risks of wound infection and pulmonary embolism were found in the corticosteroid treatment group.

NASCIS III evaluated MPSS within 8 hours of injury versus tirilazad mesylate (a 21-aminosteroid with antioxidant effect) and was the first NASCIS study to use a functional outcome measure: the Functional Independence Measure.[48] Twenty-four–hour and 48-hour infusions of corticosteroid (30 mg/kg bolus plus 5.4 mg/kg per hour) were compared with 48-hour infusion of tirilazad mesylate (2.5 mg/kg every 6 hours). No difference between tirilazad mesylate and corticosteroid treatment groups was found. Subgroup analysis showed improved neurologic function at 1 year in patients who received an MPSS bolus 3 to 8 hours after injury followed by a 48-hour infusion. Following this study, a 24-hour infusion of MPSS was suggested for patients treated within 3 hours of injury, whereas 48-hour infusions were recommended for those treated 3 to 8 hours after injury. Most who now choose to administer MPSS for acute SCI prefer 24 hours of MPSS, which was associated with a lower rate of complications.

The administration of MPSS for acute SCI remains controversial. Recent guidelines provide level I evidence against the use of corticosteroids in SCI[51]; however, a meta-analysis of 8 randomized controlled trials evaluating MPSS showed efficacy when it was used within 8 hours of injury.[52] This review emphasized the lack of other treatment options and that MPSS is the only drug that has been evaluated in phase III trials. The most important concerns with corticosteroids are the limited efficacy and the increased risk of complications, such as sepsis and pneumonia. A recent survey of 77 patients who had an SCI found that most would prefer to receive corticosteroids at time of injury despite the risks and limited efficacy.[53] Whereas 59.4% believed that a small chance of neurologic recovery was worth the risks of corticosteroid administration, only a small number (1.4%) thought it was inappropriate to administer steroids following injury. These results should be considered by practitioners caring for victims of acute SCI.[54,55] Moreover, an upcoming AOSpine guideline for the management of acute SCI will restore NASCIS II dosing of MPSS used within 3 to 8 hours of injury to a level III treatment option (personal communication).

Minocycline

Minocycline is a synthetic tetracycline class antibiotic evaluated in an array of conditions, including neurologic disorders, such as stroke, Alzheimer disease, neuro-oncology, and SCI.[56] The mechanism of action is thought to be via the anti-inflammatory, antioxidant, and antiapoptotic properties of the drug. Minocycline was evaluated in a phase II randomized controlled trial of 52 patients with SCI randomized to treatment or placebo 12 hours after injury for up to 7 days.[57] Although this study failed to show a difference in recovery from lumbar injury (6 points, $P = .2$), there was a significant improvement in cervical injury (14 points, $P = .05$). A phase III trial by Casha and colleagues[57] began enrollment in 2013.

Glyburide

Glyburide, or glibenclamide, is a sulfonylurea receptor 1 (SUR1)–regulated, TRPM4-channel, Ca^{2+}-activated nonspecific cation channel blocker used in the treatment of diabetes by promoting insulin release.[58] The compound also has been shown to be effective in models of ischemic

and hemorrhagic stroke and traumatic brain injury. Glyburide is thought to act on microvessels to reduce hemorrhagic necrosis, edema, and inflammation in SCI.[58–61] Of note, the SUR1-TRPM4 channel is also inhibited by riluzole, which has also been implicated as a potential treatment for SCI with similar in vivo efficacy.[62] In animal models, glyburide was shown to reduce hemorrhage at 24 hours after injury and diminished lesion size at 1 and 6 weeks.[60,61] Functional improvements after SCI were also shown with glyburide treatment up to 6 weeks after injury; however, in one animal study, glyburide treatment showed more limited improvement with bilateral injury (33% reduced lesion volume) compared with unilateral injury (57% reduced lesion volume) at 6 weeks.[63] These results suggest that the severity of injury may play an important role in the degree of recovery after glyburide treatment. Preparation is being made to evaluate glyburide in a multicenter trial for acute SCI following a recent demonstration of benefit in reducing edema and morbidity after ischemic stroke.[64]

Magnesium

Magnesium has been evaluated as a potential neuroprotective agent for a variety of CNS insults, including cerebral palsy.[65,66] Magnesium acts by blocking N-methyl-D-aspartate receptors, thus preventing glutamatergic excitotoxicity.[65] Multiple animal studies have shown improved white matter preservation, reduced apoptosis, improved vascular permeability, reduced inflammation, and improved functional outcome[67]; however, not all studies have had positive results, with some failing to show improvement with magnesium treatment. Unfortunately, magnesium administration was ineffective in improving outcome in a human traumatic brain injury trial.[68] A polyethylene glycol–bound magnesium compound (AC105; Accorda Therapeutics, Ardsley, NY) thought to improve biodelivery has been evaluated in vivo and is currently being evaluated in a human phase II trial.

Riluzole

Riluzole (Rilutek; Sano-Aventis, Bridgewater, NJ) is a benzothiazole-class anticonvulsant used for treatment of amyotrophic lateral sclerosis. Interestingly, riluzole is the only medication currently approved for use as a neuroprotectant; it acts by blocking voltage-sensitive calcium channels, inhibiting intracellular sodium entry and glutamate excitotoxicity.[69,70] Of note, some animal studies showed synergy with MPSS during treatment of SCI.[69,71] A phase I trial in acute SCI evaluated 36 patients treated with riluzole (50 mg orally every 12 hours for 14 days) and showed a significant increase motor recovery after cervical injury at 3 months compared with matched registry control patients (15.5 points, $P = .021$)[72]; however, improved motor scores were not seen at 6-month follow-up. A phase II/III multicenter randomized controlled trial of riluzole is currently under way by the AOSpine North America Research Network.[73]

Granulocyte colony-stimulating factor

G-CSF is a potent mitogen that stimulates leukocyte proliferation and differentiation along granulocyte lineages. G-CSF is currently approved for administration to patients with severe bone marrow suppression so safety testing of this agent in humans has already been completed.[74] G-CSF has been shown to induce mobilization of bone marrow stromal cells to SCI sites, as well as functional improvement in an animal model.[75] In addition, G-CSF has exhibited neuroprotective properties in neurodegenerative disorders.[74] G-CSF has been evaluated with stem cell treatment approaches in animal models of SCI.[76] Two studies in patients with SCI have evaluated granulocyte macrophage colony-stimulating factor (GM-CSF) in conjunction with autologous bone marrow stem cells; the patients demonstrated improvement of ASIA scores at follow-up.[77,78] No decrement in neurologic function or toxicity was noted after treatment, although there was no comparison with control patients.

Neuroregenerative Treatments in Spinal Cord Injury

Myelin-associated inhibitor targeting

Nogo was discovered and characterized during a screen of myelin inhibitory proteins using the monoclonal antibody, IN-1.[19] Subsequent in vitro and in vivo studies showed that IN-1 could improve axonal sprouting, long-distance axonal regeneration, and functional recovery.[79] Later evaluation of the humanized anti-Nogo monoclonal antibody, namely ATI-355 (Novartis Pharmaceuticals Corporation, East Hanover, NJ), was shown to induce axonal sprouting and functional recovery in primates.[80,81] The compound was evaluated in a phase I trial by continuous infusion with a programmable pump but results have not yet been published. A phase II trial is currently under way.[81]

VX-210, formerly known as Cethrin (R) (Vertex Pharmaceuticals, Boston, MA), is another promising therapeutic studied in SCI. The molecule is a modified version of C3 transferase, which is derived from *Clostridium botulinum* and inhibits guanosine triphosphatase Rho. Furthermore, this therapeutic mechanism has been shown to

facilitate axonal growth and functional recovery and has shown antiapoptotic effects.[82] VX-210 is a recombinant version of C3 transferase modified for enhanced tissue penetration and mixed with the fibrin sealant Tisseel (Baxter Healthcare Corporation, Deerfield, IL) to allow direct application to the injured spinal cord during decompressive surgery. A phase I/IIa multicenter trial of VX-210 in patients with ASIA A cervical or thoracic SCI showed improvement of 1.8 ± 5.1 points along the ASIA motor score for thoracic injury and 18.6 ± 19.3 points for cervical injury. In addition, 31% and 6% of patients showed improvement to ASIA C or D grades for cervical or thoracic injury, respectively. The largest improvement was with 3 mg of Cethrin treatment in cervical-injured patients at 12 months (27.3 points).[83] Of note, RhoA inhibition with subsequent functional improvement also has been seen in treatment with nonsteroidal anti-inflammatory drugs (eg, ibuprofen), suggesting cyclooxygenase targeting may be possible strategy.[84] A new multicenter, phase III trial examining VX-210 in patients with acute SCI is scheduled to start shortly (personal communication).

Fibroblast growth factor

FGF is a family of 22 proteins that signal through distinct tyrosine receptor kinases, including FGF receptors.[85] FGFs are potent mitogens inducing cellular proliferation and stem cell self-renewal. FGF may augment stem cell proliferation and be useful in combined approaches of SCI treatment. In addition, FGF may also have an impact in promoting angiogenesis after SCI, as shown in one animal study.[86] SUN13837 (Asubio Pharmaceuticals, Inc, Edison, NJ), is an FGF analog that has demonstrated neuroprotective and angiogenic properties.[87–89] Currently, the drug is in phase II trials, but no results in humans have yet been reported. Another phase I trial of SC0806 (BioArctic Neuroscience AB, Stockholm, Sweden), an FGF impregnated device, is also being evaluated in humans (NCT02490501).

CELLULAR TRANSPLANTATION APPROACHES FOR ACUTE SPINAL CORD INJURY

There is great hope that cellular transplantation approaches may prove a successful means of improving neurologic recovery from SCI (**Fig. 1**). Recent studies provide evidence for the presence of stem cells in the CNS capable of self-renewal, differentiation, regeneration, and response to injury, but the response of these endogenous cells is insufficient.[90,91] Cellular transplantation strategies for SCI have had various goals, including replacement of damaged neurons, secretion of

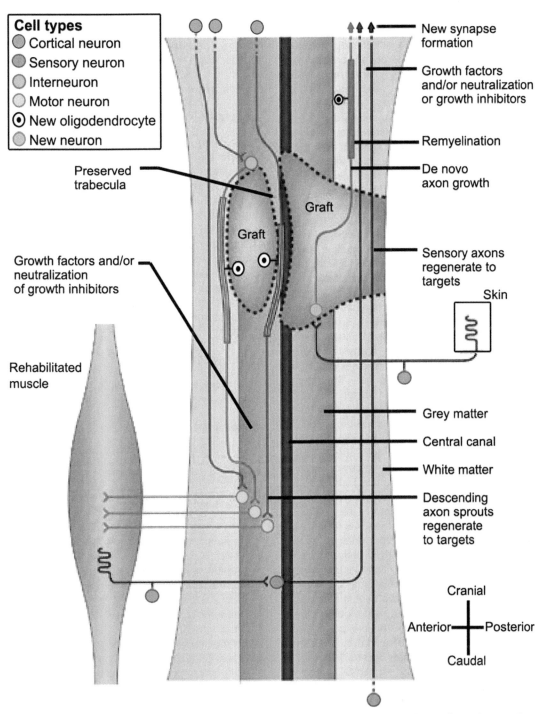

Fig. 1. Injured spinal cord after combination treatments. Schematic showing a sagittal view through injured cervical spinal cord after a hypothetical combination of potential therapies. Cysts are filled by vascularized grafts and trabeculae are spared. Grafts provide remyelinating cells, and inhibitory molecules in the scar regions and in intact spinal cord are neutralized using antibodies, peptides, or enzymes. Grafted neurons allow the formation of new relay circuits or the regeneration of injured axons back to their original targets. Furthermore, rehabilitation may allow correct synapses to be stabilized and reverses muscle atrophy. Areas of targeted molecular treatment can involve both neuroprotective and neuroregenerative mechanisms. (*From* Thuret S, Moon LD, Gage FH. Therapeutic interventions after spinal cord injury. Nat Rev Neurosci 2006;7(8):631; with permission.)

trophic factors, and/or regulation of the injured microenvironment.[92] Cell types studied in transplantation strategies for SCI include neural stem/progenitor cells, oligodendrocyte precursors, Schwann cells and olfactory ensheathing cells, and bone marrow stromal cells, as well as others.[93]

The first human cell type transplanted into human patients in a scientific trial was autologous macrophages. The phase I trial showed adequate safety and promising results.[94] Unfortunately, the phase II trial was terminated early because of funding issues and harm was suggested when the analysis of enrolled patients was published.[95] A later trial by the Geron Corporation was the first to implant oligodendrocyte precursor cells for SCI, but this study was terminated after enrolling only a couple of patients because of financial issues and criticism that the study cohort, which included patients with complete injury close to the time of injury (7–14 days), was not appropriate to demonstrate the desired endpoint.

A major advance in the cellular transplantation field has been the discovered ability to "reprogram" adult cells into pluripotent stem cells that can then form any of the cells found in the human body. This technology allows the generation of stem cells from a source other than human embryos, thus eliminating an important ethical concern.[96] In addition, because this allows transplantation of the patient's own cells, the need for immunosuppression is avoided. A study of chronic SCI in rats treated with induced pluripotent stem cell (iPSC)–derived neural progenitor cells showed differentiation into NeuN/Fox3-expressing neuronal cells, but these neuronal cells did not integrate with the spinal cord or affect function.[97] Another study of iPSC-derived astrocytes transplanted in a cervical injury model showed neuronal differentiation at 2 days, 2 weeks, and 4 weeks and some improvement in diaphragmatic function as assessed by electrophysiological recording.[98] Other studies have expanded on the role of iPSCs in various animal models, but exploration in humans remains limited.[96]

Use of stem cell therapy in human SCI remains limited to small trials with varied results.[1,40,99] Some studies show improved patient outcome, whereas others have not shown significant effect. In addition, concerns regarding the neoplastic potential of implanted stem cells and limited functional integration in current studies remain unanswered questions. The combined use of pharmacologic adjuvant therapies may aid in improving patient outcome. Combinations of stem cell treatment with neurotrophin, such as brain-derived neurotrophic factor, NT-3, FGF, epidermal growth factor, and G-CSF, have been proposed.[100–102] Pharmacologic regulation of implanted stem cells may be a feasible method to improve outcome. Various trials have attempted combined treatments[77,78,91]; however, stem cell treatment of SCI remains an area of active investigation.

SUMMARY

Better understanding of the secondary injury cascade that follows SCI, as well as a clearer appreciation of the inhibitors of regeneration, has led to new experimental treatments. With many promising therapeutic agents and strategies being studied in ongoing trials for SCI, there is great hope among physicians and patients alike. An efficacious therapy would be a major advance for acute SCI and could also benefit patients affected by other neurologic conditions. Combined stem cell treatment with pharmacologic manipulation may be another possible avenue to improve patient outcome and alter the poor natural history of SCI.

ACKNOWLEDGMENTS

We thank Kristin Kraus, MSc, for her editorial assistance with this article.

REFERENCES

1. Hawryluk G, Fehlings M. Current status and future direction of management of spinal cord injury. In: Winn R, editor. Youman's neurological surgery. 6th edition. Philadelphia: Elsevier; 2006. p. 2730–40.
2. Wyndaele M, Wyndaele JJ. Incidence, prevalence and epidemiology of spinal cord injury: what learns a worldwide literature survey? Spinal Cord 2006; 44(9):523–9.
3. Allen A. Surgery of experimental lesion of spinal cord equivalent to crush injury of fracture dislocation of spinal column. JAMA 1911;LVII(11):878–80.
4. Balentine JD. Pathology of experimental spinal cord trauma. I. The necrotic lesion as a function of vascular injury. Lab Invest 1978;39(3):236–53.
5. Kwon BK, Tetzlaff W, Grauer JN, et al. Pathophysiology and pharmacological treatment of acute spinal cord injury. Spine J 2004;4(4):451–64.
6. Ning GZ, Wu Q, Li YL, et al. Epidemiology of traumatic spinal cord injury in Asia: a systematic review. J Spinal Cord Med 2012;35(4):229–39.
7. Amar AP, Levy ML. Pathogenesis and pharmacological strategies for mitigating secondary damage in acute spinal cord injury. Neurosurgery 1999; 44(5):1027–39 [discussion 1039–40].
8. Hagg T, Oudega M. Degenerative and spontaneous regenerative processes after spinal cord injury. J Neurotrauma 2006;23(3–4):264–80.

9. Yanagawa Y, Marcillo A, Garcia-Rojas R, et al. Influence of posttraumatic hypoxia on behavioral recovery and histopathological outcome following moderate spinal cord injury in rats. J Neurotrauma 2001;18(6):635–44.

10. Tator CH, Koyanagi I. Vascular mechanisms in the pathophysiology of human spinal cord injury. J Neurosurg 1997;86(3):483–92.

11. Beattie MS, Farooqui AA, Bresnahan JC. Review of current evidence for apoptosis after spinal cord injury. J Neurotrauma 2000;17(10):915–25.

12. Juurlink BH, Paterson PG. Review of oxidative stress in brain and spinal cord injury: suggestions for pharmacological and nutritional management strategies. J Spinal Cord Med 1998;21(4):309–34.

13. Frantseva M, Perez Velazquez JL, Tonkikh A, et al. Neurotrauma/neurodegeneration and mitochondrial dysfunction. Prog Brain Res 2002;137:171–6.

14. Popovich PG. Immunological regulation of neuronal degeneration and regeneration in the injured spinal cord. Prog Brain Res 2000;128: 43–58.

15. David S, Aguayo AJ. Axonal elongation into peripheral nervous system "bridges" after central nervous system injury in adult rats. Science 1981; 214(4523):931–3.

16. Inoue T, Manley GT, Patel N, et al. Medical and surgical management after spinal cord injury: vasopressor usage, early surgeries, and complications. J Neurotrauma 2014;31(3):284–91.

17. Richardson PM, McGuinness UM, Aguayo AJ. Axons from CNS neurons regenerate into PNS grafts. Nature 1980;284(5753):264–5.

18. Ma QH, Yang WL, Nie DY, et al. Physiological roles of neurite outgrowth inhibitors in myelinated axons of the central nervous system–implications for the therapeutic neutralization of neurite outgrowth inhibitors. Curr Pharm Des 2007;13(24):2529–37.

19. Chen MS, Huber AB, van der Haar ME, et al. Nogo-A is a myelin-associated neurite outgrowth inhibitor and an antigen for monoclonal antibody IN-1. Nature 2000;403(6768):434–9.

20. McKerracher L, Rosen KM. MAG, myelin and overcoming growth inhibition in the CNS. Front Mol Neurosci 2015;8:51.

21. Wang KC, Koprivica V, Kim JA, et al. Oligodendrocyte-myelin glycoprotein is a Nogo receptor ligand that inhibits neurite outgrowth. Nature 2002; 417(6892):941–4.

22. Moreau-Fauvarque C, Kumanogoh A, Camand E, et al. The transmembrane semaphorin Sema4D/CD100, an inhibitor of axonal growth, is expressed on oligodendrocytes and upregulated after CNS lesion. J Neurosci 2003;23(27):9229–39.

23. Benson MD, Romero MI, Lush ME, et al. Ephrin-B3 is a myelin-based inhibitor of neurite outgrowth. Proc Natl Acad Sci U S A 2005;102(30):10694–9.

24. Hata K, Fujitani M, Yasuda Y, et al. RGMa inhibition promotes axonal growth and recovery after spinal cord injury. J Cell Biol 2006;173(1):47–58.

25. Low K, Culbertson M, Bradke F, et al. Netrin-1 is a novel myelin-associated inhibitor to axon growth. J Neurosci 2008;28(5):1099–108.

26. Akbik F, Cafferty WB, Strittmatter SM. Myelin associated inhibitors: a link between injury-induced and experience-dependent plasticity. Exp Neurol 2012; 235(1):43–52.

27. Fournier AE, GrandPre T, Strittmatter SM. Identification of a receptor mediating Nogo-66 inhibition of axonal regeneration. Nature 2001;409(6818): 341–6.

28. McKerracher L, Guertin P. Rho as a target to promote repair: translation to clinical studies with cethrin. Curr Pharm Des 2013;19(24):4400–10.

29. Dumont RJ, Verma S, Okonkwo DO, et al. Acute spinal cord injury, part II: contemporary pharmacotherapy. Clin Neuropharmacol 2001;24(5):265–79.

30. Pitts LH, Ross A, Chase GA, et al. Treatment with thyrotropin-releasing hormone (TRH) in patients with traumatic spinal cord injuries. J Neurotrauma 1995;12(3):235–43.

31. Gaviria M, Privat A, d'Arbigny P, et al. Neuroprotective effects of a novel NMDA antagonist, Gacyclidine, after experimental contusive spinal cord injury in adult rats. Brain Res 2000;874(2):200–9.

32. Hirbec H, Gaviria M, Vignon J. Gacyclidine: a new neuroprotective agent acting at the N-methyl-D-aspartate receptor. CNS Drug Rev 2001;7(2): 172–98.

33. Tadie M, d'Arbigny P, Mathé J. Acute spinal cord injury: early care and treatment in a multicenter study with gacyclidine. Soc Neurosci Abstr 1999; 25:1090.

34. Mocchetti I. Exogenous gangliosides, neuronal plasticity and repair, and the neurotrophins. Cell Mol Life Sci 2005;62(19–20):2283–94.

35. Geisler FH, Dorsey FC, Coleman WP. Recovery of motor function after spinal-cord injury–a randomized, placebo-controlled trial with GM-1 ganglioside. N Engl J Med 1991;324(26):1829–38.

36. Geisler FH, Coleman WP, Grieco G, et al. The Sygen multicenter acute spinal cord injury study. Spine (Phila Pa 1976) 2001;26(24 Suppl):S87–98.

37. Zhai HW, Gong ZK, Sun J, et al. Ganglioside with nerve growth factor for the recovery of extremity function following spinal cord injury and somatosensory evoked potential. Eur Rev Med Pharmacol Sci 2015;19(12):2282–6.

38. Chinnock P, Roberts I. Gangliosides for acute spinal cord injury. Cochrane Database Syst Rev 2005;(2):CD004444.

39. Hurlbert RJ, Hadley MN, Walters BC, et al. Pharmacological therapy for acute spinal cord injury. Neurosurgery 2013;72(Suppl 2):93–105.

40. Hawryluk GW, Rowland J, Kwon BK, et al. Protection and repair of the injured spinal cord: a review of completed, ongoing, and planned clinical trials for acute spinal cord injury. Neurosurg Focus 2008;25(5):E14.

41. Consortium for Spinal Cord Medicine. Early acute management in adults with spinal cord injury: a clinical practice guideline for health-care professionals. J Spinal Cord Med 2008;31(4):403–79.

42. Hadley MN, Walters BC. Introduction to the guidelines for the management of acute cervical spine and spinal cord injuries. Neurosurgery 2013; 72(Suppl 2):5–16.

43. Hawryluk G, Whetstone W, Saigal R, et al. Mean arterial blood pressure correlates with neurological recovery after human spinal cord injury: Analysis of high frequency physiologic data. J Neurotrauma 2015;32(24):1958–67.

44. Martin ND, Kepler C, Zubair M, et al. Increased mean arterial pressure goals after spinal cord injury and functional outcome. J Emerg Trauma Shock 2015;8(2):94–8.

45. Coutinho AE, Chapman KE. The anti-inflammatory and immunosuppressive effects of glucocorticoids, recent developments and mechanistic insights. Mol Cell Endocrinol 2011;335(1):2–13.

46. Bracken MB, Shepard MJ, Collins WF, et al. A randomized, controlled trial of methylprednisolone or naloxone in the treatment of acute spinal-cord injury. Results of the Second National Acute Spinal Cord Injury Study. N Engl J Med 1990; 322(20):1405–11.

47. Bracken MB, Shepard MJ, Hellenbrand KG, et al. Methylprednisolone and neurological function 1 year after spinal cord injury. Results of the National Acute Spinal Cord Injury Study. J Neurosurg 1985; 63(5):704–13.

48. Bracken MB, Shepard MJ, Holford TR, et al. Administration of methylprednisolone for 24 or 48 hours or tirilazad mesylate for 48 hours in the treatment of acute spinal cord injury. Results of the third National Acute Spinal Cord Injury Randomized Controlled Trial. National Acute Spinal Cord Injury Study. JAMA 1997;277(20):1597–604.

49. Flamm ES, Young W, Collins WF, et al. A phase I trial of naloxone treatment in acute spinal cord injury. J Neurosurg 1985;63(3):390–7.

50. Long JB, Kinney RC, Malcolm DS, et al. Intrathecal dynorphin A (1-13) and (3-13) reduce spinal cord blood flow by non-opioid mechanisms. NIDA Res Monogr 1986;75:524–6.

51. Hurlbert RJ, Hadley MN, Walters BC, et al. Pharmacological therapy for acute spinal cord injury. Neurosurgery 2015;76(Suppl 1):S71–83.

52. Bracken MB. Steroids for acute spinal cord injury. Cochrane Database Syst Rev 2012;(1): CD001046.

53. Bowers CA, Kundu B, Rosenbluth J, et al. Patients with spinal cord injuries favor administration of methylprednisolone. PLoS One 2016;11(1): e0145991.

54. Fehlings MG. Editorial: recommendations regarding the use of methylprednisolone in acute spinal cord injury: making sense out of the controversy. Spine (Phila Pa 1976) 2001;26(24 Suppl): S56–7.

55. Hall ED, Springer JE. Neuroprotection and acute spinal cord injury: a reappraisal. NeuroRx 2004; 1(1):80–100.

56. Plane JM, Shen Y, Pleasure DE, et al. Prospects for minocycline neuroprotection. Arch Neurol 2010; 67(12):1442–8.

57. Casha S, Zygun D, McGowan MD, et al. Results of a phase II placebo-controlled randomized trial of minocycline in acute spinal cord injury. Brain 2012;135(Pt 4):1224–36.

58. Kurland DB, Tosun C, Pampori A, et al. Glibenclamide for the treatment of acute CNS injury. Pharmaceuticals (Basel) 2013;6(10):1287–303.

59. Popovich PG, Lemeshow S, Gensel JC, et al. Independent evaluation of the effects of glibenclamide on reducing progressive hemorrhagic necrosis after cervical spinal cord injury. Exp Neurol 2012; 233(2):615–22.

60. Simard JM, Tsymbalyuk O, Ivanov A, et al. Endothelial sulfonylurea receptor 1-regulated NC Ca-ATP channels mediate progressive hemorrhagic necrosis following spinal cord injury. J Clin Invest 2007;117(8):2105–13.

61. Simard JM, Woo SK, Norenberg MD, et al. Brief suppression of Abcc8 prevents autodestruction of spinal cord after trauma. Sci Transl Med 2010; 2(28):28ra29.

62. Simard JM, Tsymbalyuk O, Keledjian K, et al. Comparative effects of glibenclamide and riluzole in a rat model of severe cervical spinal cord injury. Exp Neurol 2012;233(1):566–74.

63. Simard JM, Popovich PG, Tsymbalyuk O, et al. Spinal cord injury with unilateral versus bilateral primary hemorrhage–effects of glibenclamide. Exp Neurol 2012;233(2):829–35.

64. Sheth KN, Kimberly WT, Elm JJ, et al. Pilot study of intravenous glyburide in patients with a large ischemic stroke. Stroke 2014;45(1):281–3.

65. Berger R, Soder S. Neuroprotection in preterm infants. Biomed Res Int 2015;2015:257139.

66. Lee JH, Roy J, Sohn HM, et al. Magnesium in a polyethylene glycol formulation provides neuroprotection after unilateral cervical spinal cord injury. Spine (Phila Pa 1976) 2010;35(23):2041–8.

67. Tator CH, Hashimoto R, Raich A, et al. Translational potential of preclinical trials of neuroprotection through pharmacotherapy for spinal cord injury. J Neurosurg Spine 2012;17(1 Suppl):157–229.

68. Temkin NR, Anderson GD, Winn HR, et al. Magnesium sulfate for neuroprotection after traumatic brain injury: a randomised controlled trial. Lancet Neurol 2007;6(1):29–38.

69. Schwartz G, Fehlings MG. Evaluation of the neuroprotective effects of sodium channel blockers after spinal cord injury: improved behavioral and neuroanatomical recovery with riluzole. J Neurosurg 2001;94(2 Suppl):245–56.

70. Wang SJ, Wang KY, Wang WC. Mechanisms underlying the riluzole inhibition of glutamate release from rat cerebral cortex nerve terminals (synaptosomes). Neuroscience 2004;125(1):191–201.

71. Nagoshi N, Nakashima H, Fehlings MG. Riluzole as a neuroprotective drug for spinal cord injury: from bench to bedside. Molecules 2015;20(5):7775–89.

72. Grossman RG, Fehlings MG, Frankowski RF, et al. A prospective, multicenter, phase I matched-comparison group trial of safety, pharmacokinetics, and preliminary efficacy of riluzole in patients with traumatic spinal cord injury. J Neurotrauma 2014; 31(3):239–55.

73. Fehlings MG, Nakashima H, Nagoshi N, et al. Rationale, design and critical end points for the riluzole in acute spinal cord injury study (RISCIS): a randomized, double-blinded, placebo-controlled parallel multi-center trial. Spinal Cord 2016;54(1): 8–15.

74. Xiao BG, Lu CZ, Link H. Cell biology and clinical promise of G-CSF: immunomodulation and neuroprotection. J Cell Mol Med 2007;11(6):1272–90.

75. Koda M, Nishio Y, Kamada T, et al. Granulocyte colony-stimulating factor (G-CSF) mobilizes bone marrow-derived cells into injured spinal cord and promotes functional recovery after compression-induced spinal cord injury in mice. Brain Res 2007;1149:223–31.

76. Pan HC, Cheng FC, Lai SZ, et al. Enhanced regeneration in spinal cord injury by concomitant treatment with granulocyte colony-stimulating factor and neuronal stem cells. J Clin Neurosci 2008; 15(6):656–64.

77. Park HC, Shim YS, Ha Y, et al. Treatment of complete spinal cord injury patients by autologous bone marrow cell transplantation and administration of granulocyte-macrophage colony stimulating factor. Tissue Eng 2005;11(5–6):913–22.

78. Yoon SH, Shim YS, Park YH, et al. Complete spinal cord injury treatment using autologous bone marrow cell transplantation and bone marrow stimulation with granulocyte macrophage-colony stimulating factor: Phase I/II clinical trial. Stem Cells 2007;25(8):2066–73.

79. Schnell L, Schwab ME. Axonal regeneration in the rat spinal cord produced by an antibody against myelin-associated neurite growth inhibitors. Nature 1990;343(6255):269–72.

80. Freund P, Schmidlin E, Wannier T, et al. Nogo-A-specific antibody treatment enhances sprouting and functional recovery after cervical lesion in adult primates. Nat Med 2006;12(7):790–2.

81. Zorner B, Schwab ME. Anti-Nogo on the go: from animal models to a clinical trial. Ann N Y Acad Sci 2010;1198(Suppl 1):E22–34.

82. Dergham P, Ellezam B, Essagian C, et al. Rho signaling pathway targeted to promote spinal cord repair. J Neurosci 2002;22(15):6570–7.

83. Fehlings MG, Theodore N, Harrop J, et al. A phase I/IIa clinical trial of a recombinant Rho protein antagonist in acute spinal cord injury. J Neurotrauma 2011;28(5):787–96.

84. Kopp MA, Liebscher T, Niedeggen A, et al. Small-molecule-induced Rho-inhibition: NSAIDs after spinal cord injury. Cell Tissue Res 2012; 349(1):119–32.

85. Turner N, Grose R. Fibroblast growth factor signalling: from development to cancer. Nat Rev Cancer 2010;10(2):116–29.

86. De Laporte L, des Rieux A, Tuinstra HM, et al. Vascular endothelial growth factor and fibroblast growth factor 2 delivery from spinal cord bridges to enhance angiogenesis following injury. J Biomed Mater Res A 2011;98(3):372–82.

87. Shi Q, Gao W, Han X, et al. Collagen scaffolds modified with collagen-binding bFGF promotes the neural regeneration in a rat hemisected spinal cord injury model. Sci China Life Sci 2014;57(2): 232–40.

88. Zhang HY, Wang ZG, Wu FZ, et al. Regulation of autophagy and ubiquitinated protein accumulation by bFGF promotes functional recovery and neural protection in a rat model of spinal cord injury. Mol Neurobiol 2013;48(3):452–64.

89. Zhang HY, Zhang X, Wang ZG, et al. Exogenous basic fibroblast growth factor inhibits ER stress-induced apoptosis and improves recovery from spinal cord injury. CNS Neurosci Ther 2013;19(1): 20–9.

90. Antonic A, Sena ES, Lees JS, et al. Stem cell transplantation in traumatic spinal cord injury: a systematic review and meta-analysis of animal studies. PLoS Biol 2013;11(12):e1001738.

91. Yousefifard M, Rahimi-Movaghar V, Nasirinezhad F, et al. Neural stem/progenitor cell transplantation for spinal cord injury treatment; a systematic review and meta-analysis. Neuroscience 2016;322: 377–97.

92. Sahni V, Kessler JA. Stem cell therapies for spinal cord injury. Nat Rev Neurol 2010;6(7):363–72.

93. Ruff CA, Wilcox JT, Fehlings MG. Cell-based transplantation strategies to promote plasticity following spinal cord injury. Exp Neurol 2012;235(1):78–90.

94. Knoller N, Auerbach G, Fulga V, et al. Clinical experience using incubated autologous macrophages

as a treatment for complete spinal cord injury: phase I study results. J Neurosurg Spine 2005; 3(3):173–81.

95. Lammertse DP, Jones LA, Charlifue SB, et al. Autologous incubated macrophage therapy in acute, complete spinal cord injury: results of the phase 2 randomized controlled multicenter trial. Spinal Cord 2012;50(9):661–71.

96. Doulames VM, Plant GW. Induced pluripotent stem cell therapies for cervical spinal cord injury. Int J Mol Sci 2016;17(4):530.

97. Nutt SE, Chang EA, Suhr ST, et al. Caudalized human iPSC-derived neural progenitor cells produce neurons and glia but fail to restore function in an early chronic spinal cord injury model. Exp Neurol 2013;248:491–503.

98. Li K, Javed E, Scura D, et al. Human iPS cell-derived astrocyte transplants preserve respiratory function after spinal cord injury. Exp Neurol 2015; 271:479–92.

99. Donnelly EM, Lamanna J, Boulis NM. Stem cell therapy for the spinal cord. Stem Cell Res Ther 2012;3(4):24.

100. Hurtado A, Moon LD, Maquet V, et al. Poly (D,L-lactic acid) macroporous guidance scaffolds seeded with Schwann cells genetically modified to secrete a bi-functional neurotrophin implanted in the completely transected adult rat thoracic spinal cord. Biomaterials 2006;27(3):430–42.

101. Koda M, Kamada T, Hashimoto M, et al. Adenovirus vector-mediated ex vivo gene transfer of brain-derived neurotrophic factor to bone marrow stromal cells promotes axonal regeneration after transplantation in completely transected adult rat spinal cord. Eur Spine J 2007; 16(12):2206–14.

102. Lu P, Yang H, Jones LL, et al. Combinatorial therapy with neurotrophins and cAMP promotes axonal regeneration beyond sites of spinal cord injury. J Neurosci 2004;24(28):6402–9.

103. Kong CY, Hosseini AM, Belanger LM, et al. A prospective evaluation of hemodynamic management in acute spinal cord injury patients. Spinal Cord 2013;51(6):466–71.

104. Pointillart V, Petitjean ME, Wiart L, et al. Pharmacological therapy of spinal cord injury during the acute phase. Spinal Cord 2000;38(2):71–6.

105. Hurlbert RJ. The role of steroids in acute spinal cord injury: an evidence-based analysis. Spine (Phila Pa 1976) 2001;26(24 Suppl):S39–46.

Restorative Treatments for Spinal Cord Injury

Stephanie Chen, MD, Allan D. Levi, MD, PhD*

KEYWORDS

- Spinal cord injury • Neuroprotection • Cell-based therapies • Electrical stimulation

KEY POINTS

- Therapeutic hypothermia after spinal cord injury may prevent secondary damage after spinal cord injury.
- Cell transplantation with glial cells, stem cells, or a combination may enhance spinal cord regeneration and functional recovery after spinal cord injury.
- Electrical stimulation may assist in recruiting new motor circuits to improve function after spinal cord injury.

INTRODUCTION

Spinal cord injury (SCI) occurs in approximately 10,000 to 12,000 individuals per year in North America, and 250,000 individuals are living with an SCI.[1] Current treatment is focused on limiting secondary complications and maximizing residual function. However, with the life expectancy of individuals with SCI increasing, therapeutic strategies focused on restoring functional independence is becoming increasingly important. In this article, the authors discuss the range of strategies that are currently being used and researched in order to restore function after SCI.

NEUROPROTECTION

After the initial trauma of SCI, cell death and tissue loss continue over several weeks.[2,3] During this initial window the main strategies used to restrict secondary damage are surgical decompression, therapeutic hypothermia, and drugs targeting inflammation or excitotoxicity.

Therapeutic Hypothermia

Therapeutic hypothermia slows biological reactions and processes resulting in improved electrophysiologic, histologic, and motor outcomes in experimental models of SCI. The mechanism of protection includes reducing excitotoxicity,[4] vasogenic edema,[5] neuroinflammation,[6] ischemia,[7] oxidative stress,[8] and apoptosis.[9] This increasing body of evidence of efficacy has been derived primarily from animal studies and case series.[10–16]

Several case series in the 1970s described potential benefits with the use of local spinal cord cooling after SCI.[17–23] In these experimental models, cooling was performed by application of an extradural heat exchanger or perfusion of subarachnoid space with cold solution. However, the results were mixed and the procedure invasive; thus, the technique was gradually abandoned. However, in a recent case series, 20 patients with complete cervical or thoracic SCI underwent triple therapy including dexamethasone, surgical decompression, and deep cord cooling with

Disclosure: The authors do not have any conflicts of interest to disclose.
Department of Neurological Surgery, The Miami Project to Cure Paralysis, University of Miami Miller School of Medicine, 1095 Northwest 14th Terrace (D4-6), Miami, FL 33136, USA
* Corresponding author. Department of Neurological Surgery, University of Miami Miller School of Medicine, Lois Pope Life Center, 1095 Northwest 14th Terrace (D4-6), Miami, FL 33136.
E-mail address: ALevi@med.miami.edu

Neurosurg Clin N Am 28 (2017) 63–71
http://dx.doi.org/10.1016/j.nec.2016.08.004

extradural saddles (dural temperature of 6°C). At 1 year after injury, 16 patients (80%) regained some sensory or motor function.[24] Although this study is exciting, the evidence is preliminary and merits further investigation.

Systemic cooling with intravascular heat exchange cooling catheter techniques is of great modern interest as it has been shown to be safe[25–27] and potentially beneficial in a case control study (**Fig. 1**). In this study of 31 patients with complete cervical SCI (who showed no improvement within 24 hours of injury), 11 (35%) of patients regained some sensory or motor function with systemic intravascular cooling (**Fig. 2**).[28] The finding is promising as the rate of spontaneous recovery is reported to be approximately 15% to 20% in complete cervical SCI.[29,30] The surmounting body of evidence of efficacy will be further elucidated by the results of an ongoing clinical trial (NCT01739010) to test modest systemic hypothermia.

Pharmacologic Therapies

Pharmacologic therapies are also being studied to target secondary damage from inflammation and excitotoxicity. The most heavily studied pharmacotherapy agent for SCI has been methylprednisolone,

which is thought to limit the inflammatory response after SCI. However after 4 prospective blinded randomized controlled trials, there is no class I medical evidence of any benefit.[31–34] Furthermore, methylprednisolone may have harmful effects, including increased rates of wound infections, gastrointestinal hemorrhage, and hyperglycemia. Thus, the most recent guidelines from the Congress of Neurological Surgeons/American Association of Neurological Surgeons recommends against the use of methylprednisolone for the treatment of acute SCI.[32,35]

Other agents currently being studied include minocycline and riluzole. Minocycline is a semisynthetic tetracycline antibiotic, which is currently in a phase 3 clinical trial for neuroprotective benefits after acute SCI. It has been shown to reduce inflammatory cytokines, free radicals, and matrix metalloproteinases.[36–40] Riluzole is a glutamate antagonist and sodium channel blocker that is currently being tested in a phase 1 trial for acute SCI, with initial data suggesting that riluzole is well tolerated and may have neuroprotective efficacy.[41] Further discussion of the pharmacologic agents for SCI (see Michael Karsy and Gregory Hawryluk's article, "Pharmacologic Management of Acute Spinal Cord Injury," in this issue).

CELL TRANSPLANTATION AND REGROWTH

Traumatic SCI results in a disruption of axonal myelination, resulting in a loss of function. *Glial cell transplantation* has emerged as a potential target for axonal regeneration after SCI. Schwann cells are the most common glial cell in the peripheral nervous system. Their therapeutic potential is thought to be due to their ability to secrete high levels of neurotrophic growth factors and extracellular matrix molecules that promote axon growth.[42] Schwann cell grafts have been extensively studied in animal models and have been shown to increase cell survival, decrease the size of the cystic lesion after SCI, and improve locomotion scores.[43,44] However, only 3 studies have reported the use of Schwann cells in humans with SCI (**Fig. 3**).[45–47] The largest of these studies involved 33 patients with chronic American Spinal Injury Association (ASIA) grade A or B SCI in which there was a marked improvement in sensory scores but no improvement in motor function.[45] From this preclinical data, a phase 2 clinical trial of autologous Schwann cells in chronically spinal cord injured subjects is presently underway in the Miami Project to Cure Paralysis.[47]

Another cell type that is being studied for axonal regeneration after SCI is the *olfactory ensheathing cell* (OEC). OECs are a distinct population of cells that wrap the axons of olfactory receptor axons in

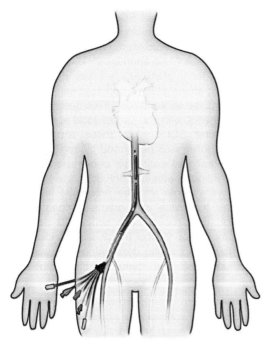

Fig. 1. An intravascular heat exchange, cooling catheter that functions by circulating ice-cold saline in balloons within the inferior vena cava in a closed circuit without adding any intravascular volume. In the University of Miami hypothermia protocol, this device is used to cool patients to a target temperature 33°C.

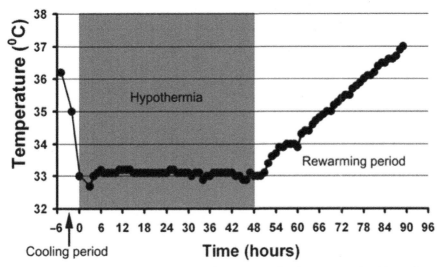

Fig. 2. The University of Miami hypothermia protocol for SCI. Hypothermia is maintained for 48 hours, and then rewarming slowly begins at the rate of 0.1°C per hour to 37°C. This rewarming takes about 24 hours. After reaching normothermia, the CoolGuard (Zoll Medical Corporation, Chelmsford, MA) catheter is removed and normothermia is maintained.

their entire length as they extend from the olfactory epithelium in the peripheral nervous system to the olfactory bulb in the central nervous system (CNS). In animal models of SCI they can limit neuronal cell death[48] and be myelinated and stimulate axonal growth.[49] Ramon-Cueto and colleagues[50] reported regeneration of corticospinal axons and improvement in motor behavior in rats after injury. Small preliminary studies of OECs have been studied in humans and have established feasibility and safety; however, results of efficacy have been mixed.[51–54] Mackay-Sim and colleagues[52] reported that only 1 of 6 patients with a chronic SCI had any neurologic improvement (ie, a mild improvement in sensation) after treatment with OECs. Lima and colleagues[51] reported that

11 of 20 patients (55%) with chronic SCI had an improvement in ASIA grade after such treatment, including 5 patients who recovered voluntary bowel control and 1 who recovered bladder control.

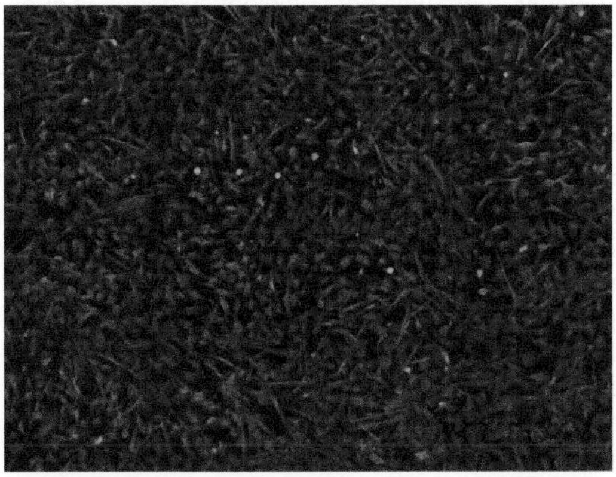

Stem Cell Transplantation

Stem cell transplantation for SCI is another area of ongoing investigation that holds great potential for tissue regeneration. Stem cells may mediate repair by secreting growth factors and replacing lost neurons, glial, or other cells. However, the progenitor cell type that is most effective has yet to be elucidated. Currently, 3 main stem cell types are being used in animal modes of SCI: human embryonic stem cells, neural stem cells, and bone marrow mesenchymal stem cells.

Embryonic stem cells are taken from blastocysts and can develop into more than 200 different cell types in the human body with an unrestricted power of self-renewal.[55] Thus, they have the highest potency but also the greatest risk for tumorigenicity as well as immune rejection. They can be directed toward multipotent neural precursors,[56] motor neurons,[57,58] and oligodendrocyte progenitor cells[59] and then transplanted. Transplantation of human embryonic stem cell derived oligodendrocyte progenitor cells into rats 7 days after injury resulted in enhanced myelination and functional recovery.[59] This finding led to the first approved clinical trial using embryonic stem cells in 2009. The Geron sponsored trial (Geron of Menlo Park, California) involved transplantation of GRNOPC1 (a treatment containing oligodendrocyte progenitor cells) into patients with complete thoracic

Fig. 3. Cultured human Schwann cells labeled with green fluorescent protein to determine cell purity before transplantation.

SCIs. Although no safety concerns were reported, in 2011 Geron stopped the trial prematurely largely because of financial reasons, raising several ethical concerns. In 2013, Asterias Bio-therapeutics acquired GRNOPC1 (now AST-OPC1) and have since initiated a phase I clinical trial transplanting AST-OPC1 in patients with complete cervical SCI (NCT02302157).

Neural stem/progenitor cells (NSC) are alternative pluripotent cells with the potential to differentiate into neurons, oligodendrocytes, and astrocytes in vitro and in vivo.[60] These cells can be obtained from the central canal of the spinal cord or subventricular zone of the brain. In most cases, in vivo transplanted NSCs preferentially differentiate into glial cells, particularly astrocytes.[61] With certain pretreatments, however, grafted NSCs can differentiate into neurons or oligodendrocytes, which may enhance synaptic contact reformation or remyelination.[62-65] In 2000, StemCells, Inc created HuCNS-SC, an adult neuro stem cell from purified human neural stem cells from a single fetal brain tissue. A phase I/II trial involving transplantation in HuCNS-SC in 12 patients (ASIA categories A and B with chronic paraplegia and an average postinjury time of 11 months) with SCI has recently been completed. Thus far, no safety concerns have been reported; early results show below-injury-level sensory improvements in several patients (**Fig. 4**).

Bone marrow–derived mesenchymal stem cells (MSCs) display broad potency, with the ability to differentiate not only into multiple mesodermal cells such as blood, bone, and muscle but also CNS cells.[66] Transplantation of MSC confers the advantage of relatively easy procurement from bone marrow aspirate and autologous transplantation, avoiding the need for immunosuppression.

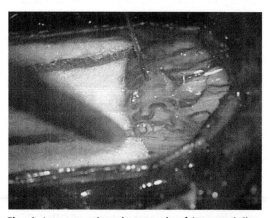

Fig. 4. Intraoperative photograph of intramedullary injection of human stem cells into the perilesional area of a patient with a cervical SCI.

Furthermore, in vivo tumor development has not been reported. A phase I clinical trial has been completed and establishes safety and potential efficacy of autologous bone marrow MSC transplantation at least 6 months after the procedure in subjects with chronic thoracic and lumbar SCI.[67] However, results regarding efficacy from clinical studies using MSCs for SCI are mixed. Park and colleagues[68] showed significant improvement in 3 of 10 subjects who received intramedullary and intrathecal injections of MSCs, whereas Bhanot and colleagues[69] reported intralesional and intrathecal injection of MSC enhanced rehabilitation in only one of 67 subjects with chronic SCI. These variable results may be due to the degree of heterogeneity in how the cells are harvested, cultured, and administered.

ELECTRICAL STIMULATION
Functional Electrical Stimulation

Functional electrical stimulation (FES) uses stimulators, surface electrodes, and frames to create purposeful contractions for the restoration of gait, upright posture, cycling, and hand movement.[70]

FES was originally designed for the restoration for walking in paraplegic patients. FES gait systems, such as the Parastep 1 (Sigmedics Inc., Fairborn, OH), consist of a multichannel stimulator, surface electrodes, and walking frames. The stand command delivers continuous stimulation to the gluteal muscles and quadriceps to maintain erect posture while pulse generators stimulate opposing muscles in order to create stepping motions.[71] Nightingale and colleagues[70] conducted a systematic review of previous published studies on patients with SCIs and the efficacy of FES gait and concluded that the use of FES gait training in incomplete SCI populations improves walking ability and overall independence in the community. However, there was not sufficient evidence to support changes in bone mineral density, joint movements, and overall reduced energy cost of gait.[72]

FES cycling has evolved as a therapeutic tool for the rehabilitation of people with paraplegia. In contrast to FES gait training exercises, FES cycling can be maintained for longer periods of time and fall risk is minimal.[73,74] In FES cycling, electrodes are placed on opposing muscle groups: the quadriceps and hamstrings and the plantar flexors and dorsiflexors of the ankle. Their legs are then placed in a rigid orthosis that restricts lateral bending movements, and a throttle on the steering handle controls electrode stimulation intensity.[73] Following an FES cycling program instituted for several weeks, Gerrits and colleagues[75] have demonstrated restoration of muscle bulk and strength, a return of the contractile properties of the quadriceps muscle toward normal, as well as increases in capillary numbers.[76] However, patients' power outputs remain too low for travel on uneven terrain.[73]

FES for the upper extremity has the potential to restore important daily hand functions to patients with quadriplegia. All of these upper extremity neuroprosthetic devices currently consist of a stimulator with electrodes that activate the muscles of the arm and hand as well as a controller. There are multiple systems available at this time wherein electrodes are placed on the surface, within a brace, or percutaneously.[77–79]

Robotic Training Strategies

Robotic training strategies use electromechanical, pneumatic, and hydraulic forces to actively move limbs or assist voluntary movement. Furthermore, these therapy robots have the potential measure therapy progress and provide feedback both to patients and therapists. Robotic-assist devices include driven (ie, motorized) gait orthoses (DGO) as well as robotic upper extremity–assist devices. DGOs, such as the Lokomat (Hocoma, Volketswil, Switzerland), generally consist of an exoskeleton that fits over patients' legs and assists the physical therapist in stabilizing the lower limbs and gait training (**Fig. 5**). Wirz and colleagues[80] conducted a multicenter study of 20 patients with incomplete SCI (ASIA grades C and D) using the Lokomat DGO wherein patients underwent an 8-week robotic training period. In this small study they concluded that the DGO resulted in significant improvement in the subjects' gait velocity, endurance, and performance of functional tasks. There were no changes, however, in the use of walking aids, orthoses, or external physical assistance following conclusion of the study.

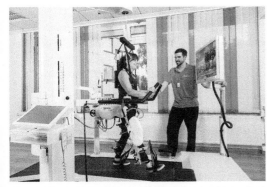

Fig. 5. The LokomatPro consists of a robotic exoskeleton that fits over the patient's leg to assist with stability and gait training. (Picture: Hocoma, Switzerland.)

Epidural Stimulation

Epidural stimulation has been used in experimental models to increase central pattern generator or lower motor neuron excitability. In one clinical case series a 16-electrode array epidural stimulator is placed over the L1-S1 cord in combination with months of intensive rehabilitation before and after implantation. Four patients with complete motor paralysis (2 ASIA-B and 2 ASIA-A) were able to execute on-command voluntary movement after implantation. With continuous stimulation, all 4 participants could stand independently with full weight bearing for several minutes, move their legs in response to cues, and recruit appropriate muscles to make specific movements in response to cues. It is thought that epidural stimulation improves lower extremity function by bringing spinal circuits closer to threshold such that the descending input form the brain or peripheral sensation is sufficient to trigger volitional movement.[81]

Intraspinal Microstimulation

Intraspinal microstimulation (ISMS) is another modality that uses targeted electrodes to recover motor circuits in patients with SCIs. Most experiments using this technology involve implanting microelectrodes distal to the site of injury in the lumbosacral spine to recover bladder control or locomotion of the hind limbs in animals.[82,83] However, recently ISMS was implanted in the cervical cord in rats with severe cervical contusions. The investigators found significant improvements in skilled forelimb reaching within the first 2 weeks of stimulation, which persisted beyond the period of stimulation.[84] These data are promising for the therapeutic and possible regenerative capacity of neuroprosthetic devices; however, further studies confirming safety and efficacy are necessary before translation to clinical use.

Brain Computer Interfaces

Brain computer interfaces (BCIs) is an emerging technology that aims to translate cerebral electrical activity into meaningful commands or movements in order to assist patients with SCI and other debilitating neurologic diseases. There are 2 general forms: invasive and noninvasive. Noninvasive BCIs derive the user's intent from scalp-recorded electroencephalographic (EEG) electrode activity, whereas invasive BCIs receive input from surgically placed electrodes directly on the brain's surface. Invasive BCIs primarily remain experimental, currently being studied in primates.[85–87]

Wolpaw and McFarland[88] demonstrated that a noninvasive BCI in 2 patients with SCIs could provide multidimensional control similar to ranges reported in invasive studies for nonhuman primates. They concluded that over multiple sessions, the user developed better EEG control and that the computer focused on those rhythms that the user was better able to control. In addition, the cursor movements over multiple sessions become more of an automatic gesture rather than the application thought produced motor imagery required in earlier sessions.

SUMMARY

Enormous advancements in therapeutic strategies for the restoration of function after SCI have arisen over the last 3 decades. However, it is clear that several questions remain unanswered. Innovations in pharmacotherapy, cellular transplantation, and technology will all undoubtedly play a role in treating this multifaceted disease. However, as we gain a greater understanding, it is crucial to maintain a critical consideration of the efficacy, cost, and ethical consequences of these findings. Only through this analysis as a community can we provide the best care for these patients who will be changed for the remainder of their lives by their injury and the rapid sequence of events that revolve around their acute hospitalization.

REFERENCES

1. Harvey C, Rothschild BB, Asmann AJ, et al. New estimates of traumatic SCI prevalence: a survey-based approach. Paraplegia 1990;28(9):537–44.
2. Tator CH. Vascular effects and blood flow in acute spinal cord injuries. J Neurosurg Sci 1984;28(3–4):115–9.
3. Management of pediatric cervical spine and spinal cord injuries. Neurosurgery 2002;50(Suppl 3):S85–99.
4. Yamamoto K, Ishikawa T, Sakabe T, et al. The hydroxyl radical scavenger Nicaraven inhibits glutamate release after spinal injury in rats. Neuroreport 1998;9(7):1655–9.
5. Westergren H, Yu WR, Farooque M, et al. Systemic hypothermia following spinal cord compression injury in the rat: axonal changes studied by beta-APP, ubiquitin, and PGP 9.5 immunohistochemistry. Spinal Cord 1999;37(10):696–704.
6. Chatzipanteli K, Yanagawa Y, Marcillo AE, et al. Posttraumatic hypothermia reduces polymorphonuclear leukocyte accumulation following spinal cord injury in rats. J Neurotrauma 2000;17(4):321–32.
7. Westergren H, Farooque M, Olsson Y, et al. Spinal cord blood flow changes following systemic hypothermia and spinal cord compression injury: an experimental study in the rat using laser-Doppler flowmetry. Spinal Cord 2001;39(2):74–84.
8. Ji X, Luo Y, Ling F, et al. Mild hypothermia diminishes oxidative DNA damage and pro-death signaling events after cerebral ischemia: a mechanism for neuroprotection. Front Biosci 2007;12:1737–47.
9. Ohmura A, Nakajima W, Ishida A, et al. Prolonged hypothermia protects neonatal rat brain against hypoxic-ischemia by reducing both apoptosis and necrosis. Brain Dev 2005;27(7):517–26.
10. Batchelor PE, Kerr NF, Gatt AM, et al. Hypothermia prior to decompression: buying time for treatment of acute spinal cord injury. J Neurotrauma 2010;27(8):1357–68.
11. Dietrich WD. Therapeutic hypothermia for acute severe spinal cord injury: ready to start large clinical trials? Crit Care Med 2012;40(2):691–2.
12. Ha KY, Kim YH. Neuroprotective effect of moderate epidural hypothermia after spinal cord injury in rats. Spine (Phila Pa 1976) 2008;33(19):2059–65.
13. Kang J, Albadawi H, Casey PJ, et al. The effects of systemic hypothermia on a murine model of thoracic aortic ischemia reperfusion. J Vasc Surg 2010;52(2):435–43.
14. Lo TP Jr, Cho KS, Garg MS, et al. Systemic hypothermia improves histological and functional outcome after cervical spinal cord contusion in rats. J Comp Neurol 2009;514(5):433–48.
15. Maybhate A, Hu C, Bazley FA, et al. Potential long-term benefits of acute hypothermia after spinal cord injury: assessments with somatosensory-evoked potentials. Crit Care Med 2012;40(2):573–9.
16. Yu CG, Jimenez O, Marcillo AE, et al. Beneficial effects of modest systemic hypothermia on locomotor function and histopathological damage following contusion-induced spinal cord injury in rats. J Neurosurg 2000;93(1 Suppl):85–93.
17. Bricolo A, Ore GD, Da Pian R, et al. Local cooling in spinal cord injury. Surg Neurol 1976;6(2):101–6.
18. Demian YK, White RJ, Yashon D, et al. Anaesthesia for laminectomy and localized cord cooling in acute cervical spine injury. Report of three cases. Br J Anaesth 1971;43(10):973–9.
19. Koons DD, Gildenberg PL, Dohn DF, et al. Local hypothermia in the treatment of spinal cord injuries. Report of seven cases. Cleve Clin Q 1972;39(3):109–17.
20. Negrin J Jr. Spinal cord hypothermia in the neurosurgical management of the acute and chronic posttraumatic paraplegic patient. Paraplegia 1973;10(4):336–43.
21. Negrin J Jr. Spinal cord hypothermia. Neurosurgical management of immediate and delayed posttraumatic neurologic sequelae. N Y State J Med 1975;75(13):2387–92.
22. Selker RG. Icewater irrigation of the spinal cord. Surg Forum 1971;22:411–3.
23. Tator CH. Acute spinal cord injury: a review of recent studies of treatment and pathophysiology. Can Med Assoc J 1972;107(2):143–5. passim.

24. Hansebout RR, Hansebout CR. Local cooling for traumatic spinal cord injury: outcomes in 20 patients and review of the literature. J Neurosurg Spine 2014; 20(5):550–61.

25. Dietrich WD, Levi AD, Wang M, et al. Hypothermic treatment for acute spinal cord injury. Neurotherapeutics 2011;8(2):229–39.

26. Levi AD, Casella G, Green BA, et al. Clinical outcomes using modest intravascular hypothermia after acute cervical spinal cord injury. Neurosurgery 2010;66(4):670–7.

27. Levi AD, Green BA, Wang MY, et al. Clinical application of modest hypothermia after spinal cord injury. J Neurotrauma 2009;26(3):407–15.

28. Dididze M, Green BA, Dietrich WD, et al. Systemic hypothermia in acute cervical spinal cord injury: a case-controlled study. Spinal Cord 2013;51(5):395–400.

29. Coleman WP, Geisler FH. Injury severity as primary predictor of outcome in acute spinal cord injury: retrospective results from a large multicenter clinical trial. Spine J 2004;4(4):373–8.

30. Fawcett JW, Curt A, Steeves JD, et al. Guidelines for the conduct of clinical trials for spinal cord injury as developed by the ICCP panel: spontaneous recovery after spinal cord injury and statistical power needed for therapeutic clinical trials. Spinal Cord 2007;45(3):190–205.

31. Bracken MB, Shepard MJ, Collins WF, et al. A randomized, controlled trial of methylprednisolone or naloxone in the treatment of acute spinal-cord injury. Results of the Second National Acute Spinal Cord Injury Study. N Engl J Med 1990;322(20): 1405–11.

32. Bracken MB, Collins WF, Freeman DF, et al. Efficacy of methylprednisolone in acute spinal cord injury. JAMA 1984;251(1):45–52.

33. Bracken MB, Shepard MJ, Holford TR, et al. Administration of methylprednisolone for 24 or 48 hours or tirilazad mesylate for 48 hours in the treatment of acute spinal cord injury. Results of the third national acute spinal cord injury randomized controlled trial. National acute spinal cord injury study. JAMA 1997; 277(20):1597–604.

34. Pointillart V, Petitjean ME, Wiart L, et al. Pharmacological therapy of spinal cord injury during the acute phase. Spinal Cord 2000;38(2):71–6.

35. Matsumoto T, Tamaki T, Kawakami M, et al. Early complications of high-dose methylprednisolone sodium succinate treatment in the follow-up of acute cervical spinal cord injury. Spine (Phila Pa 1976) 2001;26(4):426–30.

36. Tikka TM, Koistinaho JE. Minocycline provides neuroprotection against N-methyl-D-aspartate neurotoxicity by inhibiting microglia. J Immunol 2001; 166(12):7527–33.

37. Amin AR, Attur MG, Thakker GD, et al. A novel mechanism of action of tetracyclines: effects on nitric oxide synthases. Proc Natl Acad Sci U S A 1996;93(24):14014–9.

38. Yrjanheikki J, Tikka T, Keinänen R, et al. A tetracycline derivative, minocycline, reduces inflammation and protects against focal cerebral ischemia with a wide therapeutic window. Proc Natl Acad Sci U S A 1999;96(23):13496–500.

39. Chen M, Ona VO, Li M, et al. Minocycline inhibits caspase-1 and caspase-3 expression and delays mortality in a transgenic mouse model of Huntington disease. Nat Med 2000;6(7):797–801.

40. Zhu S, Stavrovskaya IG, Drozda M, et al. Minocycline inhibits cytochrome c release and delays progression of amyotrophic lateral sclerosis in mice. Nature 2002;417(6884):74–8.

41. Grossman RG, Fehlings MG, Frankowski RF, et al. A prospective, multicenter, phase I matched-comparison group trial of safety, pharmacokinetics, and preliminary efficacy of riluzole in patients with traumatic spinal cord injury. J Neurotrauma 2014; 31(3):239–55.

42. Bunge RP. The role of the Schwann cell in trophic support and regeneration. J Neurol 1994;242(1 Suppl 1):S19–21.

43. Takami T, Oudega M, Bates ML, et al. Schwann cell but not olfactory ensheathing glia transplants improve hindlimb locomotor performance in the moderately contused adult rat thoracic spinal cord. J Neurosci 2002;22(15):6670–81.

44. Guest JD, Rao A, Olson L, et al. The ability of human Schwann cell grafts to promote regeneration in the transected nude rat spinal cord. Exp Neurol 1997; 148(2):502–22.

45. Saberi H, Firouzi M, Habibi Z, et al. Safety of intramedullary Schwann cell transplantation for postrehabilitation spinal cord injuries: 2-year follow-up of 33 cases. J Neurosurg Spine 2011;15(5):515–25.

46. Zhou XH, Ning GZ, Feng SQ, et al. Transplantation of autologous activated Schwann cells in the treatment of spinal cord injury: six cases, more than five years of follow-up. Cell Transplant 2012; 21(Suppl 1):S39–47.

47. Guest J, Santamaria AJ, Benavides FD. Clinical translation of autologous Schwann cell transplantation for the treatment of spinal cord injury. Curr Opin Organ Transplant 2013;18(6):682–9.

48. Barbour HR, Plant CD, Harvey AR, et al. Tissue sparing, behavioral recovery, supraspinal axonal sparing/regeneration following sub-acute glial transplantation in a model of spinal cord contusion. BMC Neurosci 2013;14:106.

49. Witheford M, Westendorf K, Roskams AJ. Olfactory ensheathing cells promote corticospinal axonal outgrowth by a L1 CAM-dependent mechanism. Glia 2013;61(11):1873–89.

50. Ramon-Cueto A, Cordero MI, Santos-Benito FF, et al. Functional recovery of paraplegic rats and motor

axon regeneration in their spinal cords by olfactory ensheathing glia. Neuron 2000;25(2):425–35.

51. Lima C, Escada P, Pratas-Vital J, et al. Olfactory mucosal autografts and rehabilitation for chronic traumatic spinal cord injury. Neurorehabil Neural Repair 2010;24(1):10–22.

52. Mackay-Sim A, Féron F, Cochrane J, et al. Autologous olfactory ensheathing cell transplantation in human paraplegia: a 3-year clinical trial. Brain 2008;131(Pt 9):2376–86.

53. Rao Y, Zhu W, Guo Y, et al. Long-term outcome of olfactory ensheathing cell transplantation in six patients with chronic complete spinal cord injury. Cell Transplant 2013;22(Suppl 1):S21–5.

54. Tabakow P, Jarmundowicz W, Czapiga B, et al. Transplantation of autologous olfactory ensheathing cells in complete human spinal cord injury. Cell Transplant 2013;22(9):1591–612.

55. Smith AG. Embryo-derived stem cells: of mice and men. Annu Rev Cell Dev Biol 2001;17:435–62.

56. Carpenter MK, Inokuma MS, Denham J, et al. Enrichment of neurons and neural precursors from human embryonic stem cells. Exp Neurol 2001;172(2):383–97.

57. Li XJ, Du ZW, Zarnowska ED, et al. Specification of motoneurons from human embryonic stem cells. Nat Biotechnol 2005;23(2):215–21.

58. Lee H, Shamy GA, Elkabetz Y, et al. Directed differentiation and transplantation of human embryonic stem cell-derived motoneurons. Stem Cells 2007; 25(8):1931–9.

59. Keirstead HS, Nistor G, Bernal G, et al. Human embryonic stem cell-derived oligodendrocyte progenitor cell transplants remyelinate and restore locomotion after spinal cord injury. J Neurosci 2005;25(19):4694–705.

60. Reubinoff BE, Itsykson P, Turetsky T, et al. Neural progenitors from human embryonic stem cells. Nat Biotechnol 2001;19(12):1134–40.

61. Cao QL, Zhang YP, Howard RM, et al. Pluripotent stem cells engrafted into the normal or lesioned adult rat spinal cord are restricted to a glial lineage. Exp Neurol 2001;167(1):48–58.

62. Webber DJ, Bradbury EJ, McMahon SB, et al. Transplanted neural progenitor cells survive and differentiate but achieve limited functional recovery in the lesioned adult rat spinal cord. Regen Med 2007; 2(6):929–45.

63. Hwang DH, Kim BG, Kim EJ, et al. Transplantation of human neural stem cells transduced with Olig2 transcription factor improves locomotor recovery and enhances myelination in the white matter of rat spinal cord following contusive injury. BMC Neurosci 2009;10:117.

64. Yasuda A, Tsuji O, Shibata S, et al. Significance of remyelination by neural stem/progenitor cells transplanted into the injured spinal cord. Stem Cells 2011;29(12):1983–94.

65. Yan J, Xu L, Welsh AM, et al. Extensive neuronal differentiation of human neural stem cell grafts in adult rat spinal cord. PLoS Med 2007;4(2):e39.

66. Sasaki M, Honmou O, Akiyama Y, et al. Transplantation of an acutely isolated bone marrow fraction repairs demyelinated adult rat spinal cord axons. Glia 2001;35(1):26–34.

67. Mendonca MV, Larocca TF, de Freitas Souza BS, et al. Safety and neurological assessments after autologous transplantation of bone marrow mesenchymal stem cells in subjects with chronic spinal cord injury. Stem Cell Res Ther 2014;5(6):126.

68. Park JH, Kim DY, Sung IY, et al. Long-term results of spinal cord injury therapy using mesenchymal stem cells derived from bone marrow in humans. Neurosurgery 2012;70(5):1238–47 [discussion: 1247].

69. Bhanot Y, Rao S, Ghosh D, et al. Autologous mesenchymal stem cells in chronic spinal cord injury. Br J Neurosurg 2011;25(4):516–22.

70. Nightingale EJ, Raymond J, Middleton JW, et al. Benefits of FES gait in a spinal cord injured population. Spinal Cord 2007;45(10):646–57.

71. Klose KJ, Jacobs PL, Broton JG, et al. Evaluation of a training program for persons with SCI paraplegia using the Parastep 1 ambulation system: part 1. Ambulation performance and anthropometric measures. Arch Phys Med Rehabil 1997;78(8):789–93.

72. Baardman G, IJzerman MJ, Hermens HJ, et al. The influence of the reciprocal hip joint link in the Advanced Reciprocating Gait Orthosis on standing performance in paraplegia. Prosthet Orthot Int 1997;21(3):210–21.

73. Newham DJ, Donaldson Nde N. FES cycling. Acta Neurochir Suppl 2007;97(Pt 1):395–402.

74. Burnham R, Martin T, Stein R, et al. Skeletal muscle fibre type transformation following spinal cord injury. Spinal Cord 1997;35(2):86–91.

75. Gerrits HL, de Haan A, Sargeant AJ, et al. Altered contractile properties of the quadriceps muscle in people with spinal cord injury following functional electrical stimulated cycle training. Spinal Cord 2000;38(4):214–23.

76. Gerrits HL, de Haan A, Sargeant AJ, et al. Peripheral vascular changes after electrically stimulated cycle training in people with spinal cord injury. Arch Phys Med Rehabil 2001;82(6):832–9.

77. Morita I, Keith MW, Kanno T. Reconstruction of upper limb motor function using functional electrical stimulation (FES). Acta Neurochir Suppl 2007;97(Pt 1):403–7.

78. Keith MW, Peckham PH, Thrope GB, et al. Implantable functional neuromuscular stimulation in the tetraplegic hand. J Hand Surg Am 1989;14(3):524–30.

79. Peckham PH, Keith MW, Kilgore KL, et al. Efficacy of an implanted neuroprosthesis for restoring hand grasp in tetraplegia: a multicenter study. Arch Phys Med Rehabil 2001;82(10):1380–8.

80. Wirz M, Zemon DH, Rupp R, et al. Effectiveness of automated locomotor training in patients with chronic incomplete spinal cord injury: a multicenter trial. Arch Phys Med Rehabil 2005;86:672–80.

81. Edgerton VR, Harkema S. Epidural stimulation of the spinal cord in spinal cord injury: current status and future challenges. Expert Rev Neurother 2011; 11(10):1351–3.

82. Nashold BS Jr, Grimes J, Friedman H, et al. Electrical stimulation of the conus medullaris in the paraplegic. A 5-year review. Appl Neurophysiol 1977; 40(2–4):192–207.

83. Saigal R, Renzi C, Mushahwar VK. Intraspinal microstimulation generates functional movements after spinal-cord injury. IEEE Trans Neural Syst Rehabil Eng 2004;12(4):430–40.

84. Kasten MR, Sunshine MD, Secrist ES, et al. Therapeutic intraspinal microstimulation improves forelimb function after cervical contusion injury. J Neural Eng 2013;10(4):044001.

85. Wessberg J, Stambaugh CR, Kralik JD, et al. Real-time prediction of hand trajectory by ensembles of cortical neurons in primates. Nature 2000; 408(6810):361–5.

86. Chapin JK, Moxon KA, Markowitz RS, et al. Real-time control of a robot arm using simultaneously recorded neurons in the motor cortex. Nat Neurosci 1999;2(7):664–70.

87. Pesaran B, Pezaris JS, Sahani M, et al. Temporal structure in neuronal activity during working memory in macaque parietal cortex. Nat Neurosci 2002;5(8): 805–11.

88. Wolpaw JR, McFarland DJ. Control of a two-dimensional movement signal by a noninvasive brain-computer interface in humans. Proc Natl Acad Sci U S A 2004;101(51):17849–54.

Classification and Management of Pediatric Craniocervical Injuries

Hannah E. Goldstein, MD*, Richard C.E. Anderson, MD

KEYWORDS

• Craniocervical • Craniovertebral • Instability • Trauma • Fracture • Fusion

KEY POINTS

- Nearly two-thirds of pediatric injuries affect the cervical spine, and the majority affect the craniocervical junction and upper cervical spine.
- Algorithms have been developed to better screen children presenting with suspected cervical spine injury to minimize unnecessary computed tomography scans and radiation in this population.
- Most children with spinal column trauma do not require surgical intervention, and can be managed with external immobilization and follow-up imaging.
- When surgical stabilization is indicated, there are techniques available to the operating surgeon.
- It is important to keep in mind that the pediatric spine and its smaller size as well as unique biomechanical properties must be considered in operative planning.

INTRODUCTION

It is well-accepted that the pediatric spine is not just a smaller version of the adult spine; structural and biomechanical differences exist between the two. In general, the pediatric spine is much more mobile at the occipitoatlantoaxial (O–C2) complex, making it more prone to injury. The degree of mobility, as well as the fact that the pediatric spine is still growing, are important to both the understanding and proper management of traumatic pediatric craniocervical injury.

EPIDEMIOLOGY

Pediatric spine injuries overall are much less common than adult spine injuries, with an annual incidence of approximately 20 injuries per million per year.[1] Yet approximately two-thirds of pediatric spine injuries affect the cervical spine,[2,3] with craniovertebral junction (CVJ) and upper cervical injuries being 2 to 3 times as common in children

less than 3 years of age as compared with older children and adults.[3–5] Furthermore, children younger than 9 years of age are much more likely to have purely ligamentous injury without bony fractures, whereas in older children fractures are much more prevalent.[1,3,6] The degree of neurologic compromise is correlated with the presence of subluxation, rather than bony injury, with severe spinal cord injuries seen more frequently in the younger population.[3]

BIOMECHANICS

A key biomechanical difference between the pediatric and adult cervical spine is the amount of mobility at the O–C2 complex. In adults, the degree of flexion and extension at the O–C1 junction is approximately 13°. In infants and young children, however, the amount of flexion and extension at O–C1 is approximately 20°.[7–10] As a result of this and other anatomic factors, the CVJ

Department of Neurosurgery, Morgan Stanley Children's Hospital, Columbia University, 710 W. 168th Street, New York, NY 10032, USA
* Corresponding author. The Neurological Institute, Columbia University Medical Center, 710 West 168th Street, 4th Floor, New York, NY 10032.
E-mail address: heg2117@columbia.edu

Neurosurg Clin N Am 28 (2017) 73–90
http://dx.doi.org/10.1016/j.nec.2016.08.001
1042-3680/17/© 2016 Elsevier Inc. All rights reserved.

is more susceptible to injury in children as compared with adults. For instance, the major stabilizing ligaments and paraspinal muscles are structurally less developed in children, allowing for a greater degree of laxity. Additionally, the dentocentral synchondrosis between the odontoid process and the body of C2 does not fuse until approximately 8 years of age, occasionally allowing for epiphysiolysis of the growth plate.[11,12] Although beyond the scope of this report, several genetic conditions, such as Down syndrome and skeletal dysplasias, have characteristic anatomic changes at the CCJ, which can also affect the ligamentous properties and biomechanics of the pediatric spine.[13]

CLINICAL PRESENTATION

Spinal cord injury should be suspected in any child presenting with either a neurologic deficit or after an appropriate mechanism of injury (eg, motor vehicle accidents, significant falls, child abuse, etc), even in the absence of a clinical deficit. Variable based on the degree of injury, up to 20% of patients may present with a normal neurologic examination, or severe neck pain as their only complaint. More common presentations include new complaints of numbness, weakness, or signs of myelopathy, including hyperreflexia, gait instability, and other pathologic findings. Given that spinal cord injury often occurs in conjunction with widespread orthopedic injuries, it may be difficult to get a reliable neurologic examination. Any child presenting with neck or axial back pain, or decreased consciousness after injury, should be treated as if they have a spinal cord injury until proven otherwise.

PATTERNS OF INJURY
Atlantooccipital Dislocation

Atlantooccipital dislocation is defined as the traumatic separation of the occiput from C1 (**Fig. 1**). It is usually the result of high-energy acceleration–deceleration impacts, such as an auto-pedestrian accident. Twice as common in children compared with adults, it is often a fatal injury, or results in severe neurologic compromise. Usually exclusively a ligamentous injury, atlantooccipital dislocation typically results from a flexion–distraction mechanism, with rotation and lateral bending components also contributing. The abnormal

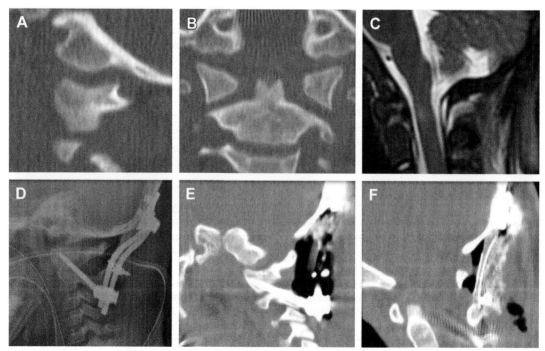

Fig. 1. Atlantooccipital dislocation. A 4-year-old girl was struck by a car while running across the street. Sagittal (*A*) and coronal (*B*) computed tomography (CT) scan and sagittal T2-weighted MRI (*C*) demonstrate traumatic atlantooccipital dislocation with spinal cord injury. The patient was intubated in the field and nonresponsive on presentation. She was taken to the operating room for occipitoatlantoaxial fusion using C1–C2 transarticular screws, an occipital plate/rod construct, and iliac crest autograft with cable. Postoperative lateral radiograph (*D*) and CT scan (*E, F*).

motion causes rupture of the O–C1 joint capsules, with occasional disruption of either or both of the tectorial membrane and alar ligaments.[14–20] In addition to spinal cord injury and compression, there may be associated brainstem injury or hemorrhage and edema in the retropharyngeal and posterior soft tissues of the neck.

Jefferson (C1) Fracture

A Jefferson fracture is defined as a fracture through the posterior ring of C1, generally incurred after an axial compression injury (**Fig. 2**).[21] It is relatively rare in children because the posterior and neurocentral synchondroses of the atlas do not fuse until around 3 and 7 years of age, respectively. Children with these fractures typically present with neck pain, muscle spasm, decreased head mobility, and head tilt. Neurologic deficits are rarely seen.

Translational Atlantoaxial Subluxation

Exceedingly rare, traumatic translational atlantoaxial subluxation is a purely ligamentous injury,

with associated compression of the spinal cord between the odontoid process and the posterior arch of C1.[22–25] More commonly seen is nontraumatic translational atlantoaxial subluxation, which is often associated with developmental disorders causing laxity of the transverse ligament or odontoid hypoplasia, such as Down syndrome, Klippel-Feil syndrome, juvenile rheumatoid arthritis, Morquio syndrome, and the skeletal dysplasias (**Fig. 3**).

Atlantoaxial Rotatory Subluxation/ Atlantoaxial Rotatory Fixation

Although more often seen after inflammatory conditions of the head and neck, approximately 30% of cases of atlantoaxial rotatory subluxation/atlantoaxial rotatory fixation are owing to trauma. Atlantoaxial rotatory subluxation/atlantoaxial rotatory fixation can result in mild rotatory subluxation all the way to complete fixation with no motion. Surprisingly, these injuries can also occur spontaneously. These are thought to be owing to

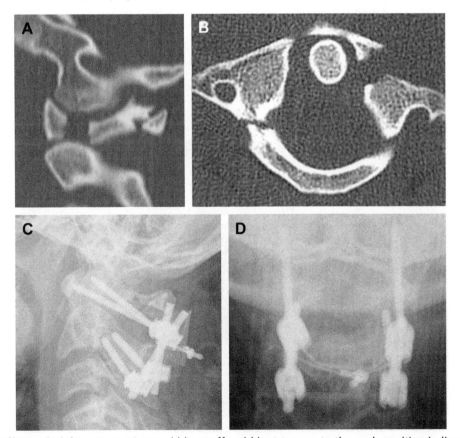

Fig. 2. Jefferson (C1) fracture. A 16-year-old boy suffered blunt trauma to the neck resulting in ligamentous injury and multiple displaced fractures of C1 that can be seen on the preoperative sagittal (*A*) and axial (*B*) computed tomography scans. He underwent posterior C1–C2 instrumentation and fusion using bilateral C1 lateral mass screws and C2 pars screws with structural allograft and cable. Postoperative lateral (*C*) and anteroposterior (*D*) radiographs.

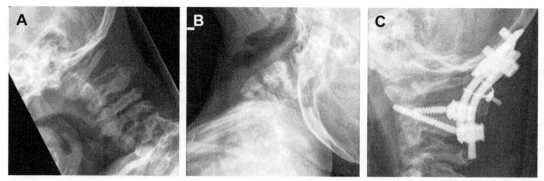

Fig. 3. Translational atlantoaxial subluxation. A 4-year-old girl presented after a fall with persistent neck pain. Flexion (*A*) and extension (*B*) lateral radiographs demonstrated excessive motion at C1–C2 with occipitalization of the atlas. She underwent occipitoatlantoaxial instrumentation and fusion with bilateral C2 pars screws and a structural allograft with cable (*C*).

physiologic hypermobility at the C1–C2 articulation or redundant synovial folds in children, which can become trapped in the C1–C2 joint spaces at the extreme of rotation. This leads to muscle spasm, thereby exacerbating the fixation. Children with atlantoaxial rotatory subluxation and atlantoaxial rotatory fixation usually present neurologically intact with neck pain and torticollis (**Fig. 4**).[25–27]

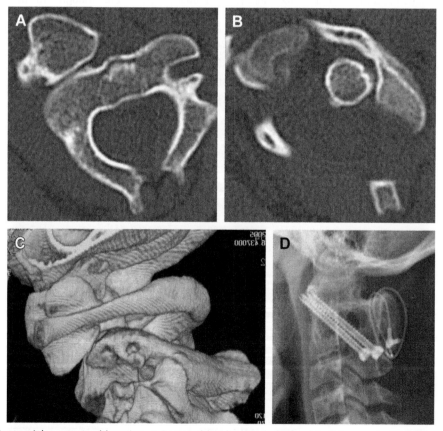

Fig. 4. Atlantoaxial rotatory subluxation. A 9-year-old girl presented after blunt trauma to the neck with C1–C2 rotatory subluxation, as seen on axial computed tomography scans (*A, B*) and 3-dimensional reconstruction (*C*) of the cervical spine. This persisted despite conservative treatment including muscle relaxants with hard collar and Halter traction with a pinless halo brace. The patient finally underwent closed reduction under general anesthesia, followed by C1–C2 posterior arthrodesis and fusion using bilateral transarticular screws with iliac crest autograft and cable. (*D*) Postoperative lateral radiograph.

Odontoid Fractures

Rare in children, translational C1–C2 subluxation may result from epiphysiolysis at the dentrocental synchondrosis. Although some C2 fractures have been associated with fatal concomitant head injury, most children present with only neck pain after minor trauma (**Fig. 5**).[28,29]

Os Odontoideum

Os odontoideum is the separation of the odontoid process from the body of the atlas. Although initially thought to be congenital or the result of a chronic odontoid nonunion, the preponderance of current evidence supports that the majority of these cases are owing to a remote fracture of the dens.[30] Although by definition it is not an acute injury, it is largely considered unstable, with a risk for catastrophic cervical spine injury (**Fig. 6**).[30]

Hangman's (C2 Pars) Fracture

Rare in children, Hangman's fractures, defined as a fracture through the C2 pars on both sides, present much the same way in the pediatric population as they do in adults. Patients complain of posttraumatic neck pain, with notable widening of the spinal canal on lateral plain radiographs (**Fig. 7**).[31,32]

RADIOGRAPHIC FINDINGS

Radiographic imaging of pediatric patients after trauma is an important topic. In an effort to better identify screening criteria for this population, Viccellio and colleagues[33] conducted the NEXUS (National Emergency X-Radiography Utilization Study) trial in 2001. In this study, 5 high-risk criteria for cervical spine injury in children less than

18 years of age were defined: (1) midline cervical tenderness, (2) evidence of intoxication, (3) altered level of alertness, (4) focal neurologic deficit, and (5) painful distracting injury. The presence of any 1 of the 5 criteria placed a patient into the high-risk group, and the absence of all criteria defined a patient as low risk. In 3065 children, 603 (19.7%) were defined as low risk. No low-risk patient suffered a cervical spine injury, whereas 0.98% of the high-risk patients were found to have injuries. The authors concluded that imaging is not necessary in the low-risk group.[33] It is estimated that this study has reduced the need for screening cervical spine radiographs in children by almost 20%.

In 2013, Rozzelle and colleagues[34] published updated guidelines for the management of acute cervical spine and spinal cord injuries. According to these guidelines, cervical spine imaging should not be pursued in trauma patients greater than 3 years old who are alert, have an intact neurologic examination, do not have midline cervical tenderness, do not have distracting injuries or toxins on board, and do not have unexplained hypotension. Similarly, cervical spine imaging is not necessary in children less than 3 years of age that meet these criteria and do not have a high-risk mechanism of injury. Cervical spine radiographs should be obtained in children who do not meet these criteria. Cervical spine computed tomography (CT) imaging is recommended in patients who have questionable radiographs or have suffered a high-energy mechanism and are at high risk for atlantooccipital dislocation.[34]

Brockmeyer and colleagues[35] looked at the prognostic value of various imaging modalities used in pediatric cervical spine clearance after

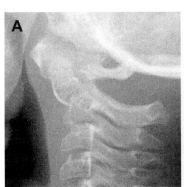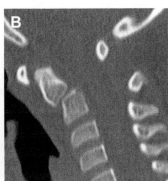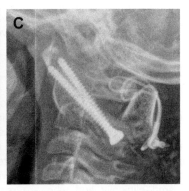

Fig. 5. Odontoid fracture. A 4-year-old girl with myopathy of unknown origin fell off a swing and suffered an angulated displaced C2 synchondrosis fracture, as visualized on lateral radiograph (*A*) and computed topography scan (*B*). After discussing the possibility of a halo, the family decided to proceed with initial surgical fixation. The patient underwent surgery using bilateral C1–C2 transarticular screw fixation with a structural iliac crest autograft and cable. (*C*) Postoperative lateral radiograph.

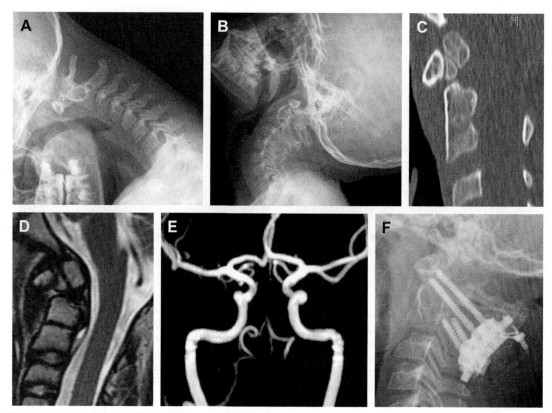

Fig. 6. Os odontoideum. A 9-year-old boy presented with transient ischemic attacks and strokes. Imaging demonstrated 15 mm of subluxation at C1–C2 on cervical spine flexion (*A*) and extension (*B*) radiographs and an os odontodeum on computed tomography scans (*C*) and MRI (*D*). MR angiogram (*E*) showed bilateral atretic vertebral arteries owing to kinking of the arteries from excessive motion. Preoperative stereotactic planning indicated that transarticular screws were not technically feasible, so bilateral C1 lateral mass and C2 pars screws were placed with connecting rods and iliac crest autograft and cable. (*F*) Postoperative lateral radiograph.

severe trauma. Even in this high-risk population, the authors found only a 4% prevalence of instability, with plain radiographs, flexion–extension films, and CT scans all showing very high rates of sensitivity and specificity in screening for instability. MRI was also shown to be very sensitive, although it had a higher false-positive rate.[35]

Imaging Modalities

Plain radiographs
Plain cervical spine radiographs, including lateral and anteroposterior views, are the initial imaging modality in any child with suspected spinal column injury. There is controversy over the usefulness of open-mouth odontoid views in children less than 5 to 9 years of age.[36,37] For children who cannot be cleared clinically and who are responsive and cooperative, cervical flexion–extension radiographs should be obtained, because ligamentous injury may be present even in the absence of bony abnormalities on upright static radiographs.

Computed tomography scans
To limit the amount of ionizing radiation exposure, cervical spine CT scans should be ordered judiciously in pediatric patients. A reasonable indication is the presence of a high-energy mechanism, such as a fall greater than 10 feet or a high-speed motor vehicle accident. When an injury is suspected on plain radiographs, a dose-limited fine-cut CT scan may be obtained through the suspicious and adjacent levels to better define the injury and aid in operative planning.

MRI
Cervical MRIs should be obtained in all children with a neurologic deficit. It should also be obtained before either closed reduction and external immobilization or open operative reduction and fixation to determine the degree of canal compromise. In noncooperative patients without neurologic deficit, fat-suppressed MRIs, preferably obtained within 48 hours of injury, can be used to evaluate for ligamentous injury.

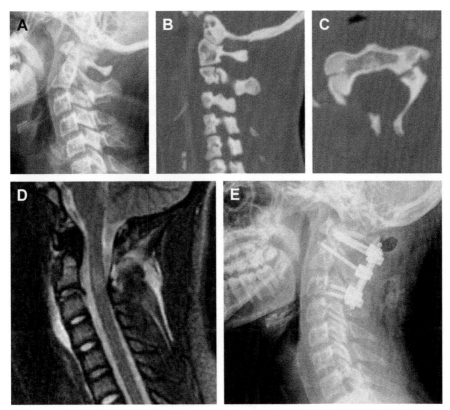

Fig. 7. Hangman's (C2 Pars) fracture. A 14-year-old girl slammed her head into a wall while playing basketball, resulting in immediate weakness and decreased sensation throughout all 4 extremities. Lateral radiograph (*A*), sagittal (*B*) and axial (*C*) computed tomography scans, and sagittal short T1 inversion recovery MRI (*D*) demonstrated a C2 hangman's fracture with spinal cord injury, gross ligamentous instability and unilateral vertebral artery injury. A C2–C3 anterior cervical discectomy and fusion was attempted, but after positioning with gentle extension, there was further separation of the fragments. She therefore underwent C1–C3 posterior instrumentation with bilateral C1 lateral mass screws, a left C2 pedicle screw traversing the fracture, and bilateral C3 lateral mass screws (*E*). Bone graft was placed only at C2–C3, allowing the possibility of subsequent removal of C1 instrumentation at a later stage.

Radiographic Determinants of Instability

Occipital condyle–C1 joint interval

The O–C1 joint interval (CCI), defined as the distance between the occipital condyle and the superior articular facet of C1, should not exceed 5 mm between any opposing points of joint articulation on plain lateral or anteroposterior radiographs.[38] However, this distance is difficult to interpret owing to the superimposition of the mastoids and the unequal overlap of the 2 O–C1 joints. Therefore, it is more commonly measured using thin-cut CT scans, with 4 mm set as the upper limit of normal for the CCI in children. In a study of 89 normal children, Pang and colleagues[39,40] found a mean combined CCI of 1.28 ± 0.26 mm, and no individual measurement of greater than 2.5 mm. In almost all children with proven atlantooccipital dislocation, at least 1 and usually both O–C1 joints are found to be separated.

Other measurements of occipital condyle–C1 instability

There are a number of other radiographic measurements that have been used to determine instability at the O–C1 joint; however, these are often less reliable in children, given the wide degree of variability, and often difficulty making the actual measurements. These include the dens–basion distance,[41,42] the basion–axial interval,[43,44] powers ratio,[25,45] the Lee X line,[46] the C1–C2;C2–C3 interspinous ratio,[47] and the atlandodental interval.[48–50]

Atlantoaxial (C1–C2) instability

Definite biomechanical studies to determine radiographic instability at C1–C2 in children have not been performed. However, owing to the biomechanical differences in young children, expert opinion has generally considered instability to exist if the atlantodens interval is greater than

5 mm in children under 8 years of age or greater than 3 mm in children more than 8 years old as measured on flexion/extension radiographs.[35,51] Owing to inherent ligamentous laxity, asymptomatic children with Down syndrome are often considered stable unless the altantodental interval is greater than 8 to 10 mm.[13,52]

MANAGEMENT AND TREATMENT

After assessing and securing the airway, breathing, and circulation after trauma, attention should be turned to the primary and secondary surveys. During initial resuscitation efforts, it is important to immobilize the child's spine to prevent additional injury. Although standard backboards and cervical collars can be used in older children and adolescents, the disproportionately large head of younger children may result in unintended flexion of the cervical spine if the child is immobilized in the supine position.[53] To avoid this, the torso can be raised with padding, or specialized boards with a recess for the occiput may be used. Furthermore, cervical collars are often too big for the pediatric patient, so temporary taping of both the head and torso to a board may be necessary.

Cervical Spine Clearance

Although there are no overarching national guidelines for the clearance of the pediatric cervical spine after trauma,[54] several published protocols are routinely followed.[35,55,56] These protocols aim to streamline the process of cervical spine clearance,[57] increase diagnostic yield,[33] and allow for nonneurosurgical medical professionals, such as emergency room doctors and trauma surgeons, to clear the cervical spine.[55,56] We have previously published a protocol, based on the NEXUS criteria, for use in communicative children between 3 and 18 years of age (**Fig. 8**).[56]

In children less than 3 years of age, or who are otherwise noncommunicative, the NEXUS criteria often cannot be applied. Clinical cervical spine clearance poses a larger challenge. Therefore, an algorithm designed specifically for clearance of the cervical spine in children less than 3 years old was developed (**Fig. 9**).[55] In a study assessing more than 500 children less than 3 years of age after trauma activations, this protocol allowed more than 80% of children to be cleared using plain radiographs, without the need for further imaging.[55]

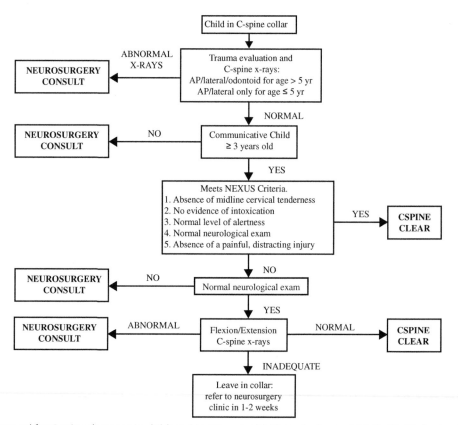

Fig. 8. Protocol for C-spine clearance in children 3 to 18 years old. (*From* Anderson RCE, Scaife ER, Fenton SJ, et al. Cervical spine clearance after trauma in children. J Neurosurg 2006;105(5 Suppl):362; with permission.)

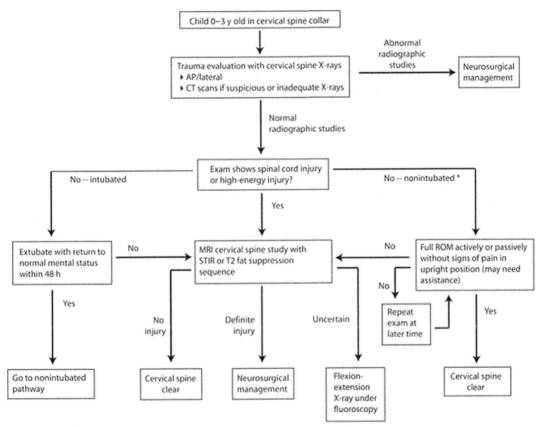

Fig. 9. C-spine clearance protocol for children less than 3 years of age. AP, anteroposterior; ROM, range of motion; STIR, short T1 inversion recovery. (*From* Anderson RCE, Kan P, Vanaman M, et al. Utility of a cervical spine clearance protocol after trauma in children between 0 and 3 years of age. J Neurosurg Pediatr 2010;5(3):294; with permission.)

External Immobilization

Most children with spinal column trauma do not require surgical intervention, and can be managed with external immobilization and follow-up imaging. Generally speaking, C1 (Jefferson) fractures with minimal ligamentous disruption and an intact transverse ligament, atlantoaxial rotatory subluxation/atlantoaxial rotary fixation, acute odontoid fractures with minimal displacement or angulation, and C2 pedicle (hangman) fractures can be managed initially with external immobilization. Contraindications to initial management with external immobilization include progressive neurologic deficits and evidence of gross instability; in these cases, surgical intervention is warranted.

Halo ring and vest

A halo ring with pins and vest is a common external orthosis technique in children with an unstable cervical injury.[58,59] It provides immobilization of the CVJ and upper cervical spine and allows for the application of traction for closed reduction. Generally applied under general anesthesia, the number of halo pins and tightness is based on age.[51] The most common complications seen with halos are pin loosening and pin site infections. Complication rates have been reported as high as 31% to 68% overall, with a direct relationship to the length of halo fixation.[60–62] A pinless halo option also exists, but good quality studies using this brace have not yet been reported.

Minerva brace

The Minerva brace is often used in children who cannot tolerate halo pin fixation. However, without the use of cranial pins, the degree of fixation is inferior to that seen with the halo ring. Furthermore, it does not allow for the possibility of cervical traction.[63] Because the brace involves placement of a rigid piece under the chin, in some children it is not tolerated owing to the inability to open the mouth to eat.

Rigid cervical collar

Although a rigid cervical collar is generally the initial stabilization method used, it provides less stability in the upper cervical levels compared with the halo vest or Minerva brace. It is often a useful adjuvant for postoperative immobilization, and often serves as a reminder for postoperative patients to limit athletic activities in the short term.

Closed Reduction

When closed reduction is used, it should be performed in the operating room, under general anesthesia, and with the use of fluoroscopy and spinal cord monitoring (if available).

SURGICAL FIXATION
Indications

Urgent surgical intervention is indicated in the setting of progressive neurologic deficit or gross instability. In certain instances, such as isolated traumatic herniated disks or apophyseal avulsion fractures, simple decompression may be all that is indicated; however, more often, internal stabilization and fusion are necessary in the setting of trauma. Types of injuries that more frequently require surgical fixation include atlantooccipital dislocation, C1 Jefferson fractures with compromise of the transverse ligament, atlantoaxial subluxation, atlantoaxial rotary subluxation, irreducible odontoid fractures with spinal cord compression, irreducible hangman fractures associated with significant ligamentous injury, or injuries that fail to fuse after a trial of external immobilization.

Preparation and Positioning

Awake fiber-optic intubation is preferred in the setting of cervical cord compression or gross instability; however, some children may not be able to tolerate awake intubation, in which case fiber-optic nasotracheal intubation can be done. Intraoperative neuromonitoring should be used whenever available, with prepositioning somatosensory evoked potentials and motor evoked potentials obtained at the start, after positioning, and throughout the duration of surgery. A cervical collar is often used to help maintain a neutral head position during patient positioning. Once positioned, alignment should be confirmed with lateral fluoroscopy.

Surgical Approach

A number of different surgical techniques can be used at the pediatric CVJ. When planning a construct, it is important to keep in mind the high degree of mobility—primarily flexion–extension at the O–C1 joint and rotation at the C1–C2 joint—in the normal cervical spine, that the construct must withstand before bony fusion.[25] Except for

rare circumstances such as odontoid screw placement, rigid internal fixation and fusion at the occipital cervical junction is typically performed from a posterior approach.

Occipital–cervical techniques
In the setting of atlantooccipital instability, occipitocervical fusion, consisting of constructs from the occiput to C2, is indicated.

Exposure After intubation and neuromonitoring setup, prepositioning somatosensory evoked potentials and motor evoked potentials are obtained. The patient is then flipped to the prone position. Although Gardner-Wells tongs and traction may be used, we prefer a Mayfield headclamp, because this allows more precise control of the head for posterior translation and reduction if needed. The patient is then prepped and draped widely to allow for percutaneous entry of transarticular or C2 pars screws and rib/iliac crest harvesting if desired. A midline incision is made through the skin, subcutaneous fat, and fascial layers. Dissection is carried out along the linea alba to minimize bleeding as well as postoperative muscle pain. Subperiosteal dissection is then carried out laterally to expose the suboccipital region, C1 lamina, and C2 bony elements.

Fixation Rigid instrumentation provides stronger and more immediate stabilization than wiring techniques alone, thereby increasing the likelihood of fusion and decreasing the duration and intensity of required postoperative immobilization. The constructs most commonly used in children are similar to those used in the adult population, consisting of C1–C2 transarticular screws, C1 lateral mass screws, C2 pars screws, C2 translaminar screws, and occasionally C2 pedicle screws. Algorithms have been described to guide the selection of rigid instrumentation at O–C2 in children (**Fig. 10**).[64–68] Given the smaller size of the pediatric spine and often unusual anatomy owing to congenital anomalies, preoperative planning on a stereotactic workstation is essential to determine the technical feasibility of screw placement and to ensure the necessary equipment (eg, screw length and diameter) is available. Typically, the smaller occipital plating systems and smallest diameter (typically 3.5 mm) and length (typically 8–10 mm) screws commercially made for adults are able to be used in the cervical spine in children as young as 1.5 to 2 years of age. Once preoperative planning is completed and the necessary equipment is available, the principles of screw placement are the same as those in the adult population.

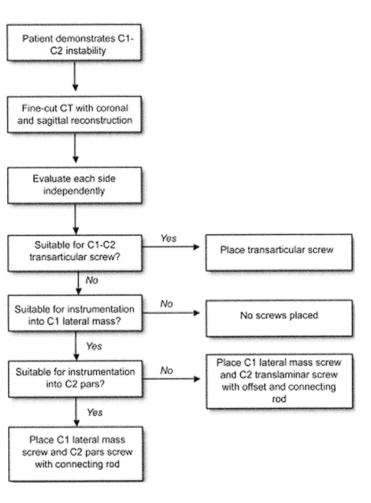

Fig. 10. Algorithm for occipitoatlantoaxial instrumentation in children. CT, computed tomography. (*From* Anderson RC, Ragel BT, Mocco J, et al. Selection of a rigid internal fixation construct for stabilization at the craniovertebral junction in pediatric patients. J Neurosurg 2007;107:36–42; with permission.)

C1–C2 transarticular screw

Initially described by Magerl and popularized by Apfelbaum and Brockmeyer in the pediatric population,[69–71] a C1–C2 transarticular screw starts just above the middle of the C2–C3 joint, passes through the C2 pars, across the C1–C2 joint, and into the C1 lateral mass (**Fig. 11**). C1–C2 transarticular screw stabilization provides excellent rotational and translational stability across the C1–C2 joint,[72] with fusion rates superior to those seen after wire-graft techniques and postoperative halo immobilization.[73–75] Familiarity with the pediatric anatomy at C1–C2, preoperative screw planning, and the use of intraoperative fluoroscopic guidance or frameless stereotaxis are imperative to placing transarticular screws safely, avoiding injury to the vertebral artery, spinal cord, or exiting nerve roots.[64,69,72,73] Even with these surgical adjuncts, vertebral artery anatomy may prevent safe transarticular screw placement unilaterally in 11% to 20% of cases, and bilaterally in 4% to 5% of cases.[69,76,77] Gluf and Brockmeyer[78] report their results in a series of 67 consecutive patients, all 16 years of age or younger, who underwent transarticular screw fixation as part of either atlantoaxial fusion or occipitocervical fusion. In all but 7 patients, bilateral transarticular screws were placed; yet even in the patients where only 1 transarticular screw could be placed safely, successful fusion was eventually achieved.[78] In another pediatric study, Wang and colleagues[79] reported a 100% fusion rate after transarticular C1–C2 screw stabilization without the use of postoperative halo immobilization, and without complications.

C1 lateral mass screw

Commonly used in the adult population, C1 lateral mass screws coupled with C2 fixation and rods provide an alternative to the C1–C2 transarticular screw for atlantoaxial constructs. C1 lateral mass screws are not typically used in occipital–C2 constructs in children because large, multicenter studies have demonstrated equivalent fusion rates with or without additional C1 fixation.[80] First described by Goel and Laheri,[81] the C1 lateral mass screw enables the surgeon to rigidly fixate C1 independent of the occiput. Although the risk of injury to the vertebral artery is probably less than with transarticular screws, vertebral artery injury in the pediatric population with C1 screws has been reported.[82,83] Preoperative planning on a stereotactic workstation is again paramount, given the significant variability that exists in the morphology of C1 not only across patients, but also between the left and right sides of a single child. The key measurement that must be made is the lateral mass width, which must be large enough to accommodate a 3.5-mm screw. A CT morphometric study in children conducted by Chamoun and colleagues[82] showed that, with proper planning, 151 of 152 lateral masses studied could accommodate a C1 lateral mass screw. When instrumenting the C1 lateral mass in children, it is important to keep in mind that there is an offset between the medial aspect of the C1 lamina and the medial surface of the C1 lateral mass not seen in adults. Once the lateral mass is properly exposed, a pilot hole is drilled at the junction of the inferior C1 lamina and the lateral mass, parallel to the plane of the posterior arch in the sagittal direction, in a straight or slightly convergent trajectory in the anterior–posterior direction, and directed toward the anterior arch of C1. A premeasured 3.5-mm screw is placed bicortically, with an 8-mm unthreaded portion remaining above the bony surface of the lateral mass to avoid irritation to the greater occipital nerve.[83,84]

C2 pars screw

Placement of a C2 pars screw is very similar to that of a C1–C2 transarticular screw, with the same starting point and trajectory, only with the use of a shorter screw that does not cross the joint space. Unlike the transarticular screw, a C2 pars screw cannot be used as a stand-alone construct and must be combined, usually with a C1 lateral mass screw and rod fixation for atlantoaxial constructs or with an occipital plate and rod for occipital constructs.

C2 translaminar screw

Originally reported on in the pediatric population by Leonard and Wright,[85] bilateral, crossing C2 translaminar screws offer a less technically challenging means of fixation, with minimal risk of injury to the vertebral artery. The entry point for a C2 translaminar screw is the junction of the C2 spinous process and lamina, near the rostral margin of the lamina on 1 side and the caudal margin of the lamina on the contralateral side to prevent screw collision. The lamina is drilled or

developed with a pediatric gearshift along its length, with the trajectory slightly less than the downslope of the lamina. The slope of the lamina can be palpated with a dental instrument for guidance. This prevents a cortical breach anteriorly into the spinal canal. Either 3.5- or 4-mm diameter screws, premeasured based on the preoperative CT scan and stereotactic planning, are then used, generally ranging in length from 16 to 28 mm in the pediatric population. Singh and Cree[86] reported their experience using C2 translaminar screws in a series of 8 pediatric patients as young as 2 years old, with a zero percent complication rate for neurologic or vascular complications, and no instances of hardware failure or screw pullout.

C2 pedicle screw

Although biomechanical studies in children comparing the stability of varying screw fixation have not been reported, placement of a C2 pedicle screw probably provides the strongest fixation point for a posterior fusion construct. The entry point for a C2 pedicle screw is rostral and lateral to that of a C2 pars screw, with a more medially directed trajectory. Screw lengths are based on premeasurements made from preoperative CT scans, and confirmed intraoperatively.[87] The disadvantages of C2 pedicle screws are that they require intraoperative stereotactic navigation for placement, the lateral entry point of the screw can be challenging to connect to the remaining construct, and in many cases the C2 pedicle is not large enough to accommodate the smallest commercially available screw (3.5 mm diameter). Although in a tomographic study looking at 75 patients all under the age of 10, Cristante and colleagues[88] reported being able to instrument greater than 90% of C2 pedicles based on anatomic measurements, Lee and colleagues[89] found that only 55.4% of patients to have a pedicle width larger than 3.5 mm, large enough to accommodate screw placement.

Occipital screws

One of the greatest challenges with instrumenting up to the occiput in the pediatric population is the relatively thin calvaria. To accommodate this, constructs using occipital plates with screw placement in the midline keel are preferred. In most cases, 6- to 10-mm occipital screws can be placed. Another less commonly used option is condylar screw fixation using stereotactic navigation. In this technique, 20- to 24-mm bicortical screws are placed through the occipital condyle and used as the cranial fixation point for O-C fusion.[90,91]

Although the specific type of instrumentation construct may have small biomechanical differences in adult studies, these differences are likely not clinically significant in the pediatric population secondary to the high overall fusion rate. Using rigid internal fixation, rather than wire constructs, fusion rates of close to 100% in children have been demonstrated, with low associated complications.[68,92–94] Contrary to convention in the adult spinal literature, where the maximum points of fixation may be critical for long term fusion, a multicenter study from the Pediatric Craniocervical Society (PCS) demonstrated equivalent rates of occipital–C2 fusion using rigid instrumentation constructs with C1–C2 transarticular screws, C1 and C2 fixation, or C2 fixation alone as the inferior anchor. This suggests that C1 fixation is not essential for optimal outcomes in children.[95]

Fusion Iliac crest and rib autograft remain the gold standards for fusion in the pediatric population at the CVJ. To maximize the biomechanical stability of the construct, these authors prefer using a structural bone graft that is decorticated and wedged between the inferior edge of the occipital plate and the superior aspect of the C2 lamina and spinous process. A cable can then be used to secure the graft and provide additional stability. Multicenter studies from the PCS have demonstrated 100% fusion rates with rigid fixation using autograft.[95] Interestingly, preliminary studies from Hankinson and colleagues[80] using national insurance databases show lower overall fusion rates, but nearly equivalent fusion rates between autograft and allograft. As in the adult population, autograft or allograft may be supplemented with biologics such as demineralized bone matrix or bone morphogenetic protein (BMP).

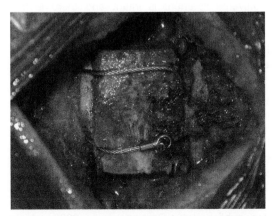

Fig. 11. Intraoperative photograph showing bilateral transarticular screws, and an iliac crest autograph held in by cable wiring.

To increase fusion rates, there has been an enormous increase in the use of BMP in both adult and pediatric populations over the last 15 years. However, after warnings from the US Food and Drug Administration were issued in 2012 regarding its safety, there has been a sharp decline in its usage. Although early reports have shown short-term safety and efficacy of BMP in the posterior cervical spine in the pediatric population, long-term data are not yet available.[96–98] Given the overall very high fusion rates in the pediatric population, BMP is unnecessary in most cases and should only be used in unusually difficult circumstances. After occipitocervical fusion with rigid instrumentation, a rigid cervical collar for 8 to 12 weeks provides sufficient immobilization in the postoperative setting in most cases.

Long-term outcomes Truly long-term outcomes after rigid instrumentation and fusion at the CVJ in children are unknown. However, data from the PCS show continued growth of the pediatric cervical spine with normal curvature and development in most children after occipital–C2 fusion, despite instrumentation even in children younger than 6 years of age.[99] Following children for a mean duration of 56 months postoperatively, Kennedy and colleagues[100] looked at vertical growth over fused levels compared with the total vertical growth of the cervical spine. After occipitocervical fusion in 31 patients, the authors reported 3 different vertical growth patterns: approximately one-half of the patients showed substantial growth across the fusion construct (13%–46% of the total growth of the cervical spine); approximately one-third of the patients had no meaningful growth; and the rest showed a decrease in height of the fused levels. This last group of patients consisted of children presenting with atlantooccipital dislocation. Overall, this study showed that most young children undergoing atlantoaxial or occipitocervical fusion have continued growth across the fused levels despite rigid internal fixation.[100]

Atlantoaxial techniques

Exposure The setup, positioning, and initial exposure are the same as that used for occipital–cervical techniques, as outlined elsewhere in this paper.

Fixation The constructs most commonly used for fixation at C1–C2 are similar to those used as anchors for O–C2 constructs as described previously. Algorithms have similarly been developed to guide the selection of rigid instrumentation at C1–C2 in children (**Fig. 12**).[65–68] As previously mentioned, C1–C2 transarticular screw stabilization provides superior rotational and translational

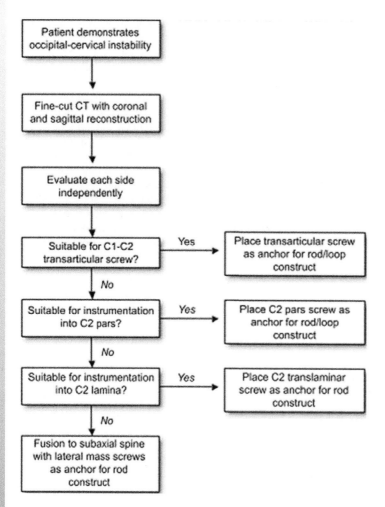

Fig. 12. Algorithm for C1–C2 instrumentation in children. CT, computed tomography. (*From* Anderson RC, Ragel BT, Mocco J, et al. Selection of a rigid internal fixation construct for stabilization at the craniovertebral junction in pediatric patients. J Neurosurg 2007;107:36–42; with permission.)

stability across the C1–C2 joint,[72] with fusion rates superior to those seen after wire-graft techniques and postoperative halo immobilization.[73–75] Another excellent option that many authors prefer over transarticular screw placement is the Goel-Harms construct, which is less technically challenging. Harms and Melcher[84] popularized the Goel-Harms construct, which uses posterior atlantoaxial fixation with bilateral C1 lateral mass and C2 pars screws linked by metallic rods. Alternatively, translaminar screws may be used in place of pars screws.[84,101] Again, preoperative screw planning on a stereotactic workstation is imperative to determine technical feasibility and allow safe screw placement in the pediatric population.

Odontoid screw

Rarely used in children owing to the late ossification of the dental synchondrosis, odontoid screws are lag screws placed from an anterior approach starting at the base of C2 just above the C2–C3 disc space, across the fracture and into the apex of the odontoid process. One or 2 screws may be used. Odontoid screws may be the screw of choice for type II odontoid fractures in which the transverse ligament is intact and there is not excessive angulation or distraction of the fracture. The main advantage of odontoid screws is that they allow for maintenance of physiologic motion at the C1–C2 joint.[51]

Wiring constructs

In rare cases, rigid instrumentation is not feasible and wiring constructs are the only option. Several techniques are available for C1–C2 wiring. Over the years, various modifications have been made to traditional wiring techniques, including the Gallie fusion,[102] the Brooks fusion,[103–105] the Dickman-Sonntag fusion, and a further modification published by Brockmeyer in 2002, which adds a multistranded cable atlantoaxial fusion as augmentation to C1–C2 transarticular screw fixation.[106] A structural bone graft is then incorporated into the wiring construct in such a way that it can sustain the rotational, translational, and flexion/extension forces exerted on the joint.

Fusion Similar to O–C2 fusion, rib and iliac crest autograft remain the gold standard in the pediatric population. However, a recent PCS study demonstrated similar fusion rates in children undergoing C1–C2 rigid instrumentation using either autograft or allograft.[95] Similar to O–C2 constructs, a structural bone graft between the posterior elements of C1 and C2 is preferred, which then can be incorporated via a wiring construct described previously.

Long-term outcomes Similar to outcomes after O–C2 fixation and fusion, recent studies show continued growth of the pediatric cervical spine after rigid instrumentation and atlantoaxial fixation.[99,100] Kennedy and colleagues[100] report a mean vertical growth of 30% of the growth of the total cervical spine after atlantoaxial fusion in 9 patients followed for an average duration of 56 months. Of these patients, 89% showed good alignment at follow-up, with straight or mildly lordotic cervical curvatures.[100]

SUMMARY

Significant differences exist between the pediatric and adult craniocervical junction, leading to greater mobility and susceptibility to injury. Any child who presents after a high-impact injury or with cervical spine pain should be considered at risk of spinal cord injury. Various radiographic screening protocols have been developed to determine who should undergo radiograph, CT, and/or MRI. These algorithms have enabled emergency medicine physicians and trauma surgeons to safely clear the cervical spine in many children after injury.

Radiographic criteria exist to determine whether posttraumatic CCJ instability is present in the pediatric patient. For those who require surgical stabilization, a number of techniques are available, including rigid internal fixation and wiring techniques with bone grafts for fusion. Overall, surgical success rates are high and long-term growth potential is maintained in the vast majority of pediatric patients.

REFERENCES

1. Hamilton MG, Myles ST. Pediatric spinal injury: review of 174 hospital admissions. J Neurosurg 1992;77:700–4.

2. Denis F. The three column spine and its significance in the classification of acute thoracolumbar spinal injuries. Spine (Phila Pa 1976) 1983;8:817–31.

3. Hadley MN, Zabramski JM, Browner CM, et al. Pediatric spinal trauma. Review of 122 cases of spinal cord and vertebral column injuries. J Neurosurg 1988;68:18–24.

4. Osenbach RK, Menezes AH. Spinal cord injury without radiographic abnormality in children. Pediatr Neurosci 1989;15:168–74 [discussion: 75].

5. Rockswold GL, Seljeskog EL. Traumatic atlantocranial dislocation with survival. Minn Med 1979;62:151–2, 154.

6. Fesmire FM, Luten RC. The pediatric cervical spine: developmental anatomy and clinical aspects. J Emerg Med 1989;7:133–42.

7. White AA, Panjabi MM. Clinical biomechanics of the spine. Philadelphia: J.B. Lippincott; 1990.

8. Baker DH, Berdon WE. Special trauma problems in children. Radiol Clin North Am 1966;4:289–305.

9. Braakman R, Penning L. The hyperflexion sprain of the cervical spine. Radiol Clin Biol 1968;37:309–20.

10. Townsend EH Jr, Rowe ML. Mobility of the upper cervical spine in health and disease. Pediatrics 1952;10:567–74.

11. Lebwohl NH, Eismont FJ. Cervical spine injuries in children. New York: Raven Press; 1994.

12. Hickman ZL, McDowell M, Anderson RCE. Principles of pediatric spinal column trauma. In: Albright AL, Pollack I, Adelson RD, editors. Principles and Practice of Pediatric Neurosurgery. New York: Thieme. p. 6040–799.

13. Hankinson TC, Anderson RC. Craniovertebral junction abnormalities in Down syndrome. Neurosurgery 2010;66:32–8.

14. Adams VI. Neck injuries: I. Occipitoatlantal dislocation–a pathologic study of twelve traffic fatalities. J Forensic Sci 1992;37:556–64.

15. Bohlman HH. Acute fractures and dislocations of the cervical spine. An analysis of three hundred hospitalized patients and review of the literature. J Bone Joint Surg Am 1979;61:1119–42.

16. Bucholz RW, Burkhead WZ. The pathological anatomy of fatal atlanto-occipital dislocations. J Bone Joint Surg Am 1979;61:248–50.

17. Davis D, Bohlman H, Walker AE, et al. The pathological findings in fatal craniospinal injuries. J Neurosurg 1971;34:603–13.

18. Dublin AB, Marks WM, Weinstock D, et al. Traumatic dislocation of the atlanto-occipital articulation (AOA) with short-term survival. With a radiographic method of measuring the AOA. J Neurosurg 1980;52:541–6.

19. Grobovschek M, Scheibelbrandner W. Atlanto-occipital dislocation. Neuroradiology 1983;25:173–4.

20. Powers B, Miller MD, Kramer RS, et al. Traumatic anterior atlanto-occipital dislocation. Neurosurgery 1979;4:12–7.

21. Judd DB, Liem LK, Petermann G. Pediatric atlas fracture: a case of fracture through a synchondrosis and review of the literature. Neurosurgery 2000;46: 991–4 [discussion: 994–5].

22. Adams VI. Neck injuries: II. Atlantoaxial dislocation–a pathologic study of 14 traffic fatalities. J Forensic Sci 1992;37:565–73.

23. Bohn D, Armstrong D, Becker L, et al. Cervical spine injuries in children. J Trauma 1990;30: 463–9.

24. McGrory BJ, Klassen RA, Chao EY, et al. Acute fractures and dislocations of the cervical spine in children and adolescents. J Bone Joint Surg Am 1993;75:988–95.

25. Pang D, Sun PP. Pediatric vertebral column and spinal cord injuries. In: Winn HR, editor. Youmans neurological surgery. Philadelphia: W.B. Saunders; 2004. p. 3515–57.

26. Birney TJ, Hanley EN Jr. Traumatic cervical spine injuries in childhood and adolescence. Spine (Phila Pa 1976) 1989;14:1277–82.

27. Fielding JW, Hawkins RJ, Hensinger RN, et al. Atlantoaxial rotary deformities. Orthop Clin North Am 1978;9:955–67.

28. Eleraky MA, Theodore N, Adams M, et al. Pediatric cervical spine injuries: report of 102 cases and review of the literature. J Neurosurg 2000;92:12–7.

29. Ware ML, Auguste KI, Gupta N, et al. Traumatic injuries of the pediatric craniocervical junction. In: Brockmeyer D, editor. Advanced pediatric craniocervical surgery. New York: Thieme Medical Publishers; 2006. p. 55–74.

30. Klimo P Jr, Kan P, Rao G, et al. Os odontoideum: presentation, diagnosis, and treatment in a series of 78 patients. J Neurosurg Spine 2008;9: 332–42.

31. Pizzutillo PD, Rocha EF, D'Astous J, et al. Bilateral fracture of the pedicle of the second cervical vertebra in the young child. J Bone Joint Surg Am 1986;68:892–6.

32. Weiss MH, Kaufman B. Hangman's fracture in an infant. Am J Dis Child 1973;126:268–9.

33. Viccellio P, Simon H, Pressman BD, et al. A prospective multicenter study of cervical spine injury in children. Pediatrics 2001;108:E20.

34. Rozzelle CJ, Aarabi B, Dhall SS, et al. Management of pediatric cervical spine and spinal cord injuries. Neurosurgery 2013;72(Suppl 2):205–26.

35. Brockmeyer DL, Ragel BT, Kestle JR. The pediatric cervical spine instability study. A pilot study assessing the prognostic value of four imaging modalities in clearing the cervical spine for children with severe traumatic injuries. Childs Nerv Syst 2012;28:699–705.

36. Buhs C, Cullen M, Klein M, et al. The pediatric trauma C-spine: is the 'odontoid' view necessary? J Pediatr Surg 2000;35:994–7.

37. Swischuk LE, John SD, Hendrick EP. Is the open-mouth odontoid view necessary in children under 5 years? Pediatr Radiol 2000;30:186–9.

38. Kaufman RA, Carroll CD, Buncher CR. Atlantooccipital junction: standards for measurement in normal children. AJNR Am J Neuroradiol 1987;8:995–9.

39. Pang D, Nemzek WR, Zovickian J. Atlanto-occipital dislocation–part 2: The clinical use of (occipital) condyle-C1 interval, comparison with other diagnostic methods, and the manifestation, management, and outcome of atlanto-occipital dislocation in children. Neurosurgery 2007;61:995–1015 [discussion: 1015].

40. Pang D, Nemzek WR, Zovickian J. Atlanto-occipital dislocation: part 1–normal occipital condyle-C1 interval in 89 children. Neurosurgery 2007;61:514–21 [discussion: 521].

41. Bulas DI, Fitz CR, Johnson DL. Traumatic atlanto-occipital dislocation in children. Radiology 1993; 188:155–8.

42. Wholey MH, Bruwer AJ, Baker HL Jr. The lateral roentgenogram of the neck; with comments on the atlanto-odontoid-basion relationship. Radiology 1958;71:350–6.

43. Harris JH Jr, Carson GC, Wagner LK. Radiologic diagnosis of traumatic occipitovertebral dissociation: 1. Normal occipitovertebral relationships on lateral radiographs of supine subjects. AJR Am J Roentgenol 1994;162:881–6.

44. Traynelis VC, Marano GD, Dunker RO, et al. Traumatic atlanto-occipital dislocation. Case report. J Neurosurg 1986;65:863–70.

45. Ware ML, Gupta N, Sun PP, et al. Clinical biomechanics of the pediatric craniocervical junction and subaxial spine. In: Brockmeyer DL, editor. Advanced pediatric craniocervical surgery. New York: Thieme Medical Publishers; 2006. p. 27–42.

46. Lee C, Woodring JH, Goldstein SJ, et al. Evaluation of traumatic atlantooccipital dislocations. AJNR Am J Neuroradiol 1987;8:19–26.

47. Sun PP, Poffenbarger GJ, Durham S, et al. Spectrum of occipitoatlantoaxial injury in young children. J Neurosurg 2000;93:28–39.

48. Copley LA, Dormans JP. Cervical spine disorders in infants and children. J Am Acad Orthop Surg 1998;6:204–14.

49. Fielding JW. Cineroentgenography of the normal cervical spine. J Bone Joint Surg Am 1957;39-A: 1280–8.

50. Spence KF Jr, Decker S, Sell KW. Bursting atlantal fracture associated with rupture of the transverse ligament. J Bone Joint Surg Am 1970;52:543–9.

51. Hickman Z, McDowell M, Anderson RCE. Principles of pediatric spinal column trauma. In: Albright AL, Pollack I, Adelson RD, editors. Principles and practice of pediatric neurosurgery. 3rd edition. New York: Thieme; 2014. p. 789–805.

52. Brockmeyer D. Down syndrome and craniovertebral instability. Topic review and treatment recommendations. Pediatr Neurosurg 1999;31:71–7.

53. Nypaver M, Treloar D. Neutral cervical spine positioning in children. Ann Emerg Med 1994;23:208–11.

54. Hadely MN. Management of pediatric cervical spine and spinal cord injuries. Neurosurgery 2002;50(Suppl):S85–99.

55. Anderson RC, Kan P, Vanaman M, et al. Utility of a cervical spine clearance protocol after trauma in children between 0 and 3 years of age. J Neurosurg Pediatr 2010;5:292–6.

56. Anderson RC, Scaife ER, Fenton SJ, et al. Cervical spine clearance after trauma in children. J Neurosurg 2006;105:361–4.

57. Frank JB, Lim CK, Flynn JM, et al. The efficacy of magnetic resonance imaging in pediatric cervical spine clearance. Spine (Phila Pa 1976) 2002;27:1176–9.

58. Chan RC, Schweigel JF, Thompson GB. Halo-thoracic brace immobilization in 188 patients with acute cervical spine injuries. J Neurosurg 1983;58:508–15.

59. Johnson RM, Owen JR, Hart DL, et al. Cervical orthoses: a guide to their selection and use. Clin Orthop Relat Res 1981;(154):34–45.

60. Baum JA, Hanley EN Jr, Pullekines J. Comparison of halo complications in adults and children. Spine (Phila Pa 1976) 1989;14:251–2.

61. Dormans JP, Criscitiello AA, Drummond DS, et al. Complications in children managed with immobilization in a halo vest. J Bone Joint Surg Am 1995;77:1370–3.

62. Garfin SR, Botte MJ, Waters RL, et al. Complications in the use of the halo fixation device. J Bone Joint Surg Am 1986;68:320–5.

63. Gaskill SJ, Marlin AE. Custom fitted thermoplastic Minerva jackets in the treatment of cervical spine instability in preschool age children. Pediatr Neurosurg 1990;16:35–9.

64. Anderson RC, Ragel BT, Mocco J, et al. Selection of a rigid internal fixation construct for stabilization at the craniovertebral junction in pediatric patients. J Neurosurg 2007;107:36–42.

65. Hedequist D. Modern instrumentation of the pediatric occiput and upper cervical spine: review article. HSS J 2015;11:9–14.

66. Hedequist DJ. Modern posterior screw techniques in the pediatric cervical spine. World J Orthop 2014;5:94–9.

67. Menezes AH. Craniocervical fusions in children. J Neurosurg Pediatr 2012;9:573–85.

68. Schultz KD Jr, Petronio J, Haid RW, et al. Pediatric occipitocervical arthrodesis. A review of current options and early evaluation of rigid internal fixation techniques. Pediatr Neurosurg 2000;33:169–81.

69. Brockmeyer DL, York JE, Apfelbaum RI. Anatomical suitability of C1-2 transarticular screw placement in pediatric patients. J Neurosurg 2000;92:7–11.

70. Suchomel P, Stulik J, Klezl Z, et al. Transarticular fixation of C1-C2: a multicenter retrospective study. Acta Chir Orthop Traumatol Cech 2004;71:6–12 [in Czech].

71. Brockmeyer DL, Apfelbaum RI. A new occipitocervical fusion construct in pediatric patients with occipitocervical instability. Technical note. J Neurosurg 1999;90:271–5.

72. Grob D, Magerl F. Surgical stabilization of C1 and C2 fractures. Orthopade 1987;16:46–54 [in German].

73. Dickman CA, Sonntag VK, Papadopoulos SM, et al. The interspinous method of posterior atlantoaxial arthrodesis. J Neurosurg 1991;74:190–8.

74. Grob D, Jeanneret B, Aebi M, et al. Atlanto-axial fusion with transarticular screw fixation. J Bone Joint Surg Br 1991;73:972–6.

75. Levy ML, McComb JG. C1-C2 fusion in children with atlantoaxial instability and spinal cord compression: technical note. Neurosurgery 1996;38:211–5 [discussion: 215–6].

76. Madawi AA, Casey AT, Solanki GA, et al. Radiological and anatomical evaluation of the atlantoaxial transarticular screw fixation technique. J Neurosurg 1997;86:961–8.

77. Paramore CG, Dickman CA, Sonntag VK. The anatomical suitability of the C1-2 complex for transarticular screw fixation. J Neurosurg 1996;85:221–4.

78. Gluf WM, Brockmeyer DL. Atlantoaxial transarticular screw fixation: a review of surgical indications, fusion rate, complications, and lessons learned in 67 pediatric patients. J Neurosurg Spine 2005;2:164–9.

79. Wang J, Vokshoor A, Kim S, et al. Pediatric atlantoaxial instability: management with screw fixation. Pediatr Neurosurg 1999;30:70–8.

80. Hankinson TC, Anderson RCE, Brockmeyer DL, et al. Comparison of fusion rates following occipitocervical and atlantoaxial instrumented arthrodesis using administrative datasets. Washington, DC: American Society of Pediatric Neurosurgeons; 2013.

81. Goel A, Laheri V. Plate and screw fixation for atlanto-axial subluxation. Acta Neurochir 1994;129:47–53.

82. Chamoun RB, Whitehead WE, Curry DJ, et al. Computed tomography morphometric analysis for C-1 lateral mass screw placement in children. Clinical article. J Neurosurg Pediatr 2009;3:20–3.

83. Jea A, Taylor MD, Dirks PB, et al. Incorporation of C-1 lateral mass screws in occipitocervical and atlantoaxial fusions for children 8 years of age or

younger. Technical note. J Neurosurg 2007;107: 178–83.

84. Harms J, Melcher RP. Posterior C1-C2 fusion with polyaxial screw and rod fixation. Spine (Phila Pa 1976) 2001;26:2467–71.

85. Leonard JR, Wright NM. Pediatric atlantoaxial fixation with bilateral, crossing C-2 translaminar screws. Technical note. J Neurosurg 2006;104: 59–63.

86. Singh B, Cree A. Laminar screw fixation of the axis in the pediatric population: a series of eight patients. Spine J 2015;15:e17–25.

87. Sattarov K, Skoch J, Abbasifard S, et al. Posterior atlantoaxial fixation: a cadaveric and fluoroscopic step-by-step technical guide. Surg Neurol Int 2015;6:S244–7.

88. Cristante AF, Torelli AG, Kohlmann RB, et al. Feasibility of intralaminar, lateral mass, or pedicle axis vertebra screws in children under 10 years of age: a tomographic study. Neurosurgery 2012;70: 835–8 [discussion: 838–9].

89. Lee H, Hong JT, Kim IS, et al. Anatomic feasibility of posterior cervical pedicle screw placement in children: computerized tomographic analysis of children under 10 years old. J Korean Neurosurg Soc 2014;56:475–81.

90. Uribe JS, Ramos E, Baaj A, et al. Occipital cervical stabilization using occipital condyles for cranial fixation: technical case report. Neurosurgery 2009; 65:E1216–7 [discussion: E1217].

91. Uribe JS, Ramos E, Vale F. Feasibility of occipital condyle screw placement for occipitocervical fixation: a cadaveric study and description of a novel technique. J Spinal Disord Tech 2008;21:540–6.

92. Brockmeyer D, Apfelbaum R, Tippets R, et al. Pediatric cervical spine instrumentation using screw fixation. Pediatr Neurosurg 1995;22:147–57.

93. Dickerman RD, Morgan JT, Mittler M. Circumferential cervical spine surgery in an 18-month-old female with traumatic disruption of the odontoid and C3 vertebrae. Case report and review of techniques. Case report and review of techniques. Pediatr Neurosurg 2005;41:88–92.

94. Fargen KM, Anderson RC, Harter DH, et al. Occipitocervicothoracic stabilization in pediatric patients. J Neurosurg Pediatr 2011;8:57–62.

95. Hankinson TC, Avellino AM, Harter D, et al. Equivalence of fusion rates after rigid internal fixation of the occiput to C-2 with or without C-1 instrumentation. J Neurosurg Pediatr 2010;5: 380–4.

96. Jain A, Kebaish KM, Sponseller PD. Factors associated with use of bone morphogenetic protein during pediatric spinal fusion surgery: an analysis of 4817 patients. J Bone Joint Surg Am 2013;95: 1265–70.

97. Mazur MD, Sivakumar W, Riva-Cambrin J, et al. Avoiding early complications and reoperation during occipitocervical fusion in pediatric patients. J Neurosurg Pediatr 2014;14:465–75.

98. Hood B, Hamilton DK, Smith JS, et al. The use of allograft and recombinant human bone morphogenetic protein for instrumented atlantoaxial fusions. World Neurosurg 2014;82(6):1369–73.

99. Anderson RC, Kan P, Gluf WM, et al. Long-term maintenance of cervical alignment after occipitocervical and atlantoaxial screw fixation in young children. J Neurosurg 2006;105:55–61.

100. Kennedy BC, D'Amico RS, Youngerman BE, et al. Long-term growth and alignment after occipitocervical and atlantoaxial fusion with rigid internal fixation in young children. J Neurosurg Pediatr 2016; 17:94–102.

101. Goel A, Desai KI, Muzumdar DP. Atlantoaxial fixation using plate and screw method: a report of 160 treated patients. Neurosurgery 2002;51: 1351–6 [discussion: 1356–7].

102. Gallie WE. Fractures and dislocations of the cervical spine. Am J Surg 1939;46:495–9.

103. Brooks AL, Jenkins EB. Atlanto-axial arthrodesis by the wedge compression method. J Bone Joint Surg Am 1978;60:279–84.

104. Griswold DM, Albright JA, Schiffman E, et al. Atlanto-axial fusion for instability. J Bone Joint Surg Am 1978;60:285–92.

105. White AA 3rd, Panjabi MM. The basic kinematics of the human spine. A review of past and current knowledge. Spine (Phila Pa 1976) 1978;3: 12–20.

106. Brockmeyer DL. A bone and cable girth-hitch technique for atlantoaxial fusion in pediatric patients. Technical note. J Neurosurg 2002;97:400–2.

Classification and Management of Pediatric Subaxial Cervical Spine Injuries

Casey J. Madura, MD, MPH, James M. Johnston Jr, MD*

KEYWORDS

- Pediatric - Subaxial cervical spine - Injury - Management - Surgery

KEY POINTS

- Management of subaxial cervical spine injury in children requires a thorough understanding of differences in anatomy, biomechanics, injury patterns, and treatment options compared with adults.
- Although a majority of cervical spine injuries can be managed nonoperatively, unstable injuries may require prompt reduction, instrumentation, and fusion, especially in cases of neurologic compromise.
- Surgical instrumentation options for pediatric cervical spine fusion have significantly increased over the past decade but must be tailored to individual children according to their age, size, and injury pattern.
- Future outcomes studies for children with subaxial cervical spine injury must use consistent, objective injury classification schema and standardized outcome measures to make meaningful recommendations about optimal treatment options for this challenging and diverse population.

INTRODUCTION

Diagnosis and management of subaxial cervical spine injuries in pediatric patients have received less attention in the published literature compared with injuries in adults. Differences in anatomy, biomechanics, fracture patterns, and management options must be taken into account and treatment must be individualized to each patient.

ANATOMY AND BIOMECHANICS

The subaxial cervical spine includes vertebral levels C3 through C7. The first 2 levels represent a typical cervical vertebral level. C7 retains the general structure of the other cervical levels but the absolute size of this level more resembles the thoracic spine. A typical cervical vertebra includes a small body connected by short pedicles to the lamina. Spinous processes are diminutive and often bifid. The spinous process of C7 is typically large and uncommonly bifid. Transverse processes of C3-6 are small and are made smaller by the presence of the foramen transversarium. The transverse process of C7 is, conversely, larger with a smaller foramen transversarium that may also be absent.[1]

Three anatomic differences between the pediatric and adult cervical spine are critical when considering a patient with a possible cervical spine injury. First, the articular processes in the cervical spine of pediatric patients retain a more axial orientation, reducing resistance to translation. Second, the vertebral bodies are more wedged anteriorly. Both allow for an increased amount of normal anatomic movement of the vertebral bodies of the subaxial cervical spine in children, especially those under 8 years old.[2] In general, at C2-3 and C3-4, up to 4.5 mm of translation of the superior vertebral body relative to the inferior

Disclosure Statement: The authors have nothing to disclose.
Division of Pediatric Neurosurgery, Department of Neurosurgery, Children's of Alabama, University of Alabama at Birmingham, 1600 7th Avenue South, Lowder Suite 400, Birmingham, Alabama 35233, USA
* Corresponding author.
E-mail address: jimj@uab.edu

Neurosurg Clin N Am 28 (2017) 91–102
http://dx.doi.org/10.1016/j.nec.2016.07.004
1042-3680/17/© 2016 Elsevier Inc. All rights reserved.

vertebral body in the sagittal plane may be considered normal, termed *pseudosubluxation*. Third, the size of the head of a child relative to the remainder of the body is proportionately larger, increasing the load borne by the cervical spine when undergoing rapids movements, such as whiplash. The fulcrum of movement in flexion injuries shifts progressively lower with increased age: C2-3 for infants and young children, C3-4 for children aged 5 to 6, and C5-6 for adolescents, similar to mature adults.[3–5]

The pediatric cervical spine is significantly more elastic than the adult spine, leading to different injury patterns. The anterior longitudinal ligament (ALL) and posterior longitudinal ligament (PLL) traverse the entirety of the spine from the sacrum up and run along the anterior and posterior faces of the vertebral bodies. The ALL attaches to the anterior tubercle of C1 (also known as the atlas) superiorly. The PLL fuses with the tectorial membrane. These 2 ligaments provide the most significant stability to the subaxial cervical spine. Other ligamentous structures with a more minor contribution include capsular ligaments surrounding the facet joints and the interspinous ligaments between spinous processes. It is important to recognize that in children, these structures are inherently more lax, allowing for greater movement of the spine than in adults.[2]

The uncovertebral joint is a joint unique to the cervical spine. Its relationship to both neural and vascular structures makes it an important anatomic landmark.[6] The uncinate process, a bony ridge projecting superiorly from the posterior and lateral aspect of each cervical vertebral body, may be absent in young children. It articulates with the inferior aspect of the vertebral body above and is encapsulated by ligamentous tissue that extends from the PLL. This ligamentous tissue also encases the nerve roots, which lie posterior to the uncovertebral joints, and the vertebral artery, which lies laterally. It is not until the age of 8 years that the joints develop to their full extent.[7] As a consequence, the normal resistance to rotation provided by this joint in the adult cervical spine is minimal in children under the age of 8 years.

Finally, the foramen transversarium represents a unique bony structure within the cervical spine. It provides protection for the vertebral artery as it traverses the neck while also leaving it vulnerable to injury in cases of cervical spine trauma. As discussed previously, it is typically smaller in C7 than the remainder of the cervical spine. Although the vertebral artery most commonly enters at C6, it has been found to enter at C5 (5%), C4 (1%), C7 (0.8%), and C3 (0.2%).[1]

EPIDEMIOLOGY AND INJURY PATTERNS

Since 2005, nationwide prevalence of traumatic pediatric cervical spine injury was 2.07%, with a mortality rate of 4.87%.[8] Motor vehicle accidents are the most common cause of pediatric cervical spine injuries (57.51%), followed by falls, sports, diving accidents, firearms, and child abuse.[2,9] Upper cervical spine injury (C1-4), cervical fracture with spinal cord injury, spinal cord injury without radiographic abnormality (SCIWORA), and dislocation vary inversely with age.[8] Obstetric complications are the primary cause of cervical spine injury in newborns, can be difficult to diagnose, and should be suspected in infants with apnea and flaccid quadriplegia after traumatic delivery. The characteristics of the cervical spine in a pediatric patient change significantly with age, with mature development not present until 8 years of age. The immaturity of the young pediatric cervical spine, including weaker ligaments and neck muscles, a relatively large head, horizontally oriented facets, and incomplete ossification expose children under the age of approximately 8 years old to an increased risk of cervical spine injury. Pure ligamentous injuries and SCIWORA are more common in children under the age of 9 whereas isolated bony injury and fracture subluxation injuries are more common in the more developed spine of older children.[2,4,10]

Relative to other parts of the spine and spinal cord, the cervical spine and spinal cord are the most susceptible to traumatic injury in children. Three-quarters of SCIWORA and fracture subluxations with all purely ligamentous injuries in children occurred in the cervical spine.[11]

CLINICAL AND RADIOGRAPHIC EVALUATION

The evaluation of children who have suffered traumatic injury, especially after blunt trauma and high-energy mechanisms, like motor vehicle accidents, can be challenging. Presenting symptoms in awake patients may include neck pain, rigidity, torticollis, numbness, radicular pain, or weakness. Unconscious patients are more difficult to evaluate and should be maintained in cervical orthosis until definitive imaging and/or examination rules out injury. Younger patients with larger heads relative to their body should have appropriate torso elevation (mean 25 mm) to preserve neutral position and avoid unintentional flexion and exacerbation of kyphotic deformity while being transported by backboard.[12]

Given the differences in shape, biomechanics, and flexibility of the pediatric cervical spine (described previously), diagnosis of cervical spine injury can be challenging. Children who have suffered significant trauma who do not meet National Emergency X-Radiography Utilization Study (NEXUS) standard criteria[13] should undergo at least anterior/posterior and lateral cervical spine radiography. In cases of ground level falls, CT imaging is generally overused, with less than 1% detection of cervical spine fractures, all identified by NEXUS and Canadian Cervical Spine Rule for radiography criteria with 100% sensitivity.[14] Adoption of standardized protocols based on NEXUS criteria has been shown to significantly reduce costs and unnecessary radiation exposure in children evaluated for cervical injury.[15–17] Studies in adults have demonstrated the significantly higher sensitivity of CT imaging for the detection of cervical spine injuries compared with plain films, especially in intubated and head-injured patients.[18] In the pediatric population, CT imaging has been recommended in cases of inadequate visualization, suspicious findings, or evidence of fracture/displacement on plain films and in obtunded children with a high-energy mechanism and blunt trauma.[15]

MRI is superior to CT in delineation of soft tissue injury and is useful in cases of neurologic deficit to evaluate for disk herniation, spinal cord contusion, nerve root compression, and epidural/subdural hematoma.[19] Despite improved soft tissue visualization, several recent studies have called into question the utility of MRI over modern-era fine-cut CT for the diagnosis of clinically relevant ligamentous instability and spinal instability in patients with head injury,[20–23] although this remains controversial.[2] Recent evaluation of the diagnostic performance of the Subaxial Cervical Spine Injury Classification (SLIC) showed improved interobserver agreement when using CT alone and limited added value for MRI in determining conservative versus surgical management.[24] Flexion extension films in awake, cooperative patients have traditionally been used for diagnosis of delayed, dynamic instability, although several studies have questioned their utility for detecting instability in the absence of abnormalities on fine-cut CT imaging.[25,26]

Multiple classification systems have been proposed to serve as a guide to rational treatment decision making in adults,[27–30] although none has been widely accepted by the world community and none has been objectively validated in pediatric populations. The Cervical Spine Injury Severity Score System (CSISS) has been demonstrated to be a reliable, comprehensive scoring system to describe subaxial cervical spine injuries, with intraobserver and interobserver intraclass correlation coefficients of 0.977 and 0.883, respectively.[27]

The CSISS uses a traditional morphologic description of fractures, which is familiar to spinal neurosurgeons (**Box 1**), combined with a 4-column model to help estimate stability based on a 20-point scale. The original SLIC included morphologic, ligamentous, and neurologic examination information in its point scale (**Table 1**)[29] and has been shown to have excellent intraobserver and interobserver reliability. The Spine Trauma Study Group published treatment

---

Box 1
Morphologic description of subaxial cervical injury

Anterior column injuries

Isolated

Compression fractures

Transverse process fractures

Traumatic disk herniations

Complex

Burst fractures

Disk distraction ± avulsion fractures

Flexion axial loading fractures

Lateral column injuries

Isolated

Superior facet fractures

Inferior facet fractures

Lateral mass pedicle fractures

Complex

Fracture separation of lateral mass

Unilateral facet dislocation ± fracture

Bilateral facet dislocation ± fracture

Posterior column injuries

Isolated

Spinous process fractures

Lamina fractures

Complex

Posterior ligamentous injuries ± fracture

Special cases

Bilateral pedicle fractures with traumatic spondylolisthesis

Fractures in ankylosed spine

SCIWORA

From Moore TA, Vaccaro AR, Anderson PA. Classification of lower cervical spine injuries. Spine 2006;31(11 Suppl):S38; [discussion: S61]; with permission.

Table 1
Subaxial injury classification system

	Points
Morphology	
No abnormality	0
Compression	1
Burst	+1 = 2
Distraction (facet perch, hyperextension)	3
Rotation/translation (facet dislocation, unstable teardrop, advanced flexion compression injury)	4
Discoligamentous complex	
Intact	0
Indeterminate (isolated interspinous widening, MRI signal change)	1
Disrupted (widening of disk space, facet perch, dislocation)	2
Neurologic status	
Intact	0
Nerve root injury	1
Complete cord injury	2
Incomplete cord injury	3
Continuous cord compression with neuro deficit	+1

Treatment recommendations of Spine Trauma Study Group[31]: SLIC score 3 or less suggests nonsurgical management; SLIC score 5 or more suggests surgical management; and SLIC score 4 is indeterminate.

From Vaccaro AR, Hulbert RJ, Patel AA, et al. The subaxial cervical spine injury classification system: a novel approach to recognize the importance of morphology, neurology, and integrity of the disco-ligamentous complex. Spine 2007;32(21):2367; with permission.

recommendations based on this scale,[31] with a score of 3 or less suggesting nonsurgical treatment and a score of 5 or more suggesting surgical treatment, with 4 being indeterminate. The few external validation studies that have been performed of the SLIC as a treatment algorithm have shown variable interobserver agreement on both classification and treatment choice,[32] with some questioning its clinical utility.[33] A new version of the SLIC that is more similar to that used for thoracolumbar fractures, the AOspine SLIC, has been recently proposed[30] and initial experience suggests moderate to substantial reliability among spine surgeons.[30,34] Despite these limitations, an accepted system, once validated in pediatric patients, could ultimately provide a useful framework to improve communication of injury patterns, determine prognosis, and suggest

appropriate treatment, while standardizing reporting of injuries for analysis in future outcome studies.

In the absence of any universally accepted classification system, the radiographic findings most commonly associated with cervical instability that are generally accepted in the pediatric literature include burst fracture, widening or subluxation of facet joints, significant separation of the spinous processes, vertebral body subluxation greater than 4.5 mm at C2-3 or C3-4 (<8 years old) or greater than 3.5 mm at any level in children greater than 8 years old,[7] angulation of the vertebral body greater than 7,[35] teardrop injury with disk disruption, and fracture dislocation (**Box 2**).

Spinal Cord Injury Without Radiographic Abnormality

In 1982, SCIWORA was first described in children as objective after trauma without evidence of fracture or ligamentous injury on plain radiographs or CT imaging.[36] As described previously, greater elasticity of the cervical spine in younger children may predispose them to this injury, although estimates of the prevalence of this entity are highly variable (4%–67%) depending on specific SCIWORA case definition.[37,38] In the past 2 decades, MRI has become indispensable in the evaluation of the children who present with normal CT imaging and neurologic deficit to rule out disk herniation, ligamentous injury, intradural or epidural hematoma, and spinal cord hemorrhage.[39] More recent work has demonstrated that those children diagnosed with SCIWORA found to have evidence of spinal cord injury on MRI were more likely to have been involved in a motor vehicle accident, require surgical intervention, and have persistent neurologic deficit at discharge than children with normal MRI.[40] Management for SCIWORA is

Box 2
Radiographic findings associated with cervical instability

Vertebral subluxation greater than 4.5 mm at C2-3 or C3-4 (<8 years old) or greater than 3.5 mm at any level (>8 years old)[7]

Angular displacement >7 degrees[35]

Tear drop injury with disk disruption

Unilateral/bilateral facet subluxation

Burst fracture

Fracture dislocation

Isolated ligamentous injury with significant facet or interspinous widening nonoperative, with most investigators advocating cervical orthosis for up to 12 weeks to minimize the risk of recurrent SCIWORA, followed by flexion-extension radiographs to rule out late instability.[7,36]

OPTIONS FOR MANAGEMENT

The options for treatment of cervical spine injuries in children are similar to those of adults, with certain important distinctions. The key determining factor remains whether the injury is believed stable or not. Stable injuries may not require any immobilization or may be dealt with via external immobilization.

Unstable injuries present more difficulty in treatment decision making. The elastic nature of the pediatric spine, especially in younger children, makes immobilization externally much more difficult. Children older than 8 and adolescents are more likely to heal successfully in external immobilization compared with children under the age of 8. Infants and neonates are especially challenging in this regard.

Closed reduction of subaxial spine fractures in children can be challenging due to noncooperativity and decreased body weight for countertraction. Surgeons must also be careful to avoid overdistraction, mandating frequent checks with lateral fluoroscopy after adding weight to verify alignment and appropriate interbody spacing. After closed reduction, halo vest fixation may provide traction in flexion or extension to allow for maintenance of proper alignment. Unfortunately, halos may be associated with significant complications and with a higher rate in younger children.[2,10,41] In the subaxial spine, cervical fracture types that are typically well managed with cervical orthosis in children without neurologic deficit include isolated compression, laminar and facet fractures without evidence of subluxation, kyphotic deformity, or instability. Proper fitting of the orthosis is mandatory and may require measurement and fabrication of custom orthotics, especially in younger children. In infants and young toddlers, a custom-fitted Minerva orthosis may be preferred over halo orthosis.

GENERAL CONSIDERATIONS REGARDING INSTRUMENTATION IN CHILDREN

Although most children with cervical spine injury are successfully managed with immobilization only, surgical stabilization remains an option and is necessary in up to 30% of patients.[2–4] Children with spinal injury and evidence of progressive neurologic deficit, deformity, and gross instability should undergo prompt closed reduction (in children older than 5) and/or surgical intervention for decompression of the neural elements, reduction of deformity, and spinal instrumentation and fusion. Internal fixation and fusion reduce the risk of progressive neurologic deficit, deformity, and pain associated with an injury. Unlike in the adult spine, however, details of instrumentation are variable and depend on the age of the child and size of the bony elements.

In general, the specific operative approach to the spine depends on the site of injury and/or compression, the experience of the surgeon, the age of the patient, and size of the bony elements. The anterior approach is typically used for cases of significant disk disruption and/or herniation in children greater than 5 years old, children with unstable burst fractures, and children with significant irreducible kyphotic deformity. The surgeon must spend some time preoperatively to define the dimensions of the involved vertebral bodies to ensure that appropriate hardware is available. In younger children (<6 years), low-profile plating systems are typically used for anterior discectomy or corpectomy and fusion, and occasionally screws must be cut to fit within the vertebral body. Recent work has shown the suitability of a single screw system for children with smaller vertebral bodies that are not amenable to standard plate/screw systems.[42]

The posterior approach is most useful for management in cases of posterior ligamentous injury, irreducible face subluxation, nerve root compression, and epidural hematoma. Options for posterior instrumentation include lateral mass screws (**Fig. 1**), sublaminar hooks (**Fig. 2**), sublaminar cables, interspinous wires (**Fig. 3**), and, in infants, sublaminar Mersilene Polyester Fiber Suture (Ethicon US, LLC) (**Fig. 4**). CT morphometric analysis of lateral masses suggests that screw instrumentation is feasible in most children older than 4 years,[43] although C7 is often significantly smaller and every child must be evaluated individually. A combined anterior/posterior approach may be required in cases of fracture dislocation with complete disruption of the anterior and posterior columns and significant distraction deformity (**Figs. 5** and **6**).

As a rule, fusion constructs should be kept as short as possible to avoid compromising spinal column growth, especially in younger patients. In a related note, given the propensity toward fusion seen in pediatric patients, surgeons must be careful to avoid exposure of uninvolved levels beyond the injured segments to avoid unintentional fusion above and below the planned construct.

Use of autograft bone (iliac crest or rib) for fusion has traditionally been the gold standard against

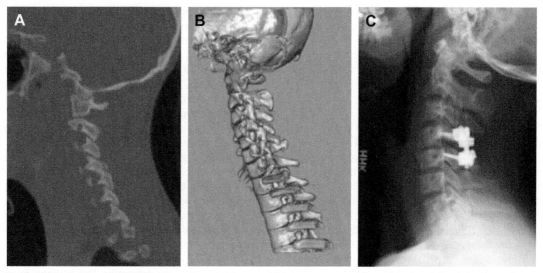

Fig. 1. Lateral mass screw instrumentation. A 16-year-old boy presents with neck pain, right deltoid weakness, and right arm pain and numbness in C5 distribution after wrestling accident. (*A*) Sagittal CT and (*B*) CT 3-D reconstruction demonstrates unilateral facet dislocation at C4-5 on the left. CTA (not shown) showed no evidence of vertebral artery injury. The child was taken to an operating room for open reduction of the facet dislocation, decompression of the right C5 nerve root, and placement of C4-5 lateral mass screws (*C*). Cancellous allograft admixed with posterior element autograft was used for fusion. Postoperatively, the patient recovered normal strength and sensation with no evidence of instability at 6 months.

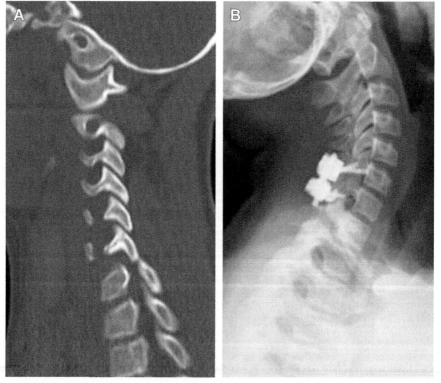

Fig. 2. Sublaminar hook variation. In cases of small or disrupted lateral masses (*A*), a sublaminar hook may be placed instead of lateral mass screws at the inferior aspect of the fusion (*B*). Careful attention must be paid to minimize compression of the dorsal spinal canal during dissection and placement.

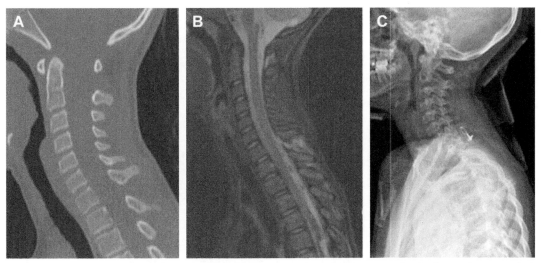

Fig. 3. Interspinous process wiring. A 6-year-old child restrained passenger involved in high-speed motor vehicle crash. The child complains of transient numbness in hands and lower extremities at accident scene, now presents with neck pain, neurologically intact. (*A*) Sagittal CT imaging shows widening of C7-T1 interspinous space without subluxation. (*B*) Sagittal T2 short-T1 inversion recovery MRI confirms isolated interspinous ligamentous injury at C7-T1 with an intact disk space, ALL, and PLL. Given the small size of C7 lateral masses and pedicles and intact C7-T1 disk space, the child underwent interspinous wiring of C7-T1 with use of rib autograft (*C*). Sublaminar cables would also be a reasonable option in this case. The child was left in a cervical collar for 6 weeks postoperatively and achieved a good fusion without evidence of cervicothoracic instability.

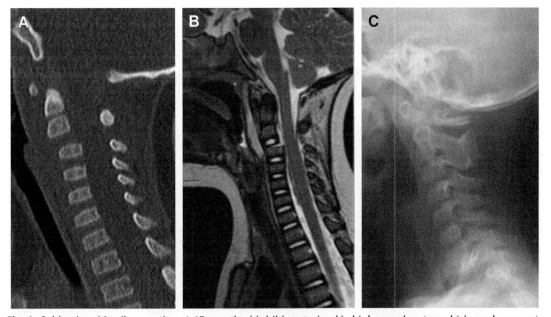

Fig. 4. Sublaminar Mersilene option. A 15-month-old child, restrained in high-speed motor vehicle crash, presents with left hemiparesis. (*A*) Sagittal CT demonstrates anterolisthesis of C2 on C3 with mild angular deformity. (*B*) T2 sagittal MRI shows shearing of the C3 superior end plate from the body through the epiphysis, resulting in angulation of C2 on C3 and widening of the C2-3 disk and interspinous spaces. The child was immediately put into halo vest with reduction of C2-3 deformity. Follow-up imaging demonstrated mild recurrent C2-3 subluxation, so the child underwent posterior C2-3 instrumentation with sublaminar Mersilene polyester fiber suture supplemented with notched rib autograft. This is a useful technique for infants and toddlers where standard screw instrumentation is not possible and sublaminar wires pull through soft cartilaginous bone.[46,47] (*C*) The child was maintained in halo vest for 3 months and demonstrated excellent reduction of deformity with robust posterior element fusion.

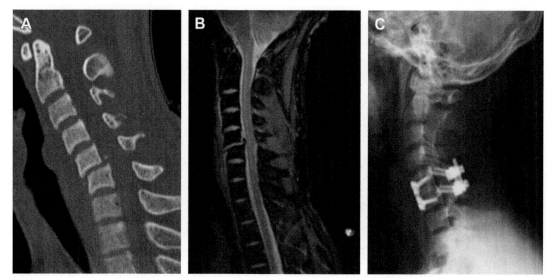

Fig. 5. Anterior cervical discectomy and fusion (ACDF) with lateral mass fixation. A 16-year-old boy presents with severe neck pain 1 day after significant flexion-type injury playing tackle football. (*A*) Sagittal CT demonstrates anterolisthesis at C5-6 with significant angulation (10°). (*B*) Sagittal T2 MRI demonstrates disruption of the C5-6 disk space with significant posterior ligamentous injury. Given disruption of the anterior column with posterior ligamentous injury, the adolescent underwent C5-6 ACDF with standard plating system and allograft followed by posterior C5-6 lateral mass instrumentation and fusion. (*C*) ACDF follow-up at 6 months shows good spinal alignment with evidence of bony fusion.

which all other grafting materials are compared and is associated with high fusion rates. Cadaveric allograft, demineralized bone matrix, and other synthetic scaffolds with calcium, phosphate, and/or hydroxyapatite are also options and have the advantage of avoiding morbidity associated with autograft harvest. Although not approved by the Food and Drug Administration for use in children, recombinant human bone morphogenetic protein 2 has also been used by experienced

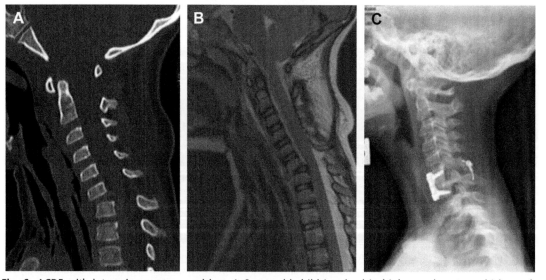

Fig. 6. ACDF with interspinous process wiring. A 6-year-old child involved in high-speed motor vehicle crash. Neurologically intact. (*A*) Sagittal CT demonstrates anterolisthesis with angulation at C6-7 disk space as well as significant widening of C6-7 spinous processes and facets. (*B*) Sagittal T2 MRI confirms highly unstable shearing of C6 inferior end plate at disk, extensive posterior ligamentous injury. Child placed in halo overnight, taken to an operating room the following day for C6-7 ACDF with smallest anterior cervical plate followed by posterior interspinous process wiring with notched rib autograft. (*C*) Follow-up at 6 months shows good alignment with anterior and posterior fusion mass.

groups for posterior cervical fusion surgery with acceptable safety and excellent fusion rates and is not associated with increased complications or cancer rates in the short term.[44,45]

SURGICAL TECHNIQUE
Anesthetic Considerations

Children with unstable cervical spine injuries should be maintained inline at all times and undergo either awake fiberoptic or fiberoptic nasotracheal intubation after induction of general anesthesia. Mean arterial pressures should be maintained at baseline range throughout the procedure. Fluoroscopy may be used to verify neutral anatomic alignment immediately after positioning. If instrumentation is placed near the cervicothoracic junction, the shoulders may be carefully taped with gentle traction to ensure adequate visualization.

Especially in cases that require reduction maneuvers, spinal cord monitoring, including somatosensory evoked potentials or motor evoked potentials, should be obtained immediately after intubation prior to positioning to establish appropriate baseline. The flip should be performed with careful attention to maintaining inline traction at all times. Postflip spinal cord monitoring data may also be obtained and monitored throughout the procedure. A standardized protocol should be developed and implemented to address intraoperative changes in spinal cord monitoring data. Increasing blood pressure, rapid confirmation of anatomic alignment with fluoroscopy, and evaluation for bony compression or hematoma are typical maneuvers that should be well understood and rapidly performed by the surgeon and supporting team.

Intraoperative adjuncts may include fluoroscopy, neuronavigation, and O-arm guidance, depending on surgeon preference. If navigation is used, it is important to keep in mind that the pediatric cervical spine is less rigid than thoracic and lumbar segments, allowing the possibility of navigation error, especially in cases of unstable fractures.

Although details of each technique are beyond the scope of this article, there are several general principles. After determination of the spinal levels to be fused, the surgeon must match the choice of instrumentation to the anatomy and relative size of the child. Size of vertebral bodies, lateral masses, and pedicles must be taken into account before surgery starts. The surgeon must also always have a plan B in case the instrumentation does not go as planned. The caveat to minimize fusion length notwithstanding, it is not advisable to stop

inferiorly at C7 with a longer multilevel construct, and T1 and T2 pedicle screws should be considered. Similarly, longer constructs to C3 should also include more robust C2 instrumentation.

For anterior pathology requiring an anterior surgical approach, in children under 6 years of age, standard ACDF plating systems cannot typically be used due to decreased height, width, and depth of the vertebral bodies. In those cases, low-profile, single-screw plate systems may be used with good results.[42] In infants under 3 years of age, use of titanium[48] and absorbable[49] craniofacial plating systems have also been described for circumferential instrumentation and fusion when standard systems cannot be used. Cervical corpectomy may be required in cases of burst fracture with significant bony deformity and/or anterior compression. Use of fibular strut grafts, polyetheretherketone cages, and expandable metal cages are all options for reconstruction of the vertebral column.

Postoperative Adjuncts

In principle, once rigid instrumentation has been placed with adequate stabilization, postoperative bracing is not necessary. In cases of nonrigid fixation (ie, sublaminar wires or interspinous wiring) placed in younger children, wearing of cervical orthosis for 6 weeks is advisable to minimize stress on the construct. Halo fixation for 6 to 12 weeks postoperatively may be required in cases of significant anterior and posterior column disruption, and nonrigid fixation should be avoided if possible given the high rate of complications in younger children.[41]

COMPLICATIONS

Complications from surgical instrumentation include injury to the vertebral artery with both anterior or posterior approaches, spinal cord injury, radicular injury, infection, unintended fusion extension, pseudarthrosis, and progressive deformity. A detailed understanding of a patient's anatomy, gleaned by careful study of the preoperative films, as well as careful surgical technique based on appropriate training and experience can help decreased the risk of technical misadventures during surgery.

OUTCOMES

Mortality rate in children with spinal injury has been reported to be significantly higher than in adults (28% vs 11%),[50] with a majority taking place at the accident scene and involving the upper cervical cord. In studies of children with spinal cord injury, the most important determinant of long-term functional outcome is initial neurologic status; 75% to 85% of children with mild to moderate incomplete spinal cord injury may improve by 1 to 2 Frankel grades, with greater than half making a full recovery.[4,5] Although there are few studies reporting long-term outcomes for either operative or nonoperative treatment of subaxial cervical spine fractures in children, use of rigid lateral mass screw instrumentation seems safe with few complications and high fusion rates.[51,52] A recent review of all pediatric cervical instrumented fusion outcomes reported in the literature included both congenital and traumatic pathologies.[53] The investigators found an increased rate of fusion (99% vs 83%, $P<.05$) and decreased complication rate (14% vs 50%, $P<.05$) associated with rigid screw instrumentation compared with traditional wiring techniques. Most complications were related to postoperative use of halo vest fixation, and a vast majority of reported cases were either occipitocervical or C1-2 fusions, making generalization of these results to subaxial cervical instrumentation problematic. More recently, pain and disability measured by the Neck Disability Index, Short Form 36, and visual analog scale for neck pain have been proposed as relevant health related quality-of-life outcomes for pediatric cohorts and have been specifically used for follow-up of children treated for unilateral facet fracture and dislocations.[54]

SUMMARY

Appropriate management of subaxial spine injury in children requires an appreciation for the differences in anatomy, biomechanics, injury patterns, and treatment options compared with adult patients. Increased flexibility, weak neck muscles, and cranial disproportion predispose younger children to upper cervical injuries and SCIWORA, whereas older children have fracture patterns more similar to adults. A majority of subaxial cervical spine injuries can be treated nonoperatively, although halo placement carries a high complication rate, especially in younger children. Surgical instrumentation options for children have significantly increased in recent years, and when anatomically feasible, rigid screw instrumentation is associated with low complication rates and high fusion rates. Future studies of outcomes for children with subaxial cervical spine injury should focus on objective injury classification and standardized outcome measures to ensure continued improvement in the quality of care for this challenging patient population.

REFERENCES

1. Bruneau M, De Witte O, Regli L, et al. Anatomical variations. In: George D, Bruneau M, Spetzler R, editors. Pathology and surgery around the vertebral artery. Paris (France): Springer Paris; 2011. p. 53–74.
2. McCall T, Fassett D, Brockmeyer D. Cervical spine trauma in children: a review. Neurosurg Focus 2006;20(2):E5.
3. Eleraky MA, Theodore N, Adams M, et al. Pediatric cervical spine injuries: report of 102 cases and review of the literature. J Neurosurg 2000;92(1 Suppl):12–7.
4. Hadley MN, Zabramski JM, Browner CM, et al. Pediatric spinal trauma. Review of 122 cases of spinal cord and vertebral column injuries. J Neurosurg 1988;68(1):18–24.
5. Hamilton MG, Myles ST. Pediatric spinal injury: review of 174 hospital admissions. J Neurosurg 1992;77(5):700–4.
6. Yilmazlar S, Kocaeli H, Uz A, et al. Clinical importance of ligamentous and osseous structures in the cervical uncovertebral foraminal region. Clin Anat 2003;16(5):404–10.
7. Pang D, Zovickian J. Vertebral column and spinal cord injuries in children. In: Richard HW, editor. Youman's neurological surgery. 6th edition. Philadelphia: Elsevier; 2011. p. 2293–332.
8. Shin JI, Lee NJ, Cho SK. Pediatric cervical spine and spinal cord injury: a national database study. Spine 2016;41(4):283–92.
9. Mann DC, Dodds JA. Spinal injuries in 57 patients 17 years or younger. Orthopedics 1993;16(2):159–64.
10. Mortazavi M, Gore PA, Chang S, et al. Pediatric cervical spine injuries: a comprehensive review. Childs Nerv Syst 2011;27(5):705–17.
11. Osenbach RK, Menezes AH. Pediatric spinal cord and vertebral column injury. Neurosurgery 1992; 30(3):385–90.
12. Nypaver M, Treloar D. Neutral cervical spine positioning in children. Ann Emerg Med 1994;23(2): 208–11.
13. Panacek EA, Mower WR, Holmes JF, et al. Test performance of the individual NEXUS low-risk clinical screening criteria for cervical spine injury. Ann Emerg Med 2001;38(1):22–5.
14. Benayoun MD, Allen JW, Lovasik BP, et al. Utility of computed tomography imaging of the cervical spine in trauma evaluation of ground level fall. J Trauma Acute Care Surg 2016;81(2):339–44.
15. Rosati SF, Maarouf R, Wolfe L, et al. Implementation of pediatric cervical spine clearance guidelines at a combined trauma center: Twelve-month impact. J Trauma Acute Care Surg 2015;78(6):1117–21.
16. Anderson RCE, Scaife ER, Fenton SJ, et al. Cervical spine clearance after trauma in children. J Neurosurg 2006;105(5 Suppl):361–4.

17. Anderson RCE, Kan P, Vanaman M, et al. Utility of a cervical spine clearance protocol after trauma in children between 0 and 3 years of age. J Neurosurg Pediatr 2010;5(3):292–6.

18. Mace SE. Emergency evaluation of cervical spine injuries: CT versus plain radiographs. Ann Emerg Med 1985;14(10):973–5.

19. Keiper MD, Zimmerman RA, Bilaniuk LT. MRI in the assessment of the supportive soft tissues of the cervical spine in acute trauma in children. Neuroradiology 1998;40(6):359–63.

20. Badhiwala JH, Lai CK, Alhazzani W, et al. Cervical spine clearance in obtunded patients after blunt traumatic injury: a systematic review. Ann Intern Med 2015;162(6):429–37.

21. Qualls D, Leonard JR, Keller M, et al. Utility of magnetic resonance imaging in diagnosing cervical spine injury in children with severe traumatic brain injury. J Trauma Acute Care Surg 2015;78(6):1122–8.

22. Plackett TP, Wright F, Baldea AJ, et al. Cervical spine clearance when unable to be cleared clinically: a pooled analysis of combined computed tomography and magnetic resonance imaging. Am J Surg 2016;211(1):115–21.

23. Khanna P, Chau C, Dublin A, et al. The value of cervical magnetic resonance imaging in the evaluation of the obtunded or comatose patient with cervical trauma, no other abnormal neurological findings, and a normal cervical computed tomography. J Trauma Acute Care Surg 2012;72(3):699–702.

24. Mascarenhas D, Dreizin D, Bodanapally UK, et al. Parsing the Utility of CT and MRI in the Subaxial Cervical Spine Injury Classification (SLIC) System: Is CT SLIC Enough? AJR Am J Roentgenol 2016;206(6):1292–7.

25. Dwek JR, Chung CB. Radiography of cervical spine injury in children: are flexion-extension radiographs useful for acute trauma? AJR Am J Roentgenol 2000;174(6):1617–9.

26. Ralston ME, Chung K, Barnes PD, et al. Role of flexion-extension radiographs in blunt pediatric cervical spine injury. Acad Emerg Med 2001;8(3):237–45.

27. Moore TA, Vaccaro AR, Anderson PA. Classification of lower cervical spine injuries. Spine 2006;31(11 Suppl):S37–43 [discussion: S61].

28. White A, Panjabi M. The problem of clinical instability in the human spine: a systematic approach. In: White A, Panjabi M, editors. Clinical biomechanics of the spine. 2nd edition. Philadelphia: JP Lippincott; 1990. p. 278–378.

29. Vaccaro AR, Hulbert RJ, Patel AA, et al. The subaxial cervical spine injury classification system: a novel approach to recognize the importance of morphology, neurology, and integrity of the disco-ligamentous complex. Spine 2007;32(21):2365–74.

30. Vaccaro AR, Koerner JD, Radcliff KE, et al. AOSpine subaxial cervical spine injury classification system. Eur Spine J 2015;25(7):2173–84.

31. Dvorak MF, Fisher CG, Fehlings MG, et al. The surgical approach to subaxial cervical spine injuries: an evidence-based algorithm based on the SLIC classification system. Spine 2007;32(23):2620–9.

32. Samuel S, Lin J-L, Smith MM, et al. Subaxial injury classification scoring system treatment recommendations: external agreement study based on retrospective review of 185 patients. Spine 2015;40(3):137–42.

33. van Middendorp JJ, Audigé L, Bartels RH, et al. The Subaxial Cervical Spine Injury Classification System: an external agreement validation study. Spine J 2013;13(9):1055–63.

34. Silva OT, Sabba MF, Lira HIG, et al. Evaluation of the reliability and validity of the newer AOSpine subaxial cervical injury classification (C-3 to C-7). J Neurosurg Spine 2016;1–6. http://dx.doi.org/10.3171/2016.2.SPINE151039.

35. Ware M, Gupta N, Sun P. Clinical biomechanics of the pediatric craniocervical junction and subaxial spine. In: Brockmeyer DL, editor. Advanced pediatric craniocervical surgery. New York: Thieme; 2005. p. 27–42.

36. Pang D, Wilberger JE. Spinal cord injury without radiographic abnormalities in children. J Neurosurg 1982;57(1):114–29.

37. Carreon LY, Glassman SD, Campbell MJ. Pediatric spine fractures: a review of 137 hospital admissions. J Spinal Disord Tech 2004;17(6):477–82.

38. Saruhashi Y, Hukuda S, Katsuura A, et al. Clinical outcomes of cervical spinal cord injuries without radiographic evidence of trauma. Spinal Cord 1998;36(8):567–73.

39. Davis PC, Reisner A, Hudgins PA, et al. Spinal injuries in children: role of MR. AJNR Am J Neuroradiol 1993;14(3):607–17.

40. Mahajan P, Jaffe DM, Olsen CS, et al. Spinal cord injury without radiologic abnormality in children imaged with magnetic resonance imaging. J Trauma Acute Care Surg 2013;75(5):843–7.

41. Baum JA, Hanley EN, Pullekines J. Comparison of halo complications in adults and children. Spine 1989;14(3):251–2.

42. Garber ST, Brockmeyer DL. Management of subaxial cervical instability in very young or small-for-age children using a static single-screw anterior cervical plate: indications, results, and long-term follow-up. J Neurosurg Spine 2016;24(6):892–6.

43. Al-Shamy G, Cherian J, Mata JA, et al. Computed tomography morphometric analysis for lateral mass screw placement in the pediatric subaxial cervical spine. J Neurosurg Spine 2012;17(5):390–6.

44. Rocque BG, Kelly MP, Miller JH, et al. Bone morphogenetic protein-associated complications in pediatric spinal fusion in the early postoperative

period: an analysis of 4658 patients and review of the literature. J Neurosurg Pediatr 2014;14(6): 635–43.

45. Sayama C, Willsey M, Chintagumpala M, et al. Routine use of recombinant human bone morphogenetic protein-2 in posterior fusions of the pediatric spine and incidence of cancer. J Neurosurg Pediatr 2015;16(1):4–13.

46. Gaines RW, Abernathie DL. Mersilene tapes as a substitute for wire in segmental spinal instrumentation for children. Spine 1986;11(9):907–13.

47. Holland CM, Kebriaei MA, Wrubel DM. Posterior cervical spinal fusion in a 3-week-old infant with a severe subaxial distraction injury. J Neurosurg Pediatr 2016;17(3):353–6.

48. Patel NB, Hazzard MA, Ackerman LL, et al. Circumferential fixation with craniofacial miniplates for a cervical spine injury in a child. J Neurosurg Pediatr 2009;4(5):429–33.

49. Lidar Z, Constantini S, Regev GJ, et al. Absorbable anterior cervical plate for corpectomy and fusion in a 2-year-old child with neurofibromatosis. Technical note. J Neurosurg Pediatr 2012;9(4): 442–6.

50. Hamilton MG, Myles ST. Pediatric spinal injury: review of 61 deaths. J Neurosurg 1992;77(5):705–8.

51. Hedequist D, Hresko T, Proctor M. Modern cervical spine instrumentation in children. Spine 2008; 33(4):379–83.

52. Hedequist D, Proctor M, Hresko T. Lateral mass screw fixation in children. J Child Orthop 2010; 4(3):197–201.

53. Hwang SW, Gressot LV, Rangel-Castilla L, et al. Outcomes of instrumented fusion in the pediatric cervical spine. J Neurosurg Spine 2012;17(5): 397–409.

54. Sellin JN, Shaikh K, Ryan SL, et al. Clinical outcomes of the surgical treatment of isolated unilateral facet fractures, subluxations, and dislocations in the pediatric cervical spine: report of eight cases and review of the literature. Childs Nerv Syst 2014; 30(7):1233–42.

Pediatric Thoracolumbar Spine Trauma

Visish Srinivasan, MD[a], Andrew Jea, MD[b],*

KEYWORDS

- Pediatric spine trauma • Thoracic • Lumbar • Fracture

KEY POINTS

- Compared with adult spine trauma, pediatric spine trauma is less likely to result in fracture due to the greater elasticity and compressibility of the pediatric spine.
- The anatomy, injury pattern, radiographic findings, and management of pediatric thoracolumbar spine trauma warrant special consideration.
- Among various thoracolumbar spine injuries, a major difference between adults and children is the occurrence of spinal cord injury (SCI) without radiographic abnormality (SCIWORA).
- The understanding of thoracolumbar spine injury in children is constantly evolving.

INTRODUCTION

Pediatric spine trauma is rare, with pediatric patients suffering only 2% to 5% of all spinal injuries.[1–5] A majority of these are in the cervical spine. This is attributed to the proportionally larger head size in children, in addition to their weaker supportive soft tissue structures in comparison to those of adults. Thus, only an estimated 0.6% to 0.9% of all spinal trauma cases are pediatric thoracic and lumbar spine injuries.[6]

Compared with adult spine trauma, pediatric spine trauma is less likely to result in fracture due to the greater elasticity and compressibility of the pediatric spine.[3,4] Radiography may show subtler signs, such as splaying of spinous processes or signs of dislocation, belying a graver injury. As a result of weaker musculature and supporting structures, traumatic forces are transferred more directly and more severely to the neural structures.[4] Fortunately, at younger ages, children have remaining plasticity of bone and neural elements that allow healing potential if treated

promptly and appropriately. Thus, the anatomy, injury pattern, radiographic findings, and management of pediatric thoracolumbar spine trauma warrant special consideration.[7]

Among various thoracolumbar spine injuries, a major difference between adults and children is the occurrence of SCIWORA. This pathology occurs almost exclusively in children under 8 years of age due to biomechanical mismatch between the hypermobility of the spine and the lack of tolerance of the spinal cord to stretch to the same degree.[8]

The understanding of thoracolumbar spine injury in children is constantly evolving. In this article, some of the common patterns of injury and their management are reviewed.

PEDIATRIC SPINAL DEVELOPMENT

Thoracolumbar spine trauma is unique in children due to consideration of the ongoing development of the spine. In the developing child, each vertebra has 3 ossification centers: a centrum and 2 neural

Disclosure: The authors have no conflicts of interest to report.
[a] Neuro-Spine Program, Division of Pediatric Neurosurgery, Department of Neurosurgery, Texas Children's Hospital, Baylor College of Medicine, 6621 Fannin Street, Suite 1230.01, Houston, TX 77030, USA; [b] Section of Pediatric Neurosurgery, Department of Neurosurgery, Goodman Campbell Brain and Spine, Indiana University School of Medicine, 705 Riley Hospital Drive, Suite 1134, Indianapolis, IN 46202, USA
* Corresponding author.
E-mail address: ajea@goodmancampbell.com

arches (ventral and dorsal) that normally fuse between ages 2 and 6 years.[5] Prior to fusion, the centrum and neural arches are connected by a cartilaginous membrane. The neural elements ascend to their normal levels in the spinal canal by the first birthday. By 6 years of age, the spinal canal attains near-adult volume. By 8 to 10 years of age, the spine is generally similar to that of the adult state. Even into early adolescence, however, the pediatric spine has greater mobility due to ligamentous laxity, shallow facet joint angulation, immature paraspinous musculature, and incomplete vertebral ossification.[1,9]

The developing spine depends on 3 cartilaginous areas for continued vertebral growth: end-plate cartilage, neurocentral cartilage, and the ring apophysis. The end-plate physeal cartilage is adjacent to the bony vertebral body. At birth, the end plate is entirely composed of cartilage; ossification islands appear by 5 years of age in the margins, eventually fusing to form the annular ring apophysis. The ring apophysis, complete by 12 years of age, encircles the full circumference of the vertebral body, providing significant strength. It remains physically separated from the vertebral body by a thin seam of cartilage until 14 to 15 years of age.

UNIQUE FEATURES OF PEDIATRIC SPINAL ANATOMY

Unlike that of an adult, the pediatric spine is dynamic; evaluation of injuries should be made in the context of a child's growth and development. Children have larger heads relative to their bodies and less neck musculature, which predisposes them to flexion and extension-type injuries.[10,11] In addition, they have inherent ligamentous laxity, elasticity, and incomplete ossification.[8,10,12,13] Children have facet joints that are small and more horizontally oriented, resulting in greater mobility and less stability.[8,10,12,14,15] As children develop a more adult-like vertebral column between 9 and 16 years of age, they gain sturdier osseoligamentous structures that provided better protection of the spinal cord. Thus, these patients tend to be subject to less severe SCI compared with those in the younger age group. Under high stress, the adult spine is more likely to suffer breakage of bones and frank rupture of ligaments in comparison the pediatric spine, where deformation and return to normal alignment are more common.[7]

EPIDEMIOLOGY

Pediatric spine fractures can occur in the thoracolumbar region, most frequently secondary to high-speed motor vehicle accidents (MVAs) or falls from significant heights. Representing 1% to 3% of all spine fractures, pediatric spine fractures occur in 2 major age groups: those younger than 5 years old and those older than 10 years old. Due to increased activity, there is a seasonal peak during the summer break from June to September and again during winter break. Whereas in younger children less than 10 years old, injuries are most frequently secondary to falls or automobile versus pedestrian accidents (75%), in children 10 to 14 years old, MVAs are more frequent (40%). As they age into late adolescence, motorcycle accidents and sports trauma increase in proportion.[8] The proportion of thoracic and lumbar fractures increases with age, because ligaments stiffen and cervical musculature matures.[16]

RISK FACTORS AND PREVENTION

Despite all efforts to optimize treatment of thoracolumbar spine trauma, the most efficacious approach is a public health one—prevention. Because motor vehicle crashes represent a majority of these injuries, prevention strategies targeted to motor vehicle crashes offer the highest yield. Risk factors for SCI include single-vehicle crashes, rollover, and ejection.[17] Before 1959, only 2-point lap belts were available in automobiles. In reality, however, only racecar drivers routinely used seat belts. The 2-point belt strapped across the torso facilitated serious abdominal injuries and thoracolumbar spine fractures in high-speed crashes, especially in small children wearing adult lap belts. Volvo was the first automobile manufacturer to include 3-point belts for front seat passengers as a standard feature. Today, Title 49 of the United States Code, Chapter 301, Motor Vehicle Safety, requires 3-point seat belts in all seating positions. Most seat belt legislation in the United States is left to the states; however, most states (28 states plus the District of Columbia) have enacted mandatory use of seat belts for all passengers. Each of the 50 states and the District of Columbia, however, have enacted their own mandatory child seat belt laws, including regulation of the use of car seats and booster seats.[18]

TYPES OF THORACOLUMBAR SPINE FRACTURES IN PEDIATRICS
Compression Fractures

Compression fractures represent the largest subtype of thoracolumbar fractures in pediatrics. They often occur around the thoracolumbar junction (**Fig. 1**). The wedge shape of the immature vertebral body and the natural kyphosis make children susceptible to compression fractures.

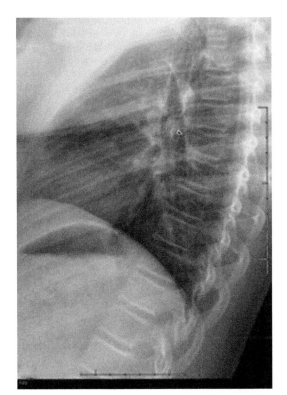

Fig. 1. T6 compression fracture in a 10-year-old girl after slipping and falling to the ground. The patient complained of midthoracic back pain. She was neurologically intact. Lateral thoracic spine radiographs and subsequent MRI show a T6 compression fracture (*arrow*) with less than 50% loss of body height and no evidence of retropulsion or canal compromise.

Lower-energy axial loading forces, such as those in minor to moderate falls or sports injuries, are associated with these fractures. Compression of the anterior column in hyperflexion injuries is also a common mechanism, with preservation of the posterior portion of the end plate(s).[5,19] Multiple levels may occasionally be affected, indicating a higher-energy injury, and should trigger evaluation for intra-abdominal injuries.[19] Most fractures result in less than 30% loss of height; loss of greater than 50% of original height should heighten concern for disruption of the posterior ligamentous complex (PLC) and prompt evaluation by MRI. A large majority of compression fractures do not require surgical intervention. Even in stable injuries, the potential for progressive deformity should be considered when the end plate is damaged and there is significant kyphosis. Fractures with minor loss of height usually recover with conservative management.[19] Thoracolumbosacral orthosis (TLSO) brace therapy can also be considered in nonoperative management of unstable fractures, usually for 6 to 8 weeks, with good results.[19]

Burst Fractures

Burst fractures, similar to compression fractures, occur after axial loading injuries to the thoracolumbar junction (**Fig. 2**). In contrast to compression fractures, burst fractures are associated with higher-energy trauma, which drives the nucleus pulposus into the vertebral body, leading to fracture of the anterior and middle columns.[7,19] In younger children, these fractures can also damage the germinal layer, leading to premature epiphyseal fusion.[7] Burst fractures are considered unstable and are more frequently associated with neurologic injury. Retropulsion of fragments of the posterior vertebral body can lead to these injuries and necessitate urgent decompression. CT is the preferred initial modality and can assess compression of canal compromise and extent of bony injury. In addition to this, MRI can provide better visualization of the neural structures, including the spinal cord, conus medullaris, and/or nerve roots that may be affected, as well as the PLC to assess for instability.[5]

Surgical management of burst fractures commonly includes decompression, in addition to stabilization, depending on the presence of a neurologic deficit or canal compromise. The extent of the instrumentation construct is a nuanced decision without clear guidelines. In adults, fusion is typically performed 2 levels above and 2 levels below the fractured vertebral level; however, in children, long fusions may lead to stunted truncal growth and crankshaft deformity. Sparing the developing spine from additional levels of fusion is important from the perspective of growth and in the pursuit of reduced operative morbidity, such as blood loss.

Although percutaneous fixation has been well described in adults, it has yet to be analyzed in great detail and studied in large series in the pediatric population. Alternatives to posterolateral fusion include anterior fusion and lateral fusion (extreme lateral interbody fusion and direct lateral interbody fusion).[19] These are less commonly used in the setting of trauma due to the common need for decompression in addition to arthrodesis. The extent of fusion is also a matter of debate.

Nonsurgical management can be pursued for biomechanically stable fractures without neurologic compromise, usually with a thoracolumbosacral brace (TLSO) for 8 to 12 weeks.

Vertebral Apophysis Fracture

Fracture of the ring apophysis, also called slipped vertebral apophysis injury, can occur in children, most commonly at L4 or L5 (**Fig. 3**). Clinical presentation is most commonly back pain and

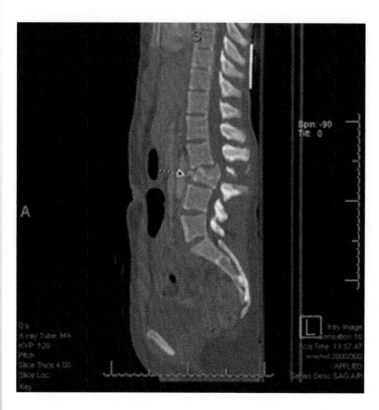

Fig. 2. Burst fracture (*arrow*) in a 17-year-old girl after an MVA. Sagittal CT scan demonstrates an L3 injury with greater than 50% loss of body height and retropulsion of bone into the canal, resulting in greater than 50% canal compromise.

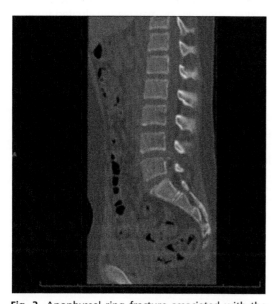

Fig. 3. Apophyseal ring fracture associated with the L5 superior end plate and L4-L5 disk herniation in a 12-year-old boy after a football injury shown on sagittal CT scan. The patient presented with intractable back and leg pain. He was taken to the operating for decompressive L4 and L5 laminectomies without discectomy.

radicular leg pain, similar to those of disk protrusion in adults, but can also include neurogenic claudication.[20] These fractures are a distinct entity that warrants awareness in children. CT is the best diagnostic imaging for this.[21] A standard approach for discectomy with fragment removal may not be necessary and may increase surgical risk; posterior laminar decompression alone at the involved levels may relieve presenting symptoms and allow for good functional outcome.[20] Overweight children may be at additional risk of this pathology.[22]

Seat Belt Injury

Seat belt injuries are a specific type of flexion-distraction injury frequently associated with severe abdominal trauma (**Fig. 4**). Classically, this includes a small bowel mesenteric tear or perforation and a compression or chance-type fracture.[23] The rib cage protects the thoracic spine against horizontal displacement but provides little protection against longitudinal distraction that can occur in these injuries. The mechanism involves migration of the lap belt toward the anterior abdominal wall, due to the tendency of children to sit further over the edge of the seat. Sudden deceleration then results in direct compression of

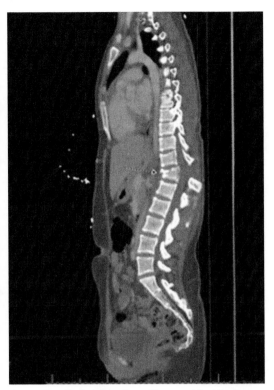

Fig. 4. Seat belt injury in a 15-year-old girl after an MVA. Sagittal CT scan shows a focal kyphosis at T12 (*arrow*) with disruption of the posterior soft tissue band and splaying of the posterior elements. The patient complained of not only back pain but also abdominal pain. Visceral and hollow organ injury was ruled out prior to taking the patient to the operating room for stabilization of her spinal column.

viscera occurring between the seat belt and the spine, with the flexion fulcrum placed at the anterior vertebral body.[23] In pediatric patients, the most commonly affected levels are L2 and L3 compared with the thoracolumbar junction in adults.[24] Further contributing to the likelihood of neurologic injury is that the elasticity of the pediatric spinal column far exceeds that of the spinal cord and the dura.[7] In their review of 28 children with seat belt syndrome, Santschi and colleagues[25] found 43% had a spinal cord injury, associated with a wide spectrum of fractures beyond the classic chance fracture. Thus, patients with this pattern of injury require special consideration, including a comprehensive trauma survey, because 50% of patients also present with significant abdominal injury (ie, the nutcracker phenomenon, where the head of the pancreas, third segment of the duodenum, and left renal vein are crushed between the superior mesenteric artery and aorta).

Slow Vehicle Crushing Injury

Slow vehicle crushing injuries, also referred to as driveway injuries, most often affect the thoracic spine and are seen in children under 5 years of age.[26] These occur most often when drivers back out slowly from a parking space, not noticing a child in the vicinity. Injury can occur when a patient's thoracic spine is upright and pinned between the car bumper and another surface, resulting in hyperextension and associated thoracoabdominal injures. Other, often younger, patients are run over by a car tire at low speeds, indicated by tire marks across the chest or abdomen, indicating potentially major thoracic or intraperitoneal injuries. Spinal injuries are most common in the former due to the presence of spinal hyperextension.[12]

Traumatic Spondylolisthesis/Spondylolysis

Traumatic spondylolisthesis/spondylolysis of the thoracic and lumbar spine can occur in several ways, some which merit special mention in the pediatric population (**Fig. 5**). In the typical nomenclature of 6 types of spondylolisthesis, type IV is designated for traumatic spondylolisthesis without injury to the pars (usually from a fracture dislocation), whereas type II indicates spondylolysis.[27] Type II spondylolisthesis is further broken down into 3 subtypes. Type IIA occurs in younger children with congenital abnormality of the lumbosacral spine, such as spina bifida occulta or variation in number of lumbosacral vertebra, predisposing them to pars articularis (pars) fatigue and microfractures. Type IIB is similar but with partial healing of the microfractures resulting in abnormally elongated pars. Type IIC, a rare type, results from high-velocity injuries that cause isolated pars fracture and resultant slip.

Spondylolisthesis/spondylolysis is of concern to pediatric athletes who may be at risk for a mechanism similar to type IIA/B. Repeated hyperextension with axial loading of the immature spine may result in fatigue and fracture of the pars in the lower lumbar spine.[28] This injury has been reported frequently in gymnastics, weight lifting, and football. As in adults, bilateral pars fracture may result in progressive spondylolisthesis. Conservative care should be the primary initial form of treatment, with avoidance of painful activities, especially repetitive hyperextension. Surgical intervention can be considered if pain persists greater than 6 months or is debilitating, for high-grade listhesis, or in the presence of a neurologic deficit.[7]

Surgical options are broad but include posterolateral arthrodesis with or without interbody

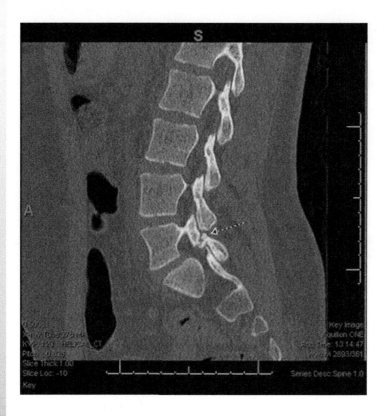

Fig. 5. Traumatic spondylolysis of the L5 pars in a 16-year-old girl after an injury while playing soccer shown on parasagittal CT scan (*arrow*). Conservative treatment was initiated for 3 months, including the use of a TLSO with leg extender. The patient failed conservative treatment, however, and eventually presented to the operating room for an L5-S1 posterior instrumented fusion.

fusion,[29] direct pars arthrodesis,[30] or pedicle screw-laminar hook constructs.[31] The latter two preserve motion at the affected segment and may be preferred in pediatric patients and, especially, athletes.[28]

SPINAL CORD INJURY WITHOUT RADIOGRAPHIC ABNORMALITY AND THE THORACIC SPINE

SCIWORA was first described by Pang and Wilberger in 1982.[14] The current consensus is that SCIWORA represents SCI in the absence of bony radiographic abnormalities.[32] SCIWORA is responsible for 6% to 19% in children and is highest among children under 8 years of age, who also have the most unfavorable prognosis. This is associated with the same factors that predispose children to SCI of all types, including heavy head, weaker neck muscles, and greater elasticity of vertebral ligaments.

The thoracic spine is much less commonly affected in SCIWORA compared with the cervical spine, comprising only 13% of all cases.[33] When affected, the upper thoracic cord is at higher risk due to watershed location in vascular supply and distribution of exiting nerve roots and dentate ligaments. High-speed MVAs, seat belt injuries, or slow-moving vehicle crush injuries can all result

in SCIWORA. A self-reducing deformity of the thoracic spine can transmit significant energy to the intrathoracic and intraabdominal compartments, causing injury to the soft tissues without fracture.

Despite the lack of fracture, SCIWORA should be considered potentially unstable, due to the potential for occult ligamentous disruptions. An analogous situation is central cord syndrome, which is most frequently managed by the placement of a cervical collar to prevent secondary injury. Two phenomena require special mention: delayed neurologic deterioration and recurrent SCIWORA.[34] In the former, progressive neurologic deficit, and even complete cord syndrome, can occur as quickly as 30 minutes to as late as 4 days after injury. Ligamentous injury may predispose to secondary SCI after initial trauma.

Recurrent Spinal Cord Injury Without Radiographic Abnormality

Recurrent SCIWORA can occur as a second set of symptoms from several days to weeks after the initial ictus. The incidence of recurrent SCIWORA is markedly reduced with timely immobilization after the initial SCIWORA presentation.[35] Similar to second concussion syndrome, recurrent

SCIWORA usually results in a more severe deficit than the initial syndrome.[7,36]

Management

Patients with thoracic SCIWORA should be evaluated for other systemic injuries, as is the practice for radiographically correlated injuries, such as fracture dislocations. Secondary SCI should be avoided by bracing and spinal precautions. Appropriate long-term immobilization can be maintained for 12 weeks with cervicothoracic, thoracolumbar, or other appropriate braces.[12] Patients and families should be counseled on strict avoidance of athletic activities.

Prognosis and Outcome

As with other subtypes of SCI, the prognosis of children who incur SCIWORA is strongly correlated with the initial neurologic status. Approximately 50% of these patients may develop subsequent neurologic deterioration after presentation. Pang[34] has also reported a trend toward more severe/complete injuries in children younger than 8 years.

MANAGEMENT OF THORACOLUMBAR SPINE TRAUMA IN CHILDREN

The authors propose just one systematic approach to the management of the most common patterns of fractures discussed thus far (**Fig. 6**).[37] The decision to intervene surgically and whether arthrodesis is needed is based on 3 factors: the need for decompression of neural elements, the stability of the injury/deformity, and the long-term potential for healing (**Table 1**). Stability, in turn, can be determined by a variety of rules, but the authors encourage use of the Thoracolumbar Injury Classification and Severity (TLICS) score, which can also help guide conservative or surgical management and has been recently been validated in children (**Table 2**).[38]

Imaging

Imaging for thoracolumbar trauma in pediatrics should be specific to the level of injury and index of suspicion for neurologic injury. Currently, no national guidelines exist.[37] In general, plain radiographs can be used to detect most osseous injuries. The authors generally recommend CT, however, whenever there is an increased

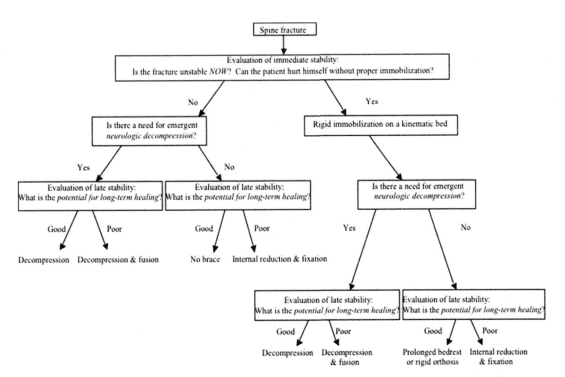

Fig. 6. A proposed algorithm to manage spine injuries. Indications for closed or open reduction and decompression and external or internal fixation are guided by 3 questions: (1) Is the injury acutely stable or unstable? (2) Is there a need for urgent neurologic decompression? and (3) What is the potential for healing with external orthosis alone?

Table 1
Common thoracic and lumbar spine injuries, association with spinal cord injury, and stability

Thoracic and Lumbar Fracture Type	Associated Spinal Cord Injury	Stability	
		Immediate	Late
Compression	Uncommon	Good	Good
Burst	Possible	Fair	Good
Fracture distraction	Possible	Fair	Good
Fracture rotation	Common	Poor	Poor

suspicion of injury and especially for surgical planning (**Fig. 7**). MRI has become the modality of choice in pediatric patients, both for reduction of radiation exposure and for its high sensitivity to detect injury. It is especially useful in ruling out operative lesions that may be missed on CT,

Table 2
Thoracolumbar Injury Classification and Severity scoring system

Feature	Score
Morphology type	
Compression	1
Burst	2
Translational/rotational	3
Distraction	4
Neurologic involvement	
Intact	0
Nerve root	2
Cord, conus medullaris (incomplete injury + 1)	2
Cauda equina	3
PLC	
Intact	0
Injury suspected/ indeterminate	2
Injured	3
Treatment recommendation	
Nonsurgical	0–3
Surgeon's choice	4
Surgical	>4

From Sellin JN, Steele WJ 3rd, Simpson L, et al. Multicenter retrospective evaluation of the validity of the Thoracolumbar Injury Classification and Severity Score system in children. J Neurosurg Pediatr 2016;18(2):165; with permission.

such as epidural hematoma or traumatic disk herniation.[37] In addition to imaging, Leroux and colleagues[39] have suggested asking patients about a sensation of "breath arrest" at the time of injury. When this sensation is absent and scans are negative, there is more assurance of no fracture.

Indications for Surgery

Clinically stable pediatric spine fractures can usually be managed nonsurgically.[3] Determination of a fracture as "stable" requires a simple approach and assessment of 3 questions. First, is there neurologic injury or progressive neurologic deficit? Second, will the fracture heal on its own? Third, is there undue pain or deformity? Various fracture classifications can serve as a guide, including the classic schema by Denis,[40] a more modern one by the AOSpine group,[41] or TLICS.[42] Specific considerations that are built into these assessments include involvement of the PLC, the presence of deformity greater than 30°, and others. Moderate injuries not necessitating surgical decompression or fixation may be considered for brace therapy, based on the extent of injury and patient age.[7] Due to the common co-occurrence of traumatic brain injury, an unconscious patient of any age should be assumed as possibly having a SCI until complete assessment is possible.[37]

THORACOLUMBAR INJURY CLASSIFICATION SCORE

The TLICS score is commonly used to determine fracture stability and guide surgical decision making, specifically with regards to the need for arthrodesis. In routine practice, it is difficult to apply various alternative classifications, such as the Magerl and AOSpine classifications; the TLICS is a well-validated tool in adults.[43,44] Sellin and colleagues[38] recently studied its applicability to 102 pediatric patients in a multicenter retrospective study that included the authors' group and found high concordance between surgical decision making (operative vs nonoperative) and TLICS score. Although further validation is warranted, the authors recommend the use of the TLICS score as an adjunct in operative decision making for pediatric thoracolumbar trauma.

USE OF BONE MORPHOGENETIC PROTEIN

The use of bone morphogenetic protein (BMP), once common as an adjunct in spinal fusions, is now mired in controversy. Recent studies, however, including a large meta-analysis of the use of BMP in spinal fusions, suggest that the concern over the risks of its use may be overstated.[45]

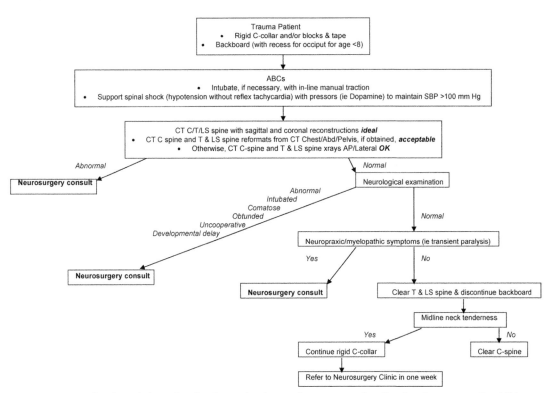

Fig. 7. A proposed CT-based algorithm for the evaluation and treatment of pediatric spine trauma. Establishment of CT-based protocols to clear the pediatric spine of suspected injury has the potential to decrease the time required to accomplish clearance and to reduce the number of missed injuries. abd, abdomen; AP, anterior-posterior; C, cervical; C-collar, cervical collar; LS, lumbosacral; SBP, systolic blood pressure; T, thoracic.

Although several of the adult series included in the meta-analysis by Cahill and colleagues found an increased or a potentially increased cancer risk associated with BMP use, no such risk has been definitively found in children. A series of 57 patients by the authors' group using recombinant human BMP-2 in the pediatric population suggested that it is a safe adjunct to posterior spine fusions of the occipitocervical, cervical, thoracic, lumbar, and lumbosacral spine, with no new cases of cancer over a mean follow-up of 48 months.[46,47] Advocates of BMP note numerous benefits over autograft or allograft, such as decreased operative time, blood loss, donor-site morbidity, transmission of infection associated with use of allograft, and rate of pseduarthrosis.[47] Its theoretically unlimited quantity and availability make it uniquely useful in pediatric spine fusions, especially in surgical management of traumatic fractures that may involve long-segment fusions but small areas of decompression. The authors also found that nationwide, greater than 10% of pediatric spinal fusions included BMP use.[48] Secondary to the variety of studies on the topic, the information available to patients on the Internet can be confusing or even misleading.[49] Thus, regardless of practice

and surgeon's choice, it is important to be familiar with the topic to appropriately counsel patients and their families.

LONG-TERM OUTCOME

The presence of a neurologic deficit at presentation is a major factor in determining long-term outcome. A large majority of lumbar spine fractures in children and younger adolescents are minor and stable and do not present with neurologic deficit.[50] In the thoracic region, it can be variable, depending on level and injury mechanism.

A systematic approach to pediatric spine fractures is needed, with attention to immediate stability, need for decompression of the neural elements, and long-term stability or propensity for healing. Because children have more laxity of the spine, physicians must keep a high suspicion for SCIWORA and, therefore, proceed with more advanced imaging (such as an MRI) when clinically indicated. Previous studies have found that between 7.5% and 30% of patients with thoracolumbar fractures require operative intervention.[50–53]

Long-term outcome after surgical treatment of pediatric thoracolumbar trauma has been studied in several series. Erfani and colleagues[54] reviewed 102 patients over 10 years and found the most common levels to be L1 (31%), L2 (19%), L3 (18%), T12 (16%), and L4 (10%). Among these, only 20% required surgical treatment, with 53.3% of patients receiving posterior spinal instrumentation and fusion for lumbar fractures. Combined anterior and posterior fusion was performed in 20%, specifically those who had lower thoracic or thoracolumbar fractures. Return to baseline neurologic function was seen in 26.7% of patients who underwent spinal stabilization after spinal injury (either cauda equina or incomplete SCI). All patients were found to be independent at follow-up.[54]

Dogan and colleagues[51] reported a similar series of 89 patients, 23 of whom underwent surgery. Lumbar fractures comprised 29.8%, whereas 19.2% were at the thoracolumbar junction. Lumbar fractures comprised a majority of operated fractures (60.9%) as well. At a mean follow-up time of 17.2 months, all patients had stable fixation and early fusion. Those who were treated with bed rest alone for mild lumbar or sacral injuries had gradual return to activity.[51]

Erfani and colleagues[54] also studied quality-of-life outcome. They reported that up to a third of patients (33.3%) noted occasional back pain in the long term. Moller and colleagues[55] noted a rate of only 21.7% of the same in their series of 23 patients. Both series reported minor or no neurologic deficits in the long term. Furthermore, Dogan and colleagues[51] reported no incidence of delayed neurologic deficit and found that 75% of the patients with incomplete spinal cord injuries recovered completely.

REFERENCES

1. Cirak B, Ziegfeld S, Knight VM, et al. Spinal injuries in children. J Pediatr Surg 2004;39(4):607–12.
2. Reynolds R. Pediatric spinal injury. Curr Opin Pediatr 2000;12(1):67–71.
3. Parisini P, Di Silvestre M, Greggi T. Treatment of spinal fractures in children and adolescents: long-term results in 44 patients. Spine (Phila Pa 1976) 2002;27(18):1989–94.
4. Hamilton MG, Myles ST. Pediatric spinal injury: review of 174 hospital admissions. J Neurosurg 1992;77(5):700–4.
5. Clark P, Letts M. Trauma to the thoracic and lumbar spine in the adolescent. Can J Surg 2001;44(5):337–45.
6. Herkowitz HN, Garfin SR, Eismont FJ, et al. Rothman-simeone, the spine. 5th edition. Philadelphia: Saunders-Elsevier; 2006.
7. Slotkin JR, Lu Y, Wood KB. Thoracolumbar spinal trauma in children. Neurosurg Clin N Am 2007;18(4):621–30.
8. Sayama C, Chen T, Trost G, et al. A review of pediatric lumbar spine trauma. Neurosurg Focus 2014;37(1):E6.
9. d'Amato C. Pediatric spinal trauma: injuries in very young children. Clin Orthop Relat Res 2005;(432):34–40.
10. Pang D. Vertebral column and spinal cord injuries in children. In: Winn HR, editor. Youmans neurological surgery. 6th edition. Philadelphia: Elsevier Saunders; 2011. p. 2293–332.
11. Reddy SP, Junewick JJ, Backstrom JW. Distribution of spinal fractures in children: does age, mechanism of injury, or gender play a significant role? Pediatr Radiol 2003;33(11):776–81.
12. Pang D, Pollack IF. Spinal cord injury without radiographic abnormality in children–the SCIWORA syndrome. J Trauma 1989;29(5):654–64.
13. Roche C, Carty H. Spinal trauma in children. Pediatr Radiol 2001;31(10):677–700.
14. Pang D, Wilberger JE Jr. Spinal cord injury without radiographic abnormalities in children. J Neurosurg 1982;57(1):114–29.
15. Swischuk LE, Swischuk PN, John SD. Wedging of C-3 in infants and children: usually a normal finding and not a fracture. Radiology 1993;188(2):523–6.
16. Piatt JH Jr. Pediatric spinal injury in the US: epidemiology and disparities. J Neurosurg Pediatr 2015;16(4):463–71.
17. Rasouli MR, Rahimi-Movaghar V, Maheronnaghsh R, et al. Preventing motor vehicle crashes related spine injuries in children. World J Pediatr 2011;7(4):311–7.
18. Wetmore JM. Delegating to the automobile: experimenting with automotive restraints in the 1970s. Technol Cult 2015;56(2):440–63.
19. Daniels AH, Sobel AD, Eberson CP. Pediatric thoracolumbar spine trauma. J Am Acad Orthop Surg 2013;21(12):707–16.
20. Thomas JG, Boatey J, Brayton A, et al. Neurogenic claudication associated with posterior vertebral rim fractures in children. J Neurosurg Pediatr 2012;10(3):241–5.
21. Sovio OM, Bell HM, Beauchamp RD, et al. Fracture of the lumbar vertebral apophysis. J Pediatr Orthop 1985;5(5):550–2.
22. Yen CH, Chan SK, Ho YF, et al. Posterior lumbar apophyseal ring fractures in adolescents: a report of four cases. J Orthop Surg (hong Kong) 2009;17(1):85–9.
23. Singla AA, Singla AA. Seatbelt syndrome with superior mesenteric artery syndrome: leave nothing to chance! J Surg Case Rep 2015;2015(11) [pii: rjv148].

24. Arkader A, Warner WC Jr, Tolo VT, et al. Pediatric chance fractures: a multicenter perspective. J Pediatr Orthop 2011;31(7):741–4.

25. Santschi M, Lemoine C, Cyr C. The spectrum of seat belt syndrome among Canadian children: results of a two-year population surveillance study. Paediatr Child Health 2008;13(4):279–83.

26. Griffin BR, Watt K, Shields LE, et al. Characteristics of low-speed vehicle run-over events in children: an 11-year review. Inj Prev 2014;20(5):302–9.

27. Congeni J, McCulloch J, Swanson K. Lumbar spondylolysis. A study of natural progression in athletes. Am J Sports Med 1997;25(2):248–53.

28. Drazin D, Shirzadi A, Jeswani S, et al. Direct surgical repair of spondylolysis in athletes: indications, techniques, and outcomes. Neurosurg Focus 2011; 31(5):E9.

29. Buttermann GR, Garvey TA, Hunt AF, et al. Lumbar fusion results related to diagnosis. Spine (Phila Pa 1976) 1998;23(1):116–27.

30. Brennan RP, Smucker PY, Horn EM. Minimally invasive image-guided direct repair of bilateral L-5 pars interarticularis defects. Neurosurg Focus 2008;25(2):E13.

31. Noggle JC, Sciubba DM, Samdani AF, et al. Minimally invasive direct repair of lumbar spondylolysis with a pedicle screw and hook construct. Neurosurg Focus 2008;25(2):E15.

32. Buldini B, Amigoni A, Faggin R, et al. Spinal cord injury without radiographic abnormalities. Eur J Pediatr 2006;165(2):108–11.

33. Henrys P, Lyne ED, Lifton C, et al. Clinical review of cervical spine injuries in children. Clin Orthop Relat Res 1977;(129):172–6.

34. Pang D. Spinal cord injury without radiographic abnormality in children, 2 decades later. Neurosurgery 2004;55(6):1325–42 [discussion: 1342–3].

35. Launay F, Leet AI, Sponseller PD. Pediatric spinal cord injury without radiographic abnormality: a meta-analysis. Clin Orthop Relat Res 2005;(433):166–70.

36. Yamaguchi S, Hida K, Akino M, et al. A case of pediatric thoracic SCIWORA following minor trauma. Childs Nerv Syst 2002;18(5):241–3.

37. Jea A, Luerssen TG. Central nervous system injury. 7th edition. Philadelphia: Elsevier Saunders; 2012.

38. Sellin JN, Steele WJ 3rd, Simpson L, et al. Multicenter retrospective evaluation of the validity of the Thoracolumbar Injury Classification and Severity Score system in children. J Neurosurg Pediatr 2016;18:164–70.

39. Leroux J, Vivier PH, Ould Slimane M, et al. Early diagnosis of thoracolumbar spine fractures in children. A prospective study. Orthop Traumatol Surg Res 2013;99(1):60–5.

40. Denis F. The three column spine and its significance in the classification of acute thoracolumbar spinal injuries. Spine (Phila Pa 1976) 1983;8(8):817–31.

41. Vaccaro AR, Oner C, Kepler CK, et al. AOSpine thoracolumbar spine injury classification system: fracture description, neurological status, and key modifiers. Spine (Phila Pa 1976) 2013;38(23): 2028–37.

42. Lee JY, Vaccaro AR, Lim MR, et al. Thoracolumbar injury classification and severity score: a new paradigm for the treatment of thoracolumbar spine trauma. J Orthop Sci 2005;10(6):671–5.

43. Joaquim AF, Fernandes YB, Cavalcante RA, et al. Evaluation of the thoracolumbar injury classification system in thoracic and lumbar spinal trauma. Spine (Phila Pa 1976) 2011;36(1):33–6.

44. Joaquim AF, Daubs MD, Lawrence BD, et al. Retrospective evaluation of the validity of the Thoracolumbar Injury Classification System in 458 consecutively treated patients. Spine J 2013; 13(12):1760–5.

45. Cahill KS, McCormick PC, Levi AD. A comprehensive assessment of the risk of bone morphogenetic protein use in spinal fusion surgery and postoperative cancer diagnosis. J Neurosurg Spine 2015;23(1):86–93.

46. Fahim DK, Whitehead WE, Curry DJ, et al. Routine use of recombinant human bone morphogenetic protein-2 in posterior fusions of the pediatric spine: safety profile and efficacy in the early postoperative period. Neurosurgery 2010;67(5):1195–204 [discussion: 1204].

47. Sayama C, Willsey M, Chintagumpala M, et al. Routine use of recombinant human bone morphogenetic protein-2 in posterior fusions of the pediatric spine and incidence of cancer. J Neurosurg Pediatr 2015;16(1):4–13.

48. Wang M, Abbah SA, Hu T, et al. Polyelectrolyte complex carrier enhances therapeutic efficiency and safety profile of bone morphogenetic protein-2 in porcine lumbar interbody fusion model. Spine (Phila Pa 1976) 2015;40(13):964–73.

49. Huang M, Briceno V, Lam SK, et al. Survey of the effectiveness of internet information on patient education for bone morphogenetic protein. World Neurosurg 2016;87:613–8.

50. Mortazavi MM, Dogan S, Civelek E, et al. Pediatric multilevel spine injuries: an institutional experience. Childs Nerv Syst 2011;27(7):1095–100.

51. Dogan S, Safavi-Abbasi S, Theodore N, et al. Thoracolumbar and sacral spinal injuries in children and adolescents: a review of 89 cases. J Neurosurg 2007;106(6 Suppl):426–33.

52. Kraus R, Stahl JP, Heiss C, et al. Fractures of the thoracic and lumbar spine in children and adolescents. Unfallchirurg 2013;116(5):435–41 [in German].

53. Puisto V, Kaariainen S, Impinen A, et al. Incidence of spinal and spinal cord injuries and their surgical treatment in children and adolescents: a

population-based study. Spine (Phila Pa 1976) 2010; 35(1):104–7.

54. Erfani MA, Pourabbas B, Nouraie H, et al. Results of fusion and instrumentation of thoracic and lumbar vertebral fractures in children: a prospective ten-year study. Musculoskelet Surg 2014;98(2): 107–14.

55. Moller A, Hasserius R, Besjakov J, et al. Vertebral fractures in late adolescence: a 27 to 47-year follow-up. Eur Spine J 2006;15(8):1247–54.

Treatment of Odontoid Fractures in the Aging Population

Jian Guan, MD, Erica F. Bisson, MD, MPH*

KEYWORDS

- Odontoid fracture • Elderly • Cervical bracing • Cervical fusion

KEY POINTS

- Odontoid fractures are the most common fracture type among the elderly population.
- Radiographic evaluation of odontoid fractures with plain films, computed tomographic imaging, and MRI plays a major role in treatment decisions.
- An array of conservative measures exists for the management of odontoid fractures ranging from semirigid orthoses to halo immobilization. Each type of brace has its own distinct risks and benefits.
- The 2 primary categories of surgical intervention for odontoid fractures are ventral odontoid screw fixation and posterior atlantoaxial arthrodesis. Fusion rates for both procedures are excellent in most patients, but pitfalls exist with both operative approaches that must be considered when selecting patients for these operations.
- There is a strong need for further high-quality research into optimal management of odontoid fractures in the elderly, a need that will only increase as the population ages worldwide.

INTRODUCTION

Nearly 20% of cervical fractures involve the odontoid process.[1] This fracture pattern most often results from a forced hyperflexion or hyperextension mechanism.[2] The elderly are especially vulnerable to this injury pattern[3] and frequently present with odontoid injury after ground-level falls with associated hyperextension.[4] The optimal management strategy for odontoid fractures remains controversial,[5] especially in the elderly,[6] because of the high morbidity and mortality with both conservative and operative intervention.[7] As the population ages, the landscape of spinal surgery is poised to shift dramatically,[8,9] and the treatment of these patients becomes an increasingly common problem among practitioners treating spinal conditions. This review discusses the management of odontoid fractures among the elderly, with a focus on the various treatment options and their outcomes.

PATIENT EVALUATION

The definition of the elderly patient is not widely agreed on, and, as in other patient populations, there is significant heterogeneity among patients of this age group.[10] Among patients who are older than 70 years, however, odontoid fractures comprise the most common cervical spine facture and in those older than 80 years the most common overall spine fracture.[11] Evaluation of patients in whom odontoid fracture is suspected consists of radiographic studies in addition to clinical evaluation. These studies can aid in definition of the fracture and in the decision on how to manage the injury.

Disclosures: Dr Bisson has stock ownership in nView. Dr Mazur has no disclosures.
Department of Neurosurgery, Clinical Neurosciences Center, University of Utah, 175 North Medical Drive East, Salt Lake City, UT 84132, USA
* Corresponding author.
E-mail address: neuropub@hsc.utah.edu

Neurosurg Clin N Am 28 (2017) 115–123
http://dx.doi.org/10.1016/j.nec.2016.07.001
1042-3680/17/© 2016 Elsevier Inc. All rights reserved.

Radiographic Evaluation

Anderson and D'Alonzo[12] defined 3 types of dens fractures based on radiographic fracture pattern. Fractures involving only the tip of the odontoid are characterized as type I, those through the base as type II, and those that extend into the vertebral body as type III (**Fig. 1**). Although most type III and almost all type I fractures eventually fuse with conservative management in a cervical collar, nonunion rates for type II injuries are significantly higher.[13]

The initial diagnostic evaluation of traumatic cervical spine injuries often includes plain radiographs, usually consisting of an anterior–posterior projection, a lateral projection, and an open-mouth view for visualization of the odontoid.[14] In cases in which a fracture is identified on plain radiographs, and in those in which the index of suspicion is high, radiographs are generally followed by computerized tomography (CT).[15] CT allows for both a confirmation of the presence of a fracture and improved definition of fracture morphology for use in subsequent management decisions.[16] Indeed, the effectiveness of CT for cervical spine trauma, combined with its ubiquity in modern practice, led some to question the need for plain radiographs in this patient population.

The role of MRI in odontoid fractures remains an area of debate. Although ligamentous injury, specifically of the transverse atlantal ligament, may be missed on plain radiographs and CT, the incidence of this seems to be low—between 0% and 10%.[17–19] Despite the rarity of this injury, the integrity of the transverse ligament is an important consideration in the treatment algorithm. Although well-aligned bony fractures may heal with orthosis, ligamentous injury in addition to the fracture has a significantly lower healing rate.[20] Additionally, if the prospect of operative intervention is entertained, odontoid screw fixation would not be appropriate in the setting of ligamentous injury.[21]

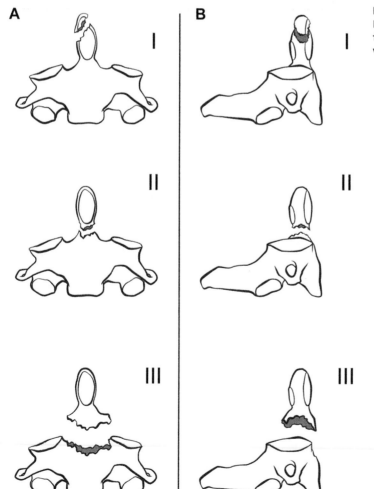

A

I

II

III

B

I

II

III

Fig. 1. The Anderson and D'Alonzo[12] odontoid fracture classification. (*A*) Anterior/posterior views. (*B*) lateral views.

Complicating decisions about the use of MRI in the elderly are that MRI findings may also be difficult to interpret in this population because of their bone composition and misinterpretation can lead to misdiagnosis.[22]

Risk Factors for Odontoid Fracture

The predilection for odontoid fractures in the elderly is believed to be secondary to progressive degenerative changes in the cervical spine as individuals age.[23] As these changes occur, motion in the subaxial cervical spine decreases, leaving the C1-2 segment as the most mobile portion of the neck. One recent study suggests that elderly individuals with severe osteoporosis and with significant degeneration of the atlanto-odontoid joint combined with a smoothened lateral atlantoaxial joint may be at higher risk for type II odontoid fractures after trauma.[24] A vascular mechanism has been implicated as well, with a watershed area at the base of the dens that is more pronounced in the elderly, contributing to fracture risk.[6]

Premorbid clinical risk factors for odontoid fractures after trauma in the elderly population have not been well studied,[7] although variables ranging from the location of the fall[25] to racial/ethnic disparities[26] have been investigated in the general trauma literature. As is the case with other traumatic injuries, worse premorbid health seems to be associated with increased morbidity and mortality in odontoid fractures regardless of management strategy,[7] as is the presence of neurologic deficit.[27]

CONSERVATIVE MANAGEMENT

Conservative management for odontoid fractures most commonly consists of rigid external fixation—with either a hard cervical collar or halo immobilization. These options are sometimes chosen in the elderly because of concerns for operative morbidity in this fragile population.[28] This risk must be counterbalanced with the higher rates of nonunion with external immobilization alone.[29]

Orthotic Types

A variety of braces are currently marketed for the management of cervical injury, falling into 4 broad categories as defined by Johnson and colleagues.[30] The least restrictive cervical collar is the so-called soft collar. Although comfortable and economical, soft collars provide little in the way of motion limitation and, therefore, play little role in the management of odontoid fractures. The second category is the semirigid orthosis, generally comprising 2 interlocking polymer segments; this category includes the Aspen (**Fig. 2**) and Miami-J collars.[31] These collars provide significantly more motion limitation—especially of rotational movement—compared with soft collars, at the cost of a lower degree of comfort.[32] The Minerva brace includes a thoracic element to the construct and commonly incorporates a posterior occipital bolster with a mandibular brace, providing further limitation of flexion and extension. The most restrictive external orthotic solution is the halo vest. Although offering the maximal movement limitation in all planes—flexion/extension, rotation, and

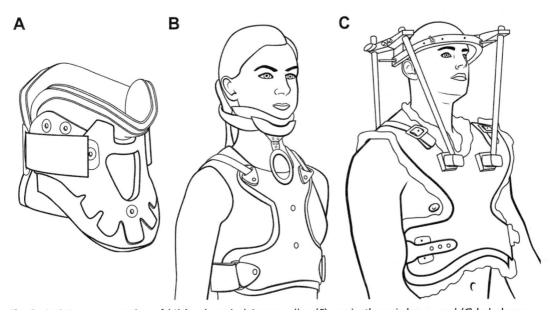

Fig. 2. Artist's representation of (A) hard cervical Aspen collar, (B) cervicothoracic brace, and (C) halo brace.

lateral bending[31,32]—the halo requires physician expertise for application.[33] The use of pins for halo vest fixation also necessitates the use of local anesthetic and can lead to various complications, including infection, nerve injury, and even fractures and durotomy.[34]

Outcomes and Complications

There remains a significant lack of high-quality evidence in the literature with regard to outcomes after conservative management of odontoid fractures in the elderly,[6] with most studies on the topic consisting of small case series. Interpretation of the results is hampered by the use of a variety of brace types between and even within individual studies.

Rates of bony fusion with external immobilization and type II fractures vary depending on the study from as low as 23% to as high as 82%.[35–37] Although osseous fusion has classically been the standard of success in the healing of odontoid fractures, a body of literature exists suggesting that in asymptomatic patients who are stable on flexion/extension imaging, so-called fibrous union should also be considered an acceptable outcome.[38,39]

As described previously, the halo brace provides the most rigid external construct available, and historically many practitioners have advocated its use as the first-line treatment for elderly patients with odontoid fractures.[37,39] Fusion rates with halo fixation can reach as high as 90%, although significant variability exists because of the heterogeneity of the literature.[6] Despite the rigidity offered by the halo, significant attention was paid in the last decade to the high rate of complications associated with their use in the elderly. Morbidity—primarily consisting of pneumonias—was reported in up to 52% of this patient population with halo vest immobilization.[40] Mortality rates are often similarly high, leading one author to deem the halo a "death sentence" for older patients with cervical fractures.[41] Despite these concerns, in carefully chosen cases, many surgeons continue to have high rates of success with halo fixation.[42]

Concerns over the use of halo fixation led some to use semirigid braces and cervicothoracic bracing systems such as the Minerva brace to treat patients with dens fractures. Sime and colleagues[43] recently did a meta-analysis of 13 studies examining differences in outcomes and complication rates between these alternative systems and the halo. With regard to achieving stability—defined as osseous fusion or fibrous nonunion without motion on flexion/extension

films—patients placed in halos had a success rate of 84%, whereas those in semirigid orthoses had a success rate of 63%, and those placed in Minerva braces had a success rate of 65%. Halo patients had an overall mortality rate of 25%, whereas those in semirigid orthoses had a mortality rate of 28%, and those with Minerva braces had a mortality rate of 25%. None of these differences, however, reached statistical significance. These findings were supported by a recent combined prospective/retrospective analysis of halo fixation versus semirigid orthoses by Patel and colleagues[44] that also found no significant difference in outcomes, although the authors noted that bony union was more common with the halo.

Although conservative measures may sometimes be the treatment option of choice for patients and their families,[45] care must be taken to avoid neurologic catastrophe. Close follow-up including surveillance radiography is necessary, as symptoms of progressive myelopathy were reported to develop years after the initial injury.[46]

SURGICAL INTERVENTION

There are many indications for surgical intervention in odontoid fractures, including instability, symptomatology, and psychosocial variables, all of which must be carefully weighed with the risks of surgery itself and tailored to the individual patient.[46] Symptoms in these patients can range from neck pain to radicular symptoms to myelopathy[45] and may worsen with time or with subsequent trauma. There is evidence that surgical intervention may reduce mortality among elderly patients with odontoid fractures compared with conservative management[47,48] and that the elderly may be at particular risk for failure of osseous healing with bracing alone.[49,50] There is also evidence that quality-of-life outcomes for elderly patients with nonoperative treatment are worse than those of patients who receive surgery.[51]

Surgical intervention for odontoid fractures can be broadly divided into 2 categories: dorsal fixation, consisting of a variety of atlantoaxial constructs, and ventral fixation, with the placement of a direct odontoid screw.

Ventral Fixation

Initially reported by Nakanishi in 1980,[52] direct screw fixation of the odontoid process was first described in the English-language literature by Böhler.[53] With proper technique, the procedure allows for stabilization of the fracture with minimal soft tissue disruption and maintenance of rotation at the atlantoaxial joint, all while avoiding the need for autograft or allograft (**Fig. 3**).[52] Rates of fusion

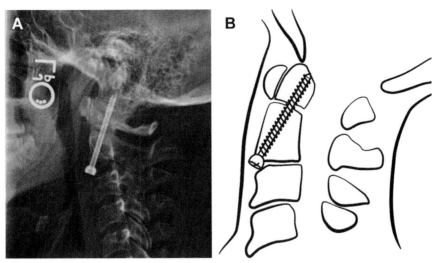

Fig. 3. (A) Lateral radiograph and (B) artist's representation of odontoid screw fixation of type II odontoid fracture.

in patients undergoing odontoid screw fixation are high, with a rate of 88% in the series of 147 cases by Apfelbaum and colleagues.[54] Complications of odontoid screw fixation in elderly patients most commonly consist of pneumonia and dysphagia,[55] although more serious complications such as intraoperative hardware failure and mortality have been reported.[56,57]

Despite favorable outcomes in many patients, there are contraindications to odontoid screw fixation that must be carefully assessed before surgery. Patients with comminuted fractures of the axis, fractures with transverse ligament disruption, and pathologic fractures are poor candidates for odontoid screw placement.[21,54] Fractures greater than 6 months of age are also a contraindication, with data showing that chronic fractures have dramatically lower rates of fusion compared with more acute injuries.[54] Historically, anteriorly oriented oblique fractures were thought to be a contraindication for odontoid screw placement, as the direction of the fracture parallels the screw trajectory and may lead to displacement during tightening of the screw, although there is some literature that suggests this may be overcome.[58] Patient body habitus, specifically a broad barrel chest or a short neck, can lead to difficulty with achieving an optimal trajectory for odontoid screw placement, although this obstacle can be overcome with experience and variations in technique.

Osteoporosis can lead to significantly decreased rates of fusion in patients who undergo ventral odontoid screw fixation.[59] This finding led to interest in the augmentation of the construct with polymethylmethacrylate-based cements. Early studies found that such augmentation significantly improves the strength of the construct,[60] and early case reports showed feasibility in patients.[61] Some have advocated the placement of 2 screws in the construct to improve biomechanical stability in patients. Although some biomechanical studies showed no difference in failure strength between 1 screw and 2 screws,[62] a study by Dailey and colleagues[63] found significant improvements in fusion rate with the 2-screw construct in the elderly population.

Dorsal Fixation

Dorsal approaches to fusion of the upper cervical spine have expanded considerably over the last several decades. Gallie[64] described one of the earliest fusion techniques in the late 1930s, using sublaminar wiring combined with iliac crest graft. In the 1970s, Tucker[65] reported the use of clamps to stabilize the C1-2 joint, attaching them to the laminae and interposing iliac crest graft between the spinous processes. Modern methods of screw fixation were developed by several practitioners, from the transarticular technique of Jeanneret and Magerl[56] to the lateral mass/pars constructs of Goel and colleagues[66] (**Fig. 4**).

Fusion rates for modern techniques of dorsal atlantoaxial fusion are excellent and in some studies approach 100%.[12] A recent meta-analysis found significantly better fusion rates for posterior fusion compared with odontoid screw fixation.[67] Morbidity associated with posterior fusion of the atlantoaxial joint includes the

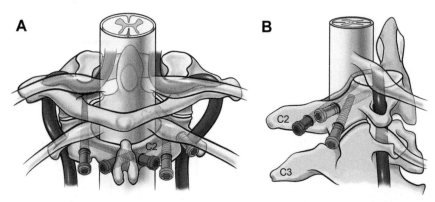

Fig. 4. (*A*) Anterior-posterior and (*B*) lateral representations of C1-C2 posterior screw fixation techniques. Ideal screw trajectories for the transarticular (*pink*), translaminar (*blue*), pars (*orange*), and pedicle (*green*) fixation techniques are shown. (Reproduced with permission from Department of Neurosurgery, University of Utah.)

elimination of all rotation at the atlantoaxial junction, thus, decreasing overall cervical rotation by as much as 50%.[68] Posterior spinal fusion also involves significantly more soft tissue dissection, thus, increasing both operating times and blood loss.[20] Posterior approaches also place the vertebral arteries at risk, possibly leading to stroke or even death.[69,70] As a result of these risks, careful evaluation of preoperative imaging—especially for possible aberrancies in the path of the vertebral artery or variations in the bony anatomy of the foramina—is crucial.[71] Any brisk bleeding encountered during the procedure should be concerning for possible vertebral injury, and instrumentation of the contralateral side should be avoided until angiographic imaging can be obtained.

Other complications of posterior cervical fusion for odontoid fractures are similar to those of anterior fixation. The most common complications are pneumonia and dysphagia, which may occur in a significant percentage of patients and may necessitate intensive care level treatment and prolonged hospitalization.[72] A less frequently described complication is a persistent occipital neuralgia secondary to transection of the C2 nerve during surgery. This neuralgia can lead to significant patient discomfort and anxiety that may be refractory to management.[73] Despite these complications, posterior spinal fusion for odontoid fractures in the elderly remains an important tool in the armamentarium for treating these patients, especially in those with contraindications for placement of an odontoid screw such as chronic fractures and transverse ligament injury.[20]

SUMMARY

With the aging of the world's population, the frequency of type II odontoid fractures will inevitably increase. Although multiple treatment options exist for these patients, morbidity and mortality from odontoid fractures remain high among the elderly. There continues to be a significant lack of high-quality evidence to guide treatment of odontoid fractures in the aged, with most of the literature consisting of small case series. Further research is needed to identify which patients benefit most from the available treatment modalities, and further refinement of operative and postoperative techniques are needed to reduce complications associated with surgical intervention.

REFERENCES

1. Hadley MN, Browner C, Sonntag VK. Axis fractures: a comprehensive review of management and treatment in 107 cases. Neurosurgery 1985;17(2):281–90.
2. Koech F, Ackland HM, Varma DK, et al. Nonoperative management of type II odontoid fractures in the elderly. Spine (Phila Pa 1976) 2008;33(26):2881–6.
3. Huybregts JG, Jacobs WC, Peul WC, et al. Rationale and design of the INNOVATE Trial: an international cooperative study on surgical versus conservative treatment for odontoid fractures in the elderly. BMC Musculoskelet Disord 2014;15:7.
4. Muller EJ, Wick M, Russe O, et al. Management of odontoid fractures in the elderly. Eur Spine J 1999;8(5):360–5.
5. Platzer P, Thalhammer G, Ostermann R, et al. Anterior screw fixation of odontoid fractures comparing younger and elderly patients. Spine (Phila Pa 1976) 2007;32(16):1714–20.
6. Pal D, Sell P, Grevitt M. Type II odontoid fractures in the elderly: an evidence-based narrative review of management. Eur Spine J 2011;20(2):195–204.
7. Woods BI, Hohl JB, Braly B, et al. Mortality in elderly patients following operative and nonoperative

management of odontoid fractures. J Spinal Disord Tech 2014;27(6):321–6.

8. O'Lynnger TM, Zuckerman SL, Morone PJ, et al. Trends for spine surgery for the elderly: implications for access to healthcare in North America. Neurosurgery 2015;77(Suppl 4):S136–41.

9. Fehlings MG, Tetreault L, Nater A, et al. The aging of the global population: the changing epidemiology of disease and spinal disorders. Neurosurgery 2015; 77(Suppl 4):S1–5.

10. Ruiz M, Bottle A, Long S, et al. Multi-morbidity in hospitalised older patients: who are the complex elderly? PLoS One 2015;10(12):e0145372.

11. Ryan MD, Henderson JJ. The epidemiology of fractures and fracture-dislocations of the cervical spine. Injury 1992;23(1):38–40.

12. Anderson LD, D'Alonzo RT. Fractures of the odontoid process of the axis. J Bone Joint Surg Am 1974;56(8):1663–74.

13. Hsu WK, Anderson PA. Odontoid fractures: update on management. J Am Acad Orthop Surg 2010; 18(7):383–94.

14. Keats TE, Dalinka MK, Alazraki N, et al. Cervical spine trauma. American College of Radiology. ACR Appropriateness Criteria. Radiology 2000; 215(Suppl):243–6.

15. Shaffer MA, Doris PE. Limitation of the cross table lateral view in detecting cervical spine injuries: a retrospective analysis. Ann Emerg Med 1981; 10(10):508–13.

16. Sanchez B, Waxman K, Jones T, et al. Cervical spine clearance in blunt trauma: evaluation of a computed tomography-based protocol. J Trauma 2005;59(1): 179–83.

17. Greene KA, Dickman CA, Marciano FF, et al. Transverse atlantal ligament disruption associated with odontoid fractures. Spine (Phila Pa 1976) 1994; 19(20):2307–14.

18. Sayama CM, Fassett DR, Apfelbaum RI. The utility of MRI in the evaluation of odontoid fractures. J Spinal Disord Tech 2008;21(7):524–6.

19. Debernardi A, D'Aliberti G, Talamonti G, et al. Traumatic (type II) odontoid fracture with transverse atlantal ligament injury: a controversial event. World Neurosurg 2013;79(5–6):779–83.

20. Joaquim AF, Patel AA. Surgical treatment of Type II odontoid fractures: anterior odontoid screw fixation or posterior cervical instrumented fusion? Neurosurg Focus 2015;38(4):E11.

21. Spence KF Jr, Decker S, Sell KW. Bursting atlantal fracture associated with rupture of the transverse ligament. J Bone Joint Surg Am 1970; 52(3):543–9.

22. Lensing FD, Bisson EF, Wiggins RH 3rd, et al. Reliability of the STIR sequence for acute type II odontoid fractures. AJNR Am J Neuroradiol 2014;35(8): 1642–6.

23. Brolin K. Neck injuries among the elderly in Sweden. Inj Control Saf Promot 2003;10(3):155–64.

24. Watanabe M, Sakai D, Yamamoto Y, et al. Analysis of predisposing factors in elderly people with type II odontoid fracture. Spine J 2014;14(6):861–6.

25. Kim SH. Risk factors for severe injury following indoor and outdoor falls in geriatric patients. Arch Gerontol Geriatr 2016;62:75–82.

26. Kiely DK, Kim DH, Gross AL, et al. Fall risk is not black and white. J Health Dispar Res Pract 2015; 8(3):72–84.

27. Patel A, Smith HE, Radcliff K, et al. Odontoid fractures with neurologic deficit have higher mortality and morbidity. Clin Orthop Relat Res 2012;470(6): 1614–20.

28. Rizk E, Kelleher JP, Zalatimo O, et al. Nonoperative management of odontoid fractures: a review of 59 cases. Clin Neurol Neurosurg 2013;115(9): 1653–6.

29. Huybregts JG, Jacobs WC, Vleggeert-Lankamp CL. The optimal treatment of type II and III odontoid fractures in the elderly: a systematic review. Eur Spine J 2013;22(1):1–13.

30. Johnson RM, Hart DL, Simmons EF, et al. Cervical orthoses. A study comparing their effectiveness in restricting cervical motion in normal subjects. J Bone Joint Surg Am 1977;59(3):332–9.

31. Lauweryns P. Role of conservative treatment of cervical spine injuries. Eur Spine J 2010;19(Suppl 1): S23–6.

32. Richter D, Latta LL, Milne EL, et al. The stabilizing effects of different orthoses in the intact and unstable upper cervical spine: a cadaver study. J Trauma 2001;50(5):848–54.

33. Botte MJ, Garfin SR, Byrne TP, et al. The halo skeletal fixator. Principles of application and maintenance. Clin Orthop Relat Res 1989;(239):12–8.

34. Garfin SR, Botte MJ, Waters RL, et al. Complications in the use of the halo fixation device. J Bone Joint Surg Am 1986;68(3):320–5.

35. Ryan MD, Taylor TK. Odontoid fractures in the elderly. J Spinal Disord 1993;6(5):397–401.

36. Muller EJ, Schwinnen I, Fischer K, et al. Non-rigid immobilisation of odontoid fractures. Eur Spine J 2003;12(5):522–5.

37. Stoney J, O'Brien J, Wilde P. Treatment of type-two odontoid fractures in halothoracic vests. J Bone Joint Surg Br 1998;80(3):452–5.

38. Lieberman IH, Webb JK. Cervical spine injuries in the elderly. J Bone Joint Surg Br 1994;76(6):877–81.

39. Ekong CE, Schwartz ML, Tator CH, et al. Odontoid fracture: management with early mobilization using the halo device. Neurosurgery 1981;9(6): 631–7.

40. Horn EM, Theodore N, Feiz-Erfan I, et al. Complications of halo fixation in the elderly. J Neurosurg Spine 2006;5(1):46–9.

41. Majercik S, Tashjian RZ, Biffl WL, et al. Halo vest immobilization in the elderly: a death sentence? J Trauma 2005;59(2):350–6 [discussion: 356–8].

42. van Middendorp JJ, Slooff WB, Nellestein WR, et al. Incidence of and risk factors for complications associated with halo-vest immobilization: a prospective, descriptive cohort study of 239 patients. J Bone Joint Surg Am 2009;91(1):71–9.

43. Sime D, Pitt V, Pattuwage L, et al. Non-surgical interventions for the management of type 2 dens fractures: a systematic review. ANZ J Surg 2014;84(5):320–5.

44. Patel A, Zakaria R, Al-Mahfoudh R, et al. Conservative management of type II and III odontoid fractures in the elderly at a regional spine centre: A prospective and retrospective cohort study. Br J Neurosurg 2015;29(2):249–53.

45. Momin E, Harsh V, Fridley J, et al. Reliability of treating asymptomatic traumatic type II dens fractures in patients over age 80: A retrospective series. J Craniovertebr Junction Spine 2015;6(4):166–72.

46. Crockard HA, Heilman AE, Stevens JM. Progressive myelopathy secondary to odontoid fractures: clinical, radiological, and surgical features. J Neurosurg 1993;78(4):579–86.

47. Smith JS, Kepler CK, Kopjar B, et al. Effect of type II odontoid fracture nonunion on outcome among elderly patients treated without surgery: based on the AOSpine North America geriatric odontoid fracture study. Spine (Phila Pa 1976) 2013;38(26):2240–6.

48. Chapman J, Smith JS, Kopjar B, et al. The AOSpine North America Geriatric Odontoid Fracture Mortality Study: a retrospective review of mortality outcomes for operative versus nonoperative treatment of 322 patients with long-term follow-up. Spine (Phila Pa 1976) 2013;38(13):1098–104.

49. Polin RS, Szabo T, Bogaev CA, et al. Nonoperative management of Types II and III odontoid fractures: the Philadelphia collar versus the halo vest. Neurosurgery 1996;38(3):450–6 [discussion: 456–7].

50. Lennarson PJ, Mostafavi H, Traynelis VC, et al. Management of type II dens fractures: a case-control study. Spine (Phila Pa 1976) 2000;25(10):1234–7.

51. Vaccaro AR, Kepler CK, Kopjar B, et al. Functional and quality-of-life outcomes in geriatric patients with type-II dens fracture. J Bone Joint Surg Am 2013;95(8):729–35.

52. Nakanishi T. Internal fixation of the odontoid fracture. Cent Jpn J Orthop Traumatic Surg 1980;23:399–406.

53. Böhler J. Anterior stabilization for acute fractures and non-unions of the dens. J Bone Joint Surg Am 1982;64(1):18–27.

54. Apfelbaum RI, Lonser RR, Veres R, et al. Direct anterior screw fixation for recent and remote odontoid fractures. J Neurosurg 2000;93(2 Suppl):227–36.

55. Vasudevan K, Grossberg JA, Spader HS, et al. Age increases the risk of immediate postoperative dysphagia and pneumonia after odontoid screw fixation. Clin Neurol Neurosurg 2014;126:185–9.

56. Jeanneret B, Magerl F. Primary posterior fusion C1/2 in odontoid fractures: indications, technique, and results of transarticular screw fixation. J Spinal Disord 1992;5(4):464–75.

57. Jeanneret B, Vernet O, Frei S, et al. Atlantoaxial mobility after screw fixation of the odontoid: a computed tomographic study. J Spinal Disord 1991;4(2):203–11.

58. Cho DC, Sung JK. Is all anterior oblique fracture orientation really a contraindication to anterior screw fixation of type II and rostral shallow type III odontoid fractures? J Korean Neurosurg Soc 2011;49(6):345–50.

59. Chiba K, Fujimura Y, Toyama Y, et al. Anterior screw fixation for odontoid fracture: clinical results in 45 cases. Eur Spine J 1993;2(2):76–81.

60. Waschke A, Berger-Roscher N, Kielstein H, et al. Cement augmented anterior odontoid screw fixation is biomechanically advantageous in osteoporotic patients with Anderson Type II fractures. J Spinal Disord Tech 2015;28(3):E126–32.

61. Terreaux L, Loubersac T, Hamel O, et al. Odontoid balloon kyphoplasty associated with screw fixation for Type II fracture in 2 elderly patients. J Neurosurg Spine 2015;22(3):246–52.

62. Sasso R, Doherty BJ, Crawford MJ, et al. Biomechanics of odontoid fracture fixation. Comparison of the one- and two-screw technique. Spine (Phila Pa 1976) 1993;18(14):1950–3.

63. Dailey AT, Hart D, Finn MA, et al. Anterior fixation of odontoid fractures in an elderly population. J Neurosurg Spine 2010;12(1):1–8.

64. Gallie W. Fractures and dislocations of the cervical spine. Am J Surg 1939;3:495–9.

65. Tucker HH. Technical report: method of fixation of subluxed or dislocated cervical spine below C1-C2. Can J Neurol Sci 1975;2(4):381–2.

66. Goel A, Desai KI, Muzumdar DP. Atlantoaxial fixation using plate and screw method: a report of 160 treated patients. Neurosurgery 2002;51(6):1351–6 [discussion: 1356–7].

67. Shen Y, Miao J, Li C, et al. A meta-analysis of the fusion rate from surgical treatment for odontoid fractures: anterior odontoid screw versus posterior C1-C2 arthrodesis. Eur Spine J 2015;24(8):1649–57.

68. Smith HE, Vaccaro AR, Maltenfort M, et al. Trends in surgical management for type II odontoid fracture: 20 years of experience at a regional spinal cord injury center. Orthopedics 2008;31(7):650.

69. Prabhu VC, France JC, Voelker JL, et al. Vertebral artery pseudoaneurysm complicating posterior C1-2 transarticular screw fixation: case report. Surg Neurol 2001;55(1):29–33 [discussion: 33–4].

70. Yoon KW, Ko JH, Cho CS, et al. Endovascular treatment of vertebral artery injury during cervical posterior fusion (C1 lateral mass screw). A case report. Interv Neuroradiol 2013;19(3):370–6.

71. Elliott RE, Tanweer O. The prevalence of the ponticulus posticus (arcuate foramen) and its importance in the Goel-Harms procedure: meta-analysis and review of the literature. World Neurosurg 2014;82(1–2):e335–43.

72. Ryang YM, Torok E, Janssen I, et al. Early morbidity and mortality in 50 very elderly patients after posterior atlantoaxial fusion for traumatic odontoid fractures. World Neurosurg 2016;87:381–91.

73. Yeom JS, Buchowski JM, Kim HJ, et al. Postoperative occipital neuralgia with and without C2 nerve root transection during atlantoaxial screw fixation: a post-hoc comparative outcome study of prospectively collected data. Spine J 2013;13(7):786–95.

Treatment of Facet Injuries in the Cervical Spine

Navid Khezri, MD[a], Tamir Ailon, MD, MPH, FRCSC[b],
Brian K. Kwon, MD, PhD, FRCSC[c],*

KEYWORDS

- Cervical spine facet injury • Prereduction MRI • Closed reduction of displaced cervical facet injury
- Surgical approach

KEY POINTS

- Numerous classification schemes have been developed to characterize subaxial cervical spine injury. The most recent schemes, such as the Subaxial Cervical Spine Injury Classification System (SLIC) and the AOSpine Subaxial Cervical Spine Classification System, take into account morphology, discoligamentous integrity, and neurologic status.
- Closed reduction of facet dislocations can be performed safely in alert, examinable patients, although concerns about the small risk of neurologic injury secondary to disk herniation justify conducting a prereduction MRI.
- Unilateral facet fractures with minimal displacement and no neurologic deficit can be managed operatively or nonoperatively, although the evidence suggests that better radiographic and clinical outcomes are achieved with surgical treatment.
- Anterior and posterior approaches can both be used successfully for the surgical management of facet injuries, and each has advantages and disadvantages. The anterior approach is well tolerated, allows one to address a disk herniation, and provides a high union rate with good sagittal alignment. The posterior approach allows for easier open reduction and biomechanically superior fixation.

INTRODUCTION

Cervical spine facet injuries comprise a spectrum of injuries ranging from undisplaced unilateral facet fractures to severely displaced bilateral facet fracture-dislocations. The likelihood of neurologic deficit increases in proportion to the energy of the mechanism and the severity of injury to the spinal column. Many classification systems have been developed to characterize cervical spine injuries. The more recent AOSpine subaxial cervical

spine injury classification system is based on morphology and additional descriptors for facet injures, neurologic status, and patient-specific modifiers. Several questions remain controversial regarding the management of cervical facet fractures. These questions include the following:

- What is the risk of neurologic injury during a closed reduction of a facet dislocation?
- Is surgery or conservative management preferable for isolated facet fractures?

Disclosures: None.
[a] Division of Neurosurgery, University of British Columbia, 3100, 950 West 10th Avenue, Vancouver, British Columbia V5Z 1M9, Canada; [b] Vancouver Spine Surgery Institute, Division of Neurosurgery, Department of Surgery, University of British Columbia, 818 West 10th Avenue, Vancouver, British Columbia V5Z 1M9, Canada; [c] Vancouver Spine Surgery Institute, Department of Orthopaedics, University of British Columbia, 818 West 10th Avenue, Vancouver, British Columbia V5Z 1M9, Canada
* Corresponding author.
E-mail address: brian.kwon@ubc.ca

Neurosurg Clin N Am 28 (2017) 125–137
http://dx.doi.org/10.1016/j.nec.2016.07.005
1042-3680/17/© 2016 Elsevier Inc. All rights reserved.

- What is the optimal surgical approach (anterior, posterior, or combined) for the surgical management of facet injuries?

This article reviews the epidemiology, imaging, classification, and treatment of cervical facet injuries; controversial aspects of management are highlighted and supporting evidence is discussed.

EPIDEMIOLOGY

The annual incidence of subaxial cervical spine fracture is 10/100,000.[1] These fractures account for approximately 65% of fractures and 75% of all dislocations in the vertebral column. Within the subaxial cervical spine, most injuries occur at either C5-C6 or C6-C7.[2–4] Facet dislocations account for 5% to 10% of all cervical spine injuries.[5] Isolated, nondisplaced or minimally displaced fractures of the facets account for fewer than 5% of all cervical injuries.[6] Neurologic injury occurs in up to 85% to 90% of patients with bilateral facet dislocation.[7]

CLASSIFICATION

Reliable classification systems for spinal injuries are important for communication among care providers and for facilitating research. An ideal classification system would have the characteristics of being comprehensive, reproducible, and a guide to treatment. Establishing such a system is challenging, and as such, numerous subaxial cervical spine injury classification systems have been developed over the years. The older systems, such as that of Allen and colleagues[8] and Harris and colleagues,[9] focused on the mechanism of injury. Such systems are challenged by the difficulties in extrapolating the exact mechanism of injury from static radiographic imaging. Newer systems have focused less on mechanism and more on injury morphology and have attempted to incorporate the status of the neurologic elements, given that neurologic injury often drives treatment decisions. Such systems include the Subaxial Cervical Spine Injury Classification System (SLIC)[10] and the most recently described AOSpine subaxial cervical spine injury classification.[11]

The Allen and Ferguson system was described in 1982 and classified cervical spine injuries into 6 categories based on the mechanism of injury.[8] Each category was further subdivided into stages reflecting progressive severity of injury. A spectrum of facet injuries was included within the mechanistic category of "flexion-distraction" as follows:

Flexion-distraction stages (**Fig. 1**)

1. Facet subluxation
2. Unilateral facet dislocation
3. Bilateral facet dislocation with 50% displacement
4. Complete dislocation (100%) displacement

The SLIC was developed to facilitate treatment decisions by integrating data across the following 3 domains (**Table 1**)[10]:

1. Injury morphology
2. Integrity of the discoligamentous complex (DLC)
3. The neurologic status of the patient

The SLIC was the first classification scheme to consider the presence or absence of neurologic injury, which was recognized as being a major factor in treatment decision-making. The SLIC score is established by adding the scores from each subdomain, with the expectation that a higher score represents a more severe, unstable injury. An SLIC score of 3 or less suggested an injury amenable to nonoperative management; scores of 5 or greater suggested that surgical management was warranted. A score of 4 was "indeterminate" and represented an injury that could be managed surgically or nonsurgically depending on surgeon preference. Unilateral and bilateral facet subluxations/dislocations are technically within the "rotation/translation" injury morphology in the SLIC system and therefore get a score of at least 4; usually 2 more points are given for DLC injury, giving these injuries a score of 6 even in neurologically intact individuals. Hence, the SLIC system generally recommends surgical treatment of facet subluxations/dislocations, although in the presence of a facet fracture with little subluxation, the SLIC remains somewhat ambiguous in terms of the optimal treatment (**Fig. 2**).

Although SLIC included neurologic injury into the classification system and helped to guide treatment, it was hampered by disagreement over injury morphology (both bone and soft tissue) among practitioners.[12] With this limitation in mind, the AOSpine Trauma Knowledge Forum developed the AOSpine subaxial cervical spine injury classification system, first published in 2015.[11] This classification system is based on 3 injury morphology types: compression injuries (A), tension band injuries (B), and translational injuries (C). Unique to this system are descriptions for facet injuries, patient-specific modifiers, and neurologic status. The system has been shown to have good interobserver and intraobserver

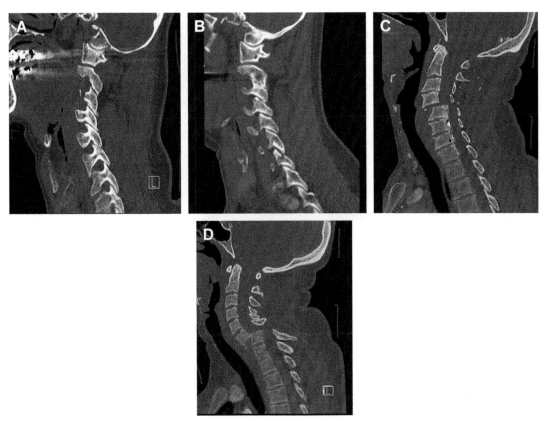

Fig. 1. The spectrum of cervical facet injuries. (*A*) C6-7 subluxed facet joint. (*B*) C6-7 unilateral facet fracture dislocation. (*C*) C4-5 bilateral facet dislocation with 50% displacement. (*D*) C6-7 bilateral facet dislocation with complete (100%) displacement.

Table 1
The Subaxial Cervical Spine Injury Classification

SLIC Three Independent Injury Domains			
1	Injury morphology	No abnormality	0
		Compression	1
		Burst	2
		Distraction	3
		Translation	4
2	DLC integrity	Intact	0
		Indeterminate	1
		Disrupted	2
3	Neurologic status	Intact	0
		Nerve root injury	1
		Complete	2
		Incomplete	3
		Persistent cord compression	+1
	Treatment option	0–3	Conservative
		4	Indeterminate
		>4	Operative management

Numeric scores are assigned in each of the 3 injury domains, that is, morphology, DLC integrity, and neurologic status. Sum score of greater than 4 warrants surgical management, whereas scores of 0 to 3 can be managed conservatively. Treatment option for patients with a score of 4 depends on surgeon's preference and other patient factors.

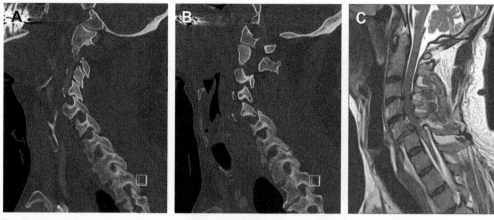

Fig. 2. SLIC and treatment decision-making. Left parasagittal CT slice (*A*), right parasagittal CT slice (*B*), and midsagittal T2-weighted MRI scan of a 54-year-old man who presented with American Spinal Injury Association impairment scale grade B after a fall from a truck. (*A*) Right-sided perched facet injury at C5-6. (*B*) Left-sided jumped facet at C5-6. (*C*) MRI shows cord signal change in the cord. This patient has an SLIC score of 10, warranting surgical intervention (morphology: rotation/translation = 4; DLC: disrupted = 2; neurology: incomplete cord injury with ongoing cord compression = 3 + 1).

reliability by the members of the AOSpine Trauma Knowledge Forum.

DIAGNOSTIC IMAGING

There is little debate at this stage that computed tomography (CT) is the initial imaging study of choice for the diagnosis of cervical spine trauma. The sensitivity of plain radiographs in detecting cervical spine injuries ranges from only 36% to 52%, whereas CT scans have a sensitivity of 98% to 100%. In the context of cervical spine facet injury, the low sensitivity of plain radiographs is attributable to nondisplaced unilateral facet fractures or minimally subluxed facet injuries, which are often impossible to visualize on radiographs (**Fig. 3**).[13–15] CT offers rapid evaluation of the entire spinal axis with excellent bony resolution. An adequate study generates axial, coronal, and sagittal reformats with both soft tissue and bone algorithms. **Figs. 4** and **5** demonstrate some of the radiological features of normal and injured facet joints.

Bilateral facet dislocation results in complete disruption of the facet joint capsules and the posterior ligamentous complex. Posterior longitudinal

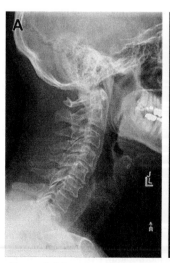
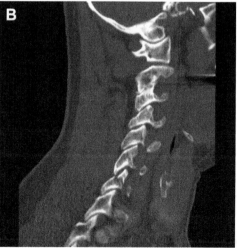

Fig. 3. Plain radiograph (*A*) and parasagittal CT scan (*B*) of a patient with left unilateral C7 facet fracture. Note normal alignment on the plain radiograph. The radiograph was interpreted as normal despite clear evidence of facet fracture on the parasagittal CT scan.

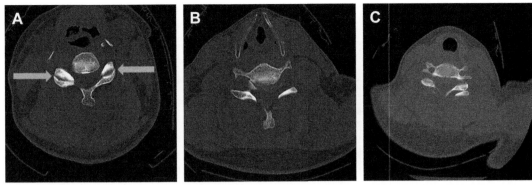

Fig. 4. (*A*) Axial CT scan demonstrating normal facet anatomy. Arrows show the "hamburger bun" sign. (*B*) "Naked facet" sign. The uncovered facet articular surfaces in bilateral facet dislocation. (*C*) "Reverse hamburger bun" sign. Note the reversed relationship of the "bun" halves in a patient with bilateral facet dislocation.

ligament (PLL) disruption is described in 40% to 100% of cases with bilateral facet joint dislocation. Traumatic disk herniation with posterior annulus disruption is described in 56% of unilateral and 82.5% of bilateral facet dislocations.[16,17] Unilateral facet joint dislocation is associated with fracture of articular processes in 75% of cases.[18] Therefore, particular attention should be paid to ruling out comminuted articular process fractures on bone windows because these may preclude closed reduction.

MRI

MRI obviously provides far superior visualization of the neural elements and the DLC than CT scanning. The extent to which MRI adds important diagnostic information in the presence of a normal helical CT scan (particularly in obtunded patients who cannot be cleared clinically) remains somewhat debatable. In a retrospective analysis,

Tomycz and colleagues[19] examined the CT and MRI scans of the cervical spine in 690 obtunded patients and found that of the 180 who had normal findings on CT scans, 38 (21.1%) had evidence of trauma on the MRI scan. None of these injuries, however, were significant enough to alter the management plan. This finding is in contrast to a study by Menaker and colleagues[20] that showed a change in management in 7.9% of 734 obtunded patients based on new findings on MRI. Aside from simply diagnosing the presence of a spinal injury, MRI is highly useful for assessing the DLC, the integrity of which is a consideration in both the SLIC and the newer AOSpine subaxial cervical spine classification systems (**Fig. 6**).

In the context of facet injuries, the use of MRI has been controversial because of the potential for a disk herniation to cause neurologic injury upon reduction/realignment of the cervical spine. After the initial description by Eismont and colleagues[21] of a patient who suffered a spinal cord

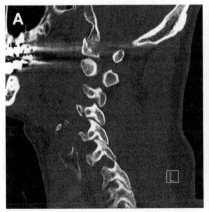
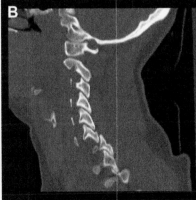

Fig. 5. (*A*) "Perched" facet joint. The inferior articular process of cephalad vertebra sits right on the superior articular process of the caudad vertebra. (*B*) "Jumped" or "locked" facet joint. The inferior articular process of the cephalad vertebra lies anterior to the superior articular process of the caudad vertebra.

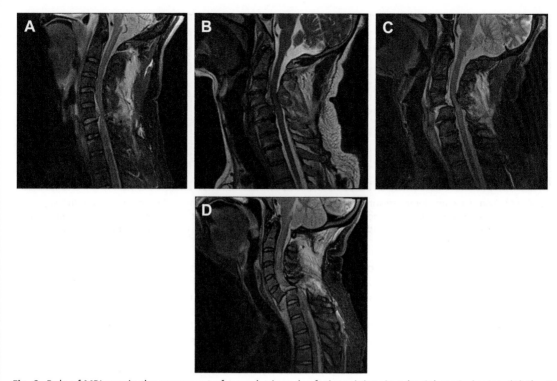

Fig. 6. Role of MRI scan in the assessment of neurologic and soft tissue injury in subaxial cervical spine. (*A*) Short tau inversion recovery (STIR) MRI shows disk herniation, posterior longitudinal ligament rupture, posterior ligamentous complex high signal. (*B*) T2-weighted MRI sequence shows a large herniated disk fragment posterior to the cephalad vertebral body. (*C*) STIR MRI sequence shows disruption of disk, anterior and posterior ligamentous complex. (*D*) STIR MRI sequence in a complete cord injury shows extensive soft tissue and cord injury.

injury during an open posterior reduction of a facet dislocation, much debate has occurred around whether, before attempting a closed reduction, an MRI scan should be performed to rule out a disk herniation. Particularly worrisome are herniations in which the disk fragment resides posterior to the displaced cephalad vertebral body (**Fig. 7**), where it might be pushed back into the cord during the realignment.[17]

Attaining a MRI study prior to cervical facet reduction, remains controversial with significant variability among practitioners.[22] Several studies have shown that closed reduction of facet dislocations can be performed safely in awake and alert patients who can be continuously examined throughout the procedure[23–26]; this was demonstrated in one small series even in patients with known disk herniations before reduction.[26] Serial MRIs conducted during the closed reduction procedure have shown that disk herniations can actually be reduced back into the intervertebral space with traction.[27] On the other hand, on a purely practical level, it can be reasonably argued that

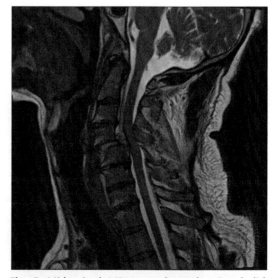

Fig. 7. Midsagittal MRI scan shows herniated disk fragment posterior to the displaced cephalad vertebral body. Closed reduction in this setting may push disk material into the spinal cord, causing further compression.

in a neurologically intact patient with a facet dislocation, there is little to lose and potentially much to gain by doing an MRI to rule out a disk herniation before attempting a closed reduction.

In the obtunded, nonexaminable patient, although there is no clear evidence to suggest that closed reduction causes neurologic injury, caution is warranted and many surgeons opt for a prereduction MRI to rule out disk herniation. The rate of transient and permanent neurologic complication from closed reduction is low: 2% to 4% and less than 1%, respectively.[28] When undertaking a closed reduction, one should recognize that it may be impossible to actually get the facets reduced. In particular, closed reductions are more likely to fail in the presence of associated facet fracture or if dislocation precedes attempted reduction by an extended period of time.[7,29] Kepler and colleagues[30] noted that closed reduction was successful in 59.1% of patients, whereas open reduction was successful in 94.9% of patients.

In summary, closed reduction can be safely performed in an awake patient that can be continuously examined. In practice, this fact is useful to acknowledge when faced with a patient with a facet dislocation and an incomplete or worsening neurologic deficit secondary to ongoing cord compression, in which there may be considerable benefit to immediately realigning the spine rather than waiting for an MRI. Also, in patients who are completely quadriplegic to begin with, the documented safety of a closed reduction would seemingly provide adequate justification for immediately realigning the spine rather than waiting for an MRI. However, in patients who are neurologically intact, there is less justification to proceeding to an urgent closed reduction without first ruling out the presence of a disk herniation on MRI. Also, if considering a posterior open reduction, confirming the absence of a disk herniation with MRI is mandatory.

DEFINITIVE MANAGEMENT

Facet fractures and dislocations represent a wide spectrum of injuries, and thus, strict guidelines for their management are difficult to establish. The goals of management are to achieve stability and maximize neurologic recovery. The guiding principles to consider are therefore: (1) the degree of instability of the injury, (2) the presence/absence of neurologic injury, and (3) unique patient factors (eg, comorbidities, body habitus, and so forth) that might influence the success or failure of surgical or nonsurgical treatment. The 2 management issues that remain somewhat controversial today include the questions: (1) what is the optimal management

(external immobilization or surgery) of the isolated unilateral facet fracture with no neurologic deficit? and (2) if surgery is indicated, what is the optimal approach (anterior, posterior, combined)?

Unilateral facet injuries that are undisplaced or minimally displaced and without neurologic deficits are often treated nonoperatively with a cervical orthosis for 6 to 12 weeks. Although these may seem like benign injuries, subsequent displacement and late chronic neck pain has prompted the question of whether some of these injuries are better treated surgically (and if so, what might help to determine this). Spector and colleagues[31] evaluated CT scans of 26 such fractures in 24 patients, managed conservatively, in order to find radiological predictors of nonoperative treatment failure. They found that patients with unilateral cervical facet fractures involving greater than 40% of the absolute height of the intact lateral mass or an absolute height greater than 1 cm are at increased risk of failure from conservative treatment.

Aarabi and colleagues[32] noted that 20% to 80% of unilateral, nondisplaced facet fractures fail nonoperative management. In their series of 25 patients with such injuries, 9 of the 15 patients treated conservatively failed, as compared with only 1 of the 10 patients treated surgically, a statistically significant difference ($P = .018$). In a recent systematic review by Kepler and colleagues,[30] patients with unilateral facet fractures treated surgically were significantly more likely to maintain successful anatomic reduction as compared with those treated nonoperatively ($P<.0001$). These results suggest that despite the undisplaced or minimally displaced nature of these injuries, there is evidence that points to improved radiographic outcomes with surgical treatment. In the case of unilateral facet dislocations with or without fracture, the clinical evidence is certainly much more strongly in favor of surgical management, as reviewed by Dvorak and colleagues.[33] Treated nonoperatively, such dislocations have a high rate of treatment failure, neurologic deterioration, and chronic neck pain.

CLOSED REDUCTION TECHNIQUES

Closed reduction of a facet dislocation as soon as possible in the emergency room setting may be advantageous in providing expeditious relief of spinal cord compression.[34] It should be recognized, however, that performing a closed reduction with traction requires analgesia and sedation, close physiologic monitoring, imaging (radiograph or fluoroscopy) to monitor progress, and patience. It should also be recognized that in a significant proportion of patients, a closed reduction is actually not possible, particularly if there is an associated facet fracture. These issues should be considered when deciding on whether it is feasible given the local emergency room environment, available personnel to assist with physiologic monitoring, and the characteristics of the facet dislocation to attempt a closed reduction.

The commonest technique used for closed reduction of a dislocated cervical facet injury is axial traction under procedural sedation. Axial traction under procedural sedation should be attempted in a high-acuity setting with close monitoring of the vital signs as well as neurologic status throughout the procedure. A portable radiograph or fluoroscopy machine is required for the assessment of reduction with incremental increase in traction force. After application of local anesthetic, Gardner-Wells tongs are applied to points located 1 cm behind and 3 cm above the external auditory canal. Initial weight of 4.5 kg is applied and increased by an average 4.5 kg sequentially at 5- to 20-minute intervals until reduction is achieved. The neurologic status of the patient is assessed immediately after each increase. Lateral radiographs 3 to 10 minutes after each weight change are used to assess displacement of vertebral bodies. Maximal safe traction weight of up to 63.5 kg has been reported. Once reduction is achieved, the traction weight can be reduced to 4.5 to 9 kg to maintain alignment.[23,35]

SURGICAL MANAGEMENT

Options for surgical management of cervical facet injuries include anterior, posterior, and combined approaches. Each of these approaches has inherent advantages and disadvantages.

Selection of surgical approach depends on a combination of factors, including surgeon preference, patient factors, injury morphology, and inherent advantages and disadvantages of any given approach. The need for decompression of a traumatic disk herniation may necessitate an anterior approach, whereas failure to achieve reduction of bilateral dislocated facets could require a direct posterior reduction.

Anterior approaches involve decompression and discectomy followed by reduction via inline traction and/or manipulation and/or application of distractor pins. Fixation is subsequently achieved with the use of interbody graft and plating. One key advantage of the anterior approach is the ability to remove the disk (whether it is herniated or not) before realigning the spinal canal. Successful reduction after disk removal can obviate posterior reduction and stabilization. The anterior approach avoids muscle-traumatizing posterior dissection and removes the need to turn the patient with an unstable C-spine injury from the supine to prone position. Another advantage of the anterior approach is the potential to limit the fusion to a single motion segment. This is in contrast to posterior approach that may require extension of the fusion to additional levels because of the inability to secure internal fixation into the fractured facet.

The main disadvantage of the anterior approach for facet dislocations is that it is more challenging to achieve a reduction, particularly in the setting of facet or pedicle fractures. Failure to reduce would therefore mandate a posterior approach and possibly revisiting the anterior approach for interbody reconstruction and plate fixation after successful posterior reduction.

An additional important consideration for anterior fixation is the presence of superior end-plate fracture or facet fractures. Johnson and colleagues[36] evaluated 87 patients with either unilateral or bilateral facet dislocation or fracture/dislocations that were treated with anterior-only discectomy, fusion, and plating. They noted a 13% incidence of radiographic loss of alignment. Significant correlation was found between radiographic failure and presence of endplate compression fracture and facet fractures. Furthermore, a somewhat rare factor to consider in addressing a facet dislocation anteriorly is the status of the ligamentum flavum; if this ligament is infolded, it may potentially cause spinal cord impingement upon reduction of the dislocation.[37] This situation should therefore be addressed with a posterior decompression to remove the infolded ligamentum flavum before reduction.

The posterior approach allows direct visualization of displaced facets. Reduction can be achieved fairly readily by direct manipulation of the posterior elements of the rostral segment. In order to disengage the facets or to remove fractured fragments, it is sometimes necessary to remove parts of the overlapping facets' joints and lamina. Care should be paid to not remove excessive facet as they contribute to stability after reduction and serve as fixation points. The spinal segment should be distracted to bring the facets back into alignment, rather than simply burring off the facets and pulling the superjacent segment posteriorly. Such a maneuver may "snow-plow" disk material back into the canal if an anterior decompression has not been performed.

A *Cochrane Review* of these 2 approaches for the treatment of unilateral facet fractures identified 2 major studies.[38] One is the randomized controlled trial by Kwon and colleagues.[39] The investigators did not find any difference in the Northern American Spine Society cervical or neurologic

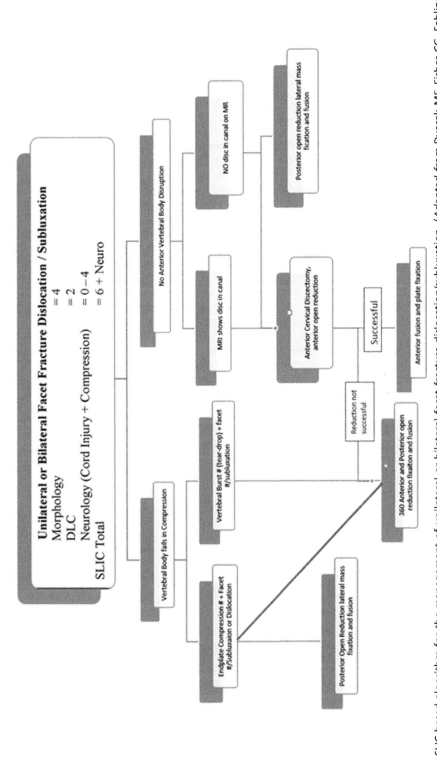

Fig. 8. SLIC-based algorithm for the management of unilateral or bilateral facet fracture dislocation/subluxation. (*Adapted from* Dvorak MF, Fisher CG, Fehlings MG, et al. The surgical approach to subaxial cervical spine injuries: an evidence-based algorithm based on the SLIC classification system. Spine (Phila Pa 1976) 2007;32(23):2624; with permission.)

scores between the 2 groups at 12 months' follow-up. Anteriorly treated patients exhibited less postoperative pain (2.6 vs 3.5; *P* = .15), lower rate of wound infection (0/20 anterior vs 4/22 posterior), higher rate of radiographically demonstrated union (100% vs 89%; *P* = .49), and better radiographic alignment (mean lordosis 8.8° vs 1.6° kyphosis; *P* = .0001). Anterior approach was accompanied by a risk of swallowing difficulty in the early postoperative period that resolved by 6 weeks in most patients. Patient-reported outcome measures did not reveal a difference between anterior and posterior fixation procedures at 12 months.

The second study is a quasi-randomized trial by Brodke and colleagues.[40] There were no significant differences between the 2 approaches in fusion rates, alignment, neurologic recovery, and long-term pain.

There remains considerable variability among practitioners with regards to surgical treatment of cervical facet dislocations. Nassr and colleagues[41] found little agreement among 25 members of the Spine Trauma Study Group in the choice of surgical approach for unilateral and bilateral facet dislocations (κ<0.1). They also noted that surgeons favored the anterior approach alone or as the first stage of a combined approach when a disk herniation was present, regardless of neurologic status of the patient. An anterior approach was preferred when a patient was neurologically intact, even if there was no disk herniation. Combined approaches were favored for the treatment of bilateral facet dislocations.

In their review, Kepler and colleagues[30] report a success rate of 87.2% in 183 patients who underwent internal fixation. The rate of maintenance of reduction for anterior approach was 90.5% as compared with 75.6% for posterior approach (odds ratio [OR] 3.1, 95% confidence interval [CI] 1.0–9.4, *P* = .05). When analyzing unilateral injuries alone, posterior approach had a 64% success rate, whereas anterior approach had a 92.6% success rate (OR 7.0, 95% CI 1.9–25.9, *P* = .0034).

Acknowledging the lack of sufficient evidence to guide the choice of surgical approach to subaxial cervical spine injuries, Dvorak and colleagues[6] used SLIC to develop algorithms for the surgical treatment of facet fracture dislocation/subluxation (**Fig. 8**) and facet subluxation or perched facet (**Fig. 9**).

As indicated in the algorithm for facet fracture dislocation, either an anterior or a posterior approach can be used if an MRI scan does not show the presence of disk material in the spinal canal. The algorithm further suggests that if the anterior decompression and open reduction are successful, an anterior fusion and plate fixation

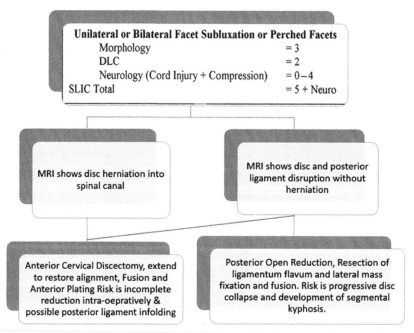

Fig. 9. SLIC-based algorithm for the management of unilateral or bilateral facet subluxation or perched facets. (*Adapted from* Dvorak MF, Fisher CG, Fehlings MG, et al. The surgical approach to subaxial cervical spine injuries: an evidence-based algorithm based on the SLIC classification system. Spine (Phila Pa 1976) 2007;32(23):2626; with permission.)

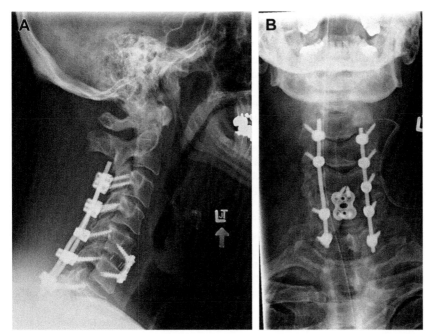

Fig. 10. Postoperative lateral (*A*) and anterior/posterior (*B*) plain C-spine radiographs of the patient in **Fig. 2**. Given the presence of both anterior and posterior abnormality, the patient received a combined anterior/posterior approach involving C5/6 anterior cervical discectomy and fusion (ACDF) and posterior C3-C7 instrumented fusion.

are sufficient for the management of the injury. In the presence of compression or burst fracture anteriorly, facet fracture/dislocation warrants a combined approach. **Fig. 10** show the same patient from **Fig. 2** who underwent a front and back combined approach.

In summary, both anterior and posterior approaches are effective in the management of cervical facet injuries. The choice of approach, including combined approaches, depends on the morphology of the injury, patient factors, and surgeon preference. Prospective controlled trials did not find any significant differences in outcome between the 2 approaches. Nevertheless, clinical practice has demonstrated that, for the most part, anterior fixation provides sufficient stability for facet injuries with the caveat that injuries with concomitant endplate or pedicle fractures should be treated posteriorly or using a combined approach.

SUMMARY

- Newer classification systems for subaxial cervical spine, such as the SLIC and the AOSpine Subaxial Cervical Spine Classification System, take into account morphology, discoligamentous integrity, and neurologic status.
- Closed reduction of facet dislocations is safe in alert and examinable patients. Given the

small risk of neurologic injury secondary to disk herniation, conducting a prereduction MRI is justified.

- The evidence suggests that better radiographic and clinical outcomes are achieved with surgical treatment of unilateral facet fractures with minimal displacement and no neurologic deficit.
- Anterior and posterior approaches can both be used successfully for the surgical management of facet injuries, and each has advantages and disadvantages. The anterior approach is well tolerated, allows one to address a disk herniation, and provides a high union rate with good sagittal alignment. The posterior approach allows for easier open reduction and biomechanically superior fixation.

REFERENCES

1. Fredo HL, Rizvi SA, Lied B, et al. The epidemiology of traumatic cervical spine fractures: a prospective population study from Norway. Scand J Trauma Resusc Emerg Med 2012;20:85.
2. Goldberg W, Mueller C, Panacek E, et al. Distribution and patterns of blunt traumatic cervical spine injury. Ann Emerg Med 2001;38(1):17–21.
3. Greenbaum J, Walters N, Levy PD. An evidenced-based approach to radiographic assessment of

cervical spine injuries in the emergency department. J Emerg Med 2009;36(1):64–71.

4. Raniga SB, Menon V, Al Muzahmi KS, et al. MDCT of acute subaxial cervical spine trauma: a mechanism-based approach. Insights Imaging 2014;5(3):321–38.

5. Maiman DJ, Barolat G, Larson SJ. Management of bilateral locked facets of the cervical spine. Neurosurgery 1986;18(5):542–7.

6. Dvorak MF, Fisher CG, Fehlings MG, et al. The surgical approach to subaxial cervical spine injuries: an evidence-based algorithm based on the SLIC classification system. Spine (Phila Pa 1976) 2007;32(23):2620–9.

7. Hadley MN, Fitzpatrick BC, Sonntag VK, et al. Facet fracture-dislocation injuries of the cervical spine. Neurosurgery 1992;30(5):661–6.

8. Allen BL Jr, Ferguson RL, Lehmann TR, et al. A mechanistic classification of closed, indirect fractures and dislocations of the lower cervical spine. Spine (Phila Pa 1976) 1982;7(1):1–27.

9. Harris JH Jr, Edeiken-Monroe B, Kopaniky DR. A practical classification of acute cervical spine injuries. Orthop Clin North Am 1986;17(1):15–30.

10. Vaccaro AR, Hulbert RJ, Patel AA, et al. The subaxial cervical spine injury classification system: a novel approach to recognize the importance of morphology, neurology, and integrity of the disco-ligamentous complex. Spine (Phila Pa 1976) 2007;32(21):2365–74.

11. Vaccaro AR, Koerner JD, Radcliff KE, et al. AOSpine subaxial cervical spine injury classification system. Eur Spine J 2016;25(7):2173–84.

12. van Middendorp JJ, Audige L, Bartels RH, et al. The subaxial cervical spine injury classification system: an external agreement validation study. Spine J 2013;13(9):1055–63.

13. Bailitz J, Starr F, Beecroft M, et al. CT should replace three-view radiographs as the initial screening test in patients at high, moderate, and low risk for blunt cervical spine injury: a prospective comparison. J Trauma 2009;66(6):1605–9.

14. McCulloch PT, France J, Jones DL, et al. Helical computed tomography alone compared with plain radiographs with adjunct computed tomography to evaluate the cervical spine after high-energy trauma. J Bone Joint Surg Am 2005;87(11):2388–94.

15. Widder S, Doig C, Burrowes P, et al. Prospective evaluation of computed tomographic scanning for the spinal clearance of obtunded trauma patients: preliminary results. J Trauma 2004;56(6):1179–84.

16. Carrino JA, Manton GL, Morrison WB, et al. Posterior longitudinal ligament status in cervical spine bilateral facet dislocations. Skeletal Radiol 2006;35(7):510–4.

17. Vaccaro AR, Madigan L, Schweitzer ME, et al. Magnetic resonance imaging analysis of soft tissue disruption after flexion-distraction injuries of the subaxial cervical spine. Spine (Phila Pa 1976) 2001;26(17):1866–72.

18. Shanmuganathan K, Mirvis SE, Levine AM. Rotational injury of cervical facets: CT analysis of fracture patterns with implications for management and neurologic outcome. AJR Am J Roentgenol 1994;163(5):1165–9.

19. Tomycz ND, Chew BG, Chang YF, et al. MRI is unnecessary to clear the cervical spine in obtunded/comatose trauma patients: the four-year experience of a level I trauma center. J Trauma 2008;64(5):1258–63.

20. Menaker J, Philp A, Boswell S, et al. Computed tomography alone for cervical spine clearance in the unreliable patient–are we there yet? J Trauma 2008;64(4):898–903 [discussion: 903–4].

21. Eismont FJ, Arena MJ, Green BA. Extrusion of an intervertebral disc associated with traumatic subluxation or dislocation of cervical facets. Case report. J Bone Joint Surg Am 1991;73(10):1555–60.

22. Arnold PM, Brodke DS, Rampersaud YR, et al. Differences between neurosurgeons and orthopedic surgeons in classifying cervical dislocation injuries and making assessment and treatment decisions: a multicenter reliability study. Am J Orthop (Belle Mead NJ) 2009;38(10):E156–61.

23. Cotler JM, Herbison GJ, Nasuti JF, et al. Closed reduction of traumatic cervical spine dislocation using traction weights up to 140 pounds. Spine (Phila Pa 1976) 1993;18(3):386–90.

24. Grant GA, Mirza SK, Chapman JR, et al. Risk of early closed reduction in cervical spine subluxation injuries. J Neurosurg 1999;90(Suppl 1):13–8.

25. Lee JY, Nassr A, Eck JC, et al. Controversies in the treatment of cervical spine dislocations. Spine J 2009;9(5):418–23.

26. Vaccaro AR, Falatyn SP, Flanders AE, et al. Magnetic resonance evaluation of the intervertebral disc, spinal ligaments, and spinal cord before and after closed traction reduction of cervical spine dislocations. Spine (Phila Pa 1976) 1999;24(12):1210–7.

27. Darsaut TE, Ashforth R, Bhargava R, et al. A pilot study of magnetic resonance imaging-guided closed reduction of cervical spine fractures. Spine (Phila Pa 1976) 2006;31(18):2085–90.

28. Gelb DE, Hadley MN, Aarabi B, et al. Initial closed reduction of cervical spinal fracture-dislocation injuries. Neurosurgery 2013;72(Suppl 2):73–83.

29. Treatment of subaxial cervical spinal injuries. Neurosurgery 2002;50(Suppl 3):S156–65.

30. Kepler CK, Vaccaro AR, Chen E, et al. Treatment of isolated cervical facet fractures: a systematic review. J Neurosurg Spine 2015;1–8. http://www.ncbi.nlm.nih.gov/pubmed/26516667.

31. Spector LR, Kim DH, Affonso J, et al. Use of computed tomography to predict failure of

nonoperative treatment of unilateral facet fractures of the cervical spine. Spine (Phila Pa 1976) 2006; 31(24):2827–35.

32. Aarabi B, Mirvis S, Shanmuganathan K, et al. Comparative effectiveness of surgical versus nonoperative management of unilateral, nondisplaced, subaxial cervical spine facet fractures without evidence of spinal cord injury: clinical article. J Neurosurg Spine 2014;20(3):270–7.

33. Dvorak M, Vaccaro AR, Hermsmeyer J, et al. Unilateral facet dislocations: is surgery really the preferred option? Evid Based Spine Care J 2010;1(1):57–65.

34. Newton D, England M, Doll H, et al. The case for early treatment of dislocations of the cervical spine with cord involvement sustained playing rugby. J Bone Joint Surg Br 2011;93(12):1646–52.

35. Star AM, Jones AA, Cotler JM, et al. Immediate closed reduction of cervical spine dislocations using traction. Spine (Phila Pa 1976) 1990;15(10):1068–72.

36. Johnson MG, Fisher CG, Boyd M, et al. The radiographic failure of single segment anterior cervical plate fixation in traumatic cervical flexion distraction injuries. Spine (Phila Pa 1976) 2004;29(24):2815–20.

37. Rhee JM, Kimmerly WS, Smucker JD. Infolding of the ligamentum flavum: a cause of spinal cord compression after reduction of cervical facet injuries. J Spinal Disord Tech 2006;19(3):208–12.

38. Del Curto D, Tamaoki MJ, Martins DE, et al. Surgical approaches for cervical spine facet dislocations in adults. Cochrane Database Syst Rev 2014;(10): CD008129.

39. Kwon BK, Fisher CG, Boyd MC, et al. A prospective randomized controlled trial of anterior compared with posterior stabilization for unilateral facet injuries of the cervical spine. J Neurosurg Spine 2007;7(1):1–12.

40. Brodke DS, Anderson PA, Newell DW, et al. Comparison of anterior and posterior approaches in cervical spinal cord injuries. J Spinal Disord Tech 2003;16(3): 229–35.

41. Nassr A, Lee JY, Dvorak MF, et al. Variations in surgical treatment of cervical facet dislocations. Spine (Phila Pa 1976) 2008;33(7):E188–93.

The Role of a Miniopen Thoracoscopic-assisted Approach in the Management of Burst Fractures Involving the Thoracolumbar Junction

Ricky Raj S. Kalra, MD, Meic H. Schmidt, MD, MBA[1],*

KEYWORDS

- Thoracoscopic surgery • Burst fractures • Vertebrectomy • Expandable cages
- Minimally invasive surgery • Thoracotomy

KEY POINTS

- Thoracoscopic miniopen access to the anterior spine should be considered as an alternative minimally invasive access approach to traditional open procedures.
- Thoracoscopy can be used along the entire thoracic spine and can be extended via transdiaphragmatic incision to the upper third of L2 in the retroperitoneal space, allowing access to the most common sites of burst fractures.
- Good single-lung ventilation with a double-lumen endotracheal tube is crucial for thoracoscopy.
- Thoracoscopic miniopen surgery can be used for vertebrectomy and anterior reconstruction of unstable fractures.

INTRODUCTION

The thoracolumbar junction (TLJ) from T11 to L2 represents a transition zone for several anatomic structures that have implications and predilections for spinal cord trauma, bony fractures, and ligamentous injuries. The spinal cord anatomy changes at the conus and cauda equina. The diaphragm inserts at T12/L1 and divides the thoracic cavity from the retroperitoneal space. The spinal column transitions from the stiff thoracic spine, with rib heads overlapping the disk spaces and ribs that attach to the sternum creating a 4-column structure, to a mobile spine, where floating ribs attach only to the vertebral body, resulting in a 3-column structure. These unique characteristics contribute to the complexity of clinical symptoms, neurologic deficits, and radiological features of burst fractures.

The management of traumatic burst fracture is a controversial topic in spine surgery because of limited high-quality outcomes data. Therapy options range from no treatment, to nonoperative treatment with bracing, to surgical instrumentation of various sorts. Stable burst fractures without neurologic deficit are often treated conservatively. For unstable burst fractures that involve the TLJ, spine surgeons often consider surgery an important option.

An unstable burst fracture involves both the anterior and the middle columns and is associated with a primarily axial load with or without flexion, rotation, or lateral flexion forces. In addition, McAfee and colleagues[1] classified burst fractures

Department of Neurosurgery, Clinical Neurosciences Center, University of Utah, 175 N. Medical Drive East, Salt Lake City, UT 84132, USA
[1] Present address: Department of Neurosurgery, New York Medical College, Valhalla, New York
* Corresponding author.
E-mail address: neuropub@hsc.utah.edu

Neurosurg Clin N Am 28 (2017) 139–145
http://dx.doi.org/10.1016/j.nec.2016.07.006
1042-3680/17/© 2016 Elsevier Inc. All rights reserved.

based on the status of the posterior elements. Unstable burst fractures should have evidence of disruption of the posterior elements, including pedicles, lamina, and ligaments.

Posterior approaches for correction of burst fracture–related kyphosis and fusion remain the most common spine surgery for unstable burst fractures; however, posterior-alone approaches for unstable burst fractures involving the TLJ can result in loss of correction, degenerative kyphosis, nonunion, and hardware failure. This outcome is likely secondary to the loss of weight-bearing capacity of the fractured vertebral body, including the end plates and the adjacent ligamentous structures. Strategies to counteract these problems include multilevel posterior fusion, transpedicular bone grafting, vertebral augmentation, screw insertion at the fracture level, and corpectomy with vertebral body replacement (VBR).[2–5]

Corpectomy and VBR can be done via a posterior lateral approach or anterior approaches alone or in combination with posterior fusion.[6] The thoracoabdominal approach consists of a thoracotomy with a transthoracic incision of the diaphragm to enter the retroperitoneal space. This traditional, open approach provides excellent access to the anterior spine but is associated with significant access-related morbidity and postoperative complications. The development of the miniopen thoracoscopic approach for anterior column surgery after a short-segment posterior fusion has decreased the access morbidity and allowed faster healing times,[7] although the learning curve related to miniopen thoracoscopic surgery has restricted its widespread appeal in treating burst fractures. This article describes the use of this procedure for addressing burst fractures at the TLJ.

SURGICAL TECHNIQUE
Anesthesia and Surgical Setup

The thoracoscopic miniopen procedure is performed under general anesthesia with double-lumen tube intubation for single-lung ventilation. Once the endotracheal tube is positioned, its placement is confirmed by bronchoscopy. An arterial line is placed before patient positioning for continuous blood pressure monitoring.

The patient is placed in a lateral decubitus position. The approach side depends on the position of the major vessels shown on the preoperative computed tomography scan. There needs to be enough distance from the aorta to allow for the placement of the anterior lateral plate to avoid direct contact between the plate and the aorta. At the TLJ, the burst fracture is most commonly

accessed from the left side, which also avoids manipulation or retraction of the liver during the transdiaphragmatic exposure.

Four supports are placed: at the sternum, between the scapulae, and at the sacrum and coccyx. An axillary roll, a Krause arm rest, and a special U-shaped cushion for the legs are also positioned to prevent obstruction during the instrumentation (**Fig. 1**A, B). Four access portals (for the endoscope, suction-irrigation, retractors, and working access) are localized. The burst fracture is displayed in the lateral projection under precise adjustment of the image intensifier, and the injured spinal section is marked onto the lateral thoracic wall. The projection of the vertebrae, whose end plates and anterior and posterior margins should be displayed in the central beam, is used as the sole reference for portal placement.

The working portal is positioned directly above the lesion, and then the location for the endoscope portal is marked approximately 2 intercostal spaces from the working portal along the axis of the spine in a cranial direction at the TLJ. The suction and irrigation and retractor portals are then located ventral from these portals.

Operation

After skin disinfection and sterile draping, single-lung ventilation is begun. The most cranial portal is opened first to reduce the risk of injury to the liver, spleen, and diaphragm. After opening, the insertion site is inspected with the fingers before the trocar is introduced and then the rigid 30° endoscope is inserted to inspect the thoracic cavity for adhesions or parenchymal lesions. The lung is visually confirmed to be deflated. The access ports for the instruments are placed under direct visualization, the instruments are introduced and the diaphragm is safely retracted, and the operating portal is opened (**Fig. 1**C).

The attachment sites of the diaphragm to the spine are at the level of the first lumbar vertebra and the lowest point of the thoracic cavity is at the level of the baseplate of the second lumbar vertebra (**Fig. 1**D). After incision of the diaphragm attachment to the spine, a trocar is placed intrathoracically in the phrenicocostal sinus to afford access to the retroperitoneal section of the TLJ down to the baseplate of the second lumbar vertebra. A 4-cm to 5-cm incision parallel to the attachment of the diaphragm is used to prevent a postoperative diaphragmatic hernia; access as far as the L1-L2 intervertebral disk can be obtained with a shorter, 2-cm to 3-cm incision.

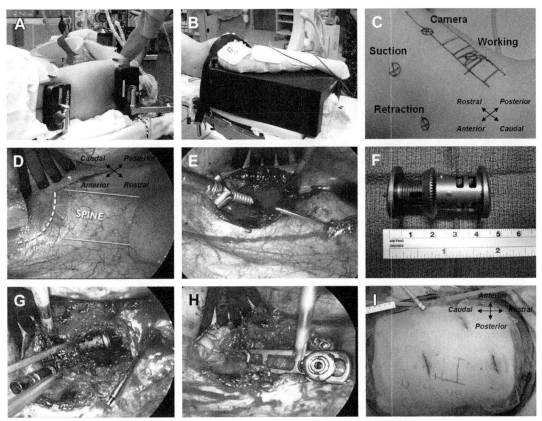

Fig. 1. (*A*) The patient is positioned on a radiolucent table in the right lateral decubitus position for a left-sided thoracoscopic approach to L1. (*B*) The independent leg is slightly flexed at the hip to facilitate iliopsoas relaxation, making it easier to dissect this muscle off the lateral aspect of the vertebral bodies at the thoracolumbar junction. (*C*) The level of interest is marked, identifying the vertebral body above and below, and the 4 chest portals are planned. (*D*) Endoscopic view of the spine (*solid lines*). The diaphragm is swept inferiorly with a fan retractor and a diaphragmatic incision is planned (*dotted lines*). (*E*) A K wire is placed above the planned corpectomy and a polyaxial screw clamp combination is placed below it. (*F*) Lateral view of a fully expanded gear-driven cage. (*G*) The cage is placed and expanded within the central corpectomy. (*H*) Final anterolateral plate construct. (*I*) Closure with chest tube exiting the retraction port. (*From* Ragel BT, Amini A, Schmidt MH. Thoracoscopic vertebral body replacement with an expandable cage after ventral spinal canal decompression. Neurosurgery 2007;61(5 Suppl 2):317–22. [discussion: 322–23]; with permission.)

Navigation in the Thorax

Landmarks are set under image intensifier control to serve as orientation points for the surgeon and camera operator. The Kirschner (K) wires associated with the implant are used for initial landmark localization and define the subsequent positioning of the cannulated screws with integrated clamping elements. They are placed near the end plates between the posterior and central thirds of the vertebra. This positioning avoids injury to the segment vessels and ensures that the screws are anchored where the bone density is higher (see **Fig. 1D; Fig. 2**).

To access burst fractures in this region, the psoas muscle must be mobilized from ventral to dorsal to avoid irritating the fibers of the lumbar plexus. Then, the pleura is opened between the K wires, and the segmental blood vessels are exposed and identified. Once the vessels are mobilized subperiosteally and ligated with titanium clips ventrally and dorsally, they are dissected with the endoscopic hook scissors. Then, the lateral aspects of the vertebral body and the disk can be exposed with the Cobb raspatory.

Screw Placement

At this point, a cannulated broach is used to over-drill the K wires, and the lateral cortex of the vertebral body is opened. The working trocar is exchanged for a speculum, and the clamping element is tightened with a screw of appropriate length. The direction of the screw is checked in

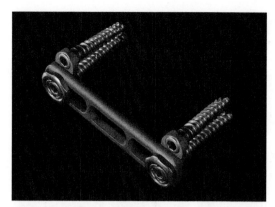

Fig. 2. The MACS-TL ventrolateral thoracolumbar spinal implant (Aesculap, Tuttlingen, Germany) is a minimally invasive rigid fixation plate designed for miniopen thoracoscopic spinal stabilization. (*From* Kalra R, Schmidt MH. Thoracoscopic corpectomy and reconstruction. In: Benzel E, editor. Spine surgery. Philadelphia: Elsevier; 2016; with permission.)

both planes under C-arm monitoring and can be adjusted after removal of the K wire. A region of safety is now defined by the connecting line between the screws and the anterior boundary of the clamping elements. Within this zone, the partial removal of the vertebral body and the disks can be safely performed (**Fig. 3**). The ventral and dorsal extent also correspond with the dimensions of the planned VBR (**Fig. 1**E).

Osteotomy and Cage Placement

Lateral incisions are made in the intervertebral disks, and the disk space is opened with a slightly offset osteotome. A straight osteotome is used for

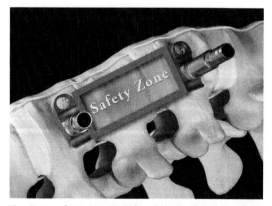

Fig. 3. A safety zone is defined by the borders of the clamps. Instruments are kept within these safe boundaries, which also define the limits of the corpectomy. (© Department of Neurosurgery, University of Utah. Reproduced with permission.)

the posterior osteotomy between the disk spaces along the connecting line between the screws. The corresponding depth is maintained at about two-thirds of the diameter of the vertebra in the anterior direction. The anterior boundary of the clamping elements serves to indicate the line of the anterior osteotomy. It is important to avoid perforation of the anterior vertebral wall and adjacent vessels; this can be aided by use of an osteotome that is slightly angled to the rear.

Because most of the fragments of the burst fracture are loose after the injury, the central section of the fractured vertebral body is easily removed with a rongeur. Resected cancellous bone is preserved for use as bone graft adjacent to the vertebral body. The intervertebral disks are resected using a curet and rongeurs, and the end plates are cleaned with box cutters to remove any cartilage to allow bone fusion across the bone graft–packed cage, but weakening of the load-bearing end plates must be avoided.

Retropulsed Fragment with Spinal Cord Injury

When compression of the spinal canal is associated with neurologic deficit, recovery of function and sensory deficits may be possible if the structures have not been severed. The authors address the retropulsed fragment most commonly with ligamentotaxis or posterior resection during the initial posterior surgery; however, if that is insufficient a thoracoscopic anterior decompression can be used. After completion of the corpectomy, the pedicle of the fractured vertebral body is identified. In traumatic burst fracture, the retropulsed fragments are usually located medially, trapped between the 2 pedicles. Because of the difficulty in removing or reducing the fragment in this position, it is often necessary to resect the ipsilateral pedicle with a punch. Resection of the ipsilateral pedicle both exposes the spinal canal and frees the retropulsed fragment from between the pedicles. The pedicle is exposed subperiosteally with a Cobb elevator, which is used to push the nerve root dorsally without separating it from the surrounding soft tissue. After the inferior margin of the pedicle is identified, the pedicle is thinned with a high-speed bur and transected with a punch. Removal of the base of the pedicle and the dorsocranial vertebral body exposes the posterior margin fragment and the dura. The retropulsed fragment can now be elevated to decompress the dura, mobilized toward the partial corpectomy, and resected. The operation concludes with the ventral instrumentation (**Fig. 4**).

The Obelisc cage (Ulrich Medical USA, Chesterfield, MO) or Hydrolift cage (Aesculap, Center

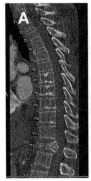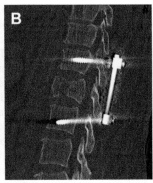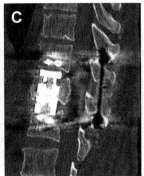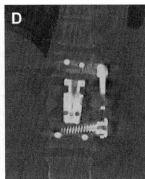

Fig. 4. A 52-year-old man involved in an off-road motor vehicle crash had a T12 burst fracture with neurologic deficits (*A*). He underwent T11 through L1 dorsal spinal fusion (*B*) followed by T12 thoracoscopic corpectomy and reconstruction with an expandable titanium cage (*C, D*).

Valley, PA) provides continuously variable distraction and adaptation of the end plates for VBR/vertebral body reconstruction. Two Langenbeck hooks are inserted into the working portal, which is widened slightly, so the VBR can be introduced and positioned over the defect. It is important to confirm that no soft tissue, in particular the ligated segment vessels, is trapped between the corpectomy defect and the VBR. The implant is then positioned into the vertebral body and distracted. The VBR device is surrounded with the harvested cancellous bone or frozen allograft bone, which can be irrigated with antibiotic. The packed corpectomy defect is covered with a piece of Surgicel fibrillar (oxidized cellulose polymer) (**Fig. 1**F–H).

The plate is now fastened to the cannulated screws and clamping elements, and the ventral screws of the 4-point fixation are inserted. A special measuring instrument is used to assess the distance between the screws, and a plate of the correct length is selected. The plate is introduced lengthwise through the working portal, laid onto the clamping elements, and definitively fixed with a starting torque of 15 Nm. The plate is brought into direct bone contact with the lateral vertebral body wall by further tightening of the bone screws. The dorsal screws are inserted after temporary fixation of a targeting device and opening of the cortex. Because of the wedge shape of the vertebral body, the ventral screws are usually 5 mm shorter than the dorsal screws. In addition, a locking screw is inserted to lock the polyaxial mechanism of the dorsal screws (see **Fig. 2**).

Closure and Postoperative Care

Before the operation is concluded, radiographs are taken with the C-arm in both planes to check the decompression and position of the implants. Any incisions of the diaphragmatic attachment

that are longer than 2 cm should be closed with 2 or 3 adapting sutures endoscopically. The thoracic cavity is inspected endoscopically, the site is irrigated, a chest tube is inserted through the suction-irrigation portal, and the remaining instruments are removed. Complete reinflation and

Table 1 Indications for mini-TAA	
Indication	**Frequency**
VBR for anterior column reconstruction after posterior short-segment fixation and fusion	Common
Load sharing score of >6 TL-AOSIS score >5	Common
Spinal canal decompression	Common
Significant spinal canal stenosis after posterior decompression ± fragment resection with: Severe radicular pain ± Significant bowel and bladder dysfunction ± Significant motor deficit	Common
Mechanical back pain and loss of correction after posterior surgery	Common
VBR for anterior column reconstruction for fusion after percutaneous screw fixation	Common
VBR for anterior column reconstruction for pincer fracture (A2)	Rare
Partial VBR for superior or inferior incomplete burst fracture (A3)	Rare

Abbreviation: TL-AOSIS, Thoracolumbar AOSpine Injury Score.

ventilation of the lung is checked endoscopically, and the endoscope is removed.

All 4 surgical incisions are closed with deep and superficial sutures. The thoracic drainage is connected to suction of 15 cm H_2O, and use of the chest tube is usually continued for 24 hours. A postoperative chest radiograph is obtained immediately and after 12 to 24 hours to confirm there is no pneumothorax.

Follow-up is scheduled for intervals of 1, 3, 6, 12, and 24 months. Office work and light duty are allowed at 3 to 4 weeks and full activity is typically obtained by 3 months.

DISCUSSION

The treatment of TLJ burst fracture will remain a controversial topic because of lack of consistent diagnosis and symptoms; however, common indications for surgical intervention are listed in **Table 1**. Once surgery is selected as a treatment option, the best approach for the patient should be selected. Anterior, posterior, and combined surgical approaches can be used to perform all possible surgical treatment goals, which are:

- Correction of the kyphotic deformity
- Stabilization and fusion of the injured segment
- Decompression neural structure
- Repair of dural injuries

Although each of these surgical goals can be accomplished with all surgical approaches, some goals are easier achieved with either the posterior or anterior approach (**Table 2**). The use of combined surgery (ie, posterior-anterior) has been discouraged because of the increased combined morbidity; however, the advent of minimally invasive surgical techniques for anterior and posterior spine surgery might make it possible to take advantage of the benefits of each approach without an increase in morbidity.

The safety and efficacy of thoracoscopic spinal surgery have been shown, with excellent outcomes compared with the open approach. Beisse[8] reported that fusion rates at 1-year radiographic follow-up were up to 90% using the MACS-TL anterolateral plating system.[8] In comparison with traditional thoracotomy procedures, which have morbidity rates of 14% to 29.5%,[9] the complication rates for thoracoscopic procedures have been between 0% and 5.4%.[9,10] In patients undergoing thoracoscopic procedures, the dosage and duration of postoperative analgesic use are 42% and 31% lower, respectively,[9] and the rate of chronic pain is between 4% and 35% (compared with 7%–55% with open thoracotomy).[9] Patients undergoing a thoracoscopic surgery also had a shorter median hospital stay (7 days vs 9 days).

The learning curve associated with the thoracoscopic technique can be a drawback of the

Table 2
Pros (P) and cons (C) of anterior and posterior approaches

Surgical Goals	Posterior	Anterior	Comments
Acute-emergent surgery	+	−	P: less complicated, fewer resources C: more resources
EBL acute surgery	+	−	P: less EBL and easier to control C: more EBL and harder to control
Decompression of neural elements	+	−	P: laminectomy alone C: not possible
Removal of burst fracture	+	−	P: more familiar approaches C: technically more difficult
Dural repair	+	−	P: suture repair more likely C: risk of CSF pleural fistula
Correction of deformity	+	−	P: easier to correct C: can be done with open technique
Stabilization with instrumentation	+	+	P: stronger pedicle screws C: plate most likely needs a brace
Anterior column support	−	+	P: more extensive exposure C: larger cage or graft
Wound infection	−	+	P: higher risk C: rare to have infection
Fusion rate	−	+	P: lower fusion rate, little autograft C: higher fusion rate, lots of autograft

Abbreviations: CSF, cerebrospinal fluid; EBL, estimated blood loss.

approach, because operative times increase initially to an average of greater than or equal to 6 hours[10] before decreasing to about 3 hours for trauma cases.[11] This drawback may be countered by a decrease in average estimated blood loss and the avoidance of most major intraoperative complications with meticulous adherence to surgical technique.[12,13]

SUMMARY

In the past 10 years, endoscopic procedures on the spine have become an alternative to open spine surgery for many procedures, including complete fracture treatment with VBR and ventral instrumentation as well as anterior decompression of the spinal canal. Through the miniopen thoracoscopic-assisted approach, the TLJ and the retroperitoneal segments of the spine can be accessed with reduced morbidity. The complication rate of the endoscopic procedure is of the same scale as that for open procedures, with clear advantages in terms of the reduced access morbidity associated with the minimally invasive technique.

ACKNOWLEDGMENTS

This article is based, in part, on previous work by the authors.[14,15] The authors thank Kristin Kraus, MSc, for excellent editorial assistance.

REFERENCES

1. McAfee PC, Regan JR, Fedder IL, et al. Anterior thoracic corpectomy for spinal cord decompression performed endoscopically. Surg Laparosc Endosc 1995;5(5):339–48.

2. Pellise F, Barastegui D, Hernandez-Fernandez A, et al. Viability and long-term survival of short-segment posterior fixation in thoracolumbar burst fractures. Spine J 2015;15(8):1796–803.

3. Alanay A, Acaroglu E, Yazici M, et al. Short-segment pedicle instrumentation of thoracolumbar burst fractures: does transpedicular intracorporeal grafting prevent early failure? Spine (Phila Pa 1976) 2001; 26(2):213–7.

4. Oner FC, Verlaan JJ, Verbout AJ, et al. Cement augmentation techniques in traumatic thoracolumbar spine fractures. Spine (Phila Pa 1976) 2006;31(Suppl 11):S89–95 [discussion: S104].

5. Verlaan JJ, Dhert WJ, Verbout AJ, et al. Balloon vertebroplasty in combination with pedicle screw instrumentation: a novel technique to treat thoracic and lumbar burst fractures. Spine (Phila Pa 1976) 2005; 30(3):E73–9.

6. Schmidt MH, Larson SJ, Maiman DJ. The lateral extracavitary approach to the thoracic and lumbar spine. Neurosurg Clin North Am Oct 2004;15(4): 437–41.

7. Beisse R. Endoscopic surgery on the thoracolumbar junction of the spine. Eur Spine J 2010;19(Suppl 1): S52–65.

8. Beisse R. Thoracoscopic decompression and fixation (MACS-TL). In: Kim D, Fessler R, Regan JJ, editors. Endoscopic spine surgery and instrumentation. New York: Thieme; 2004. p. 180–98.

9. Beisse R. Endoscopic repair in spinal trauma. In: Regan J, Lieberman IH, editors. Atlas of minimal access spine surgery. 2nd edition. St Louis (MO): Quality Medical Publishing; 2004. p. 285–320.

10. Kan P, Schmidt MH. Minimally invasive thoracoscopic approach for anterior decompression and stabilization of metastatic spine disease. Neurosurg Focus 2008;25(2):E8.

11. Ray WZ, Schmidt MH. Thoracoscopic vertebrectomy for thoracolumbar junction fractures and tumors: surgical technique and evaluation of the learning curve. Clin Spine Surg 2016;29(7):E344–50.

12. Amini A, Apfelbaum RI, Schmidt MH. Chylorrhea: a rare complication of thoracoscopic discectomy of the thoracolumbar junction. Case report. J Neurosurg Spine 2007;6(6):563–6.

13. Binning MJ, Bishop F, Schmidt MH. Splenic rupture related to thoracoscopic spine surgery. Spine (Phila Pa 1976) 2010;35(14):E654–6.

14. Kalra R, Schmidt MH, Beisse R. Thoracoscopic spine surgery. In: Winn H, editor. Youman's neurological surgery. Philadelphia: Elsevier; 2016.

15. Kalra R, Schmidt MH. Thoracoscopic corpectomy and reconstruction. In: Benzel E, editor. Spine surgery. Philadelphia: Elsevier; 2016.

Complications in the Management of Patients with Spine Trauma

CrossMark

Geoffrey Stricsek, MD[a], George Ghobrial, MD[a],
Jefferson Wilson, MD[a], Thana Theofanis, MD[a],
James S. Harrop, MD[a,b],*

KEYWORDS

- Spinal cord injury • Trauma • Complications

KEY POINTS

- More than 50% of patients diagnosed with acute traumatic spinal cord injury experience at least 1 complication during their initial hospitalizations.
- Of patients who survive the event precipitating SCI, the greatest risk of mortality is from associated complications, not SCI itself.

INTRODUCTION

The most recent estimates suggest that there are roughly 17,000 new cases of spinal cord injury (SCI) each year, with a prevalence between 243,000 to 347,000 people.[1] Lifetime costs of SCI range from $1.1 million to almost $5 million based on severity and age at time of injury.[1] Compared with patients undergoing elective spine surgery, patients admitted to the hospital with spinal trauma have significantly longer hospital stays[2,3] and a significantly increased risk of complications.[4] Previous literature has defined a complication in the setting of SCI to be any "change in a patient's physiological state or anatomic integrity that required medical or surgical treatment and/or prolonged [a] patient's hospitalization."[5]

More than 50% of patients diagnosed with an acute traumatic SCI experience at least 1 complication during their initial hospitalization.[5] Age, extent of neurologic injury at the time of hospital admission, mechanism of injury, and the presence of comorbid illness are associated with a higher likelihood of developing a complication after SCI.[6] The more severe the neurologic injury, the greater the likelihood of increasing complications: 90% of American Spinal Injury Association (ASIA) grade A patients have at least 2 complications.[5] Risk of complication is also related to the mechanism of injury (patients with penetrating trauma have a higher risk of complication) and associated traumatic brain injury (patients with Glasgow Coma Scale score <8 have a higher risk of complication).[5] However, patients with SCI are also more likely to have multiple medical comorbidities[4]: 55% of complications occur within the first 7 days of injury; 78% occur within 14 days.[5]

Of the patients with SCI who survive their initial traumatic injuries, the greatest risk of mortality comes not from spinal cord damage but from the complications that can develop over the course

a Division of Spine and Peripheral Nerve Surgery, Department of Neurologic Surgery, Thomas Jefferson University, 909 Walnut Street – Third Floor, Philadelphia, PA 19107, USA; b Department of Orthopedic Surgery, Thomas Jefferson University, 909 Walnut Street – Third Floor, Philadelphia, PA 19107, USA
* Corresponding author. Division of Spine and Peripheral Nerve Surgery, Department of Neurological Surgery, Thomas Jefferson University, 909 Walnut Street – Third Floor, Philadelphia, PA 19107.
E-mail address: James.Harrop@jefferson.edu

Neurosurg Clin N Am 28 (2017) 147–155
http://dx.doi.org/10.1016/j.nec.2016.08.007
1042-3680/17/© 2016 Elsevier Inc. All rights reserved.

of their care[7]; thus, vigilance in the identification and treatment of complications is a critical element in the care of all patients with SCI. In addition to the potential complications associated with the management of SCI, this article also discusses SCI-associated disorders that can increase the risk of those complications.

INTRACRANIAL INJURY

Any traumatic mechanism sufficient to create a traumatic SCI has the potential to cause an intracranial injury. From 5% to 23% of patients with SCI are reported to have associated intracranial disorders, including subdural or extradural hematoma, intraparenchymal contusion, or diffuse axonal injury.[5,8,9] Cranial imaging for patients with SCI should be considered to identify any process that could potentially increase a patient's risk of morbidity and mortality. Patients with intracranial pathology are significantly more likely to experience pulmonary complications as well,[10] and these pulmonary complications are responsible for more than one-quarter of SCI deaths.[7,11] Osseous element injuries, including occipital condyle fracture, can be identified on cranial imaging and these may be associated with an increased risk of atlanto-occipital dislocation (nearly 10%).[12] Undiagnosed occipital condyle fractures can lead to lower cranial nerve injury,[13] thereby increasing the risk of dysphagia, aspiration, and diaphragm dysfunction, depending on which cranial nerves are involved.

VASCULAR INJURY

From 40% to 60% of patients with SCI are diagnosed with a cervical spine injury.[14] In this SCI subgroup, there is an increased risk of vascular injury, reported at between 15% and 30%,[15–17] thus it is important to understand the mechanism of injury as well as to review all imaging for signs of vessel damage. Situations in which vascular imaging with computed tomography (CT) or magnetic resonance (MR) angiography may be warranted include subaxial cervical spine subluxation, any fracture extending through a transverse foramen, craniocervical dislocation, or penetrating mechanism of injury because these are associated with increased risk of vertebral and carotid artery damage (**Figs. 1–3**).[18,19] Early identification of vessel damage and initiation of appropriate therapy is important because it may reduce the risk of stroke (**Fig. 4**).[20]

DURAL INJURIES

Although not often identified on preoperative imaging, dural injuries are commonly associated with traumatic SCI. The thoracolumbar spine is a more common site than the cervical spine, with a quoted incidence of 9% to 36% compared with 9% to 13% for the cervical spine.[21–24] Traumatic dural injuries are more common in burst, flexion-distraction, and fracture dislocation injuries and also are more likely to be associated with neurologic injury as a result of the high-energy mechanism required to cause spinal canal disruption sufficient to disrupt the dura.[24–27] Identification and appropriate management of cerebrospinal fluid leak is important because it can reduce the risk of patient morbidity. The rate of complication associated with traumatic dural injuries is low (0%–2%)[23,24] but includes poor wound healing/wound breakdown, pseudomeningocele formation with associated headaches, and meningitis.

PREEXISTING SPINAL DISORDER

The presence of preexisting spinal disorders (eg, ankylosing spondylitis [AS]) has been shown to have a negative impact on motor recovery following SCI.[28] Approximately 2% of patients with SCI also have AS and the AS population carries an 11-fold increased risk of SCI compared with the general population.[29,30] Thus, patients

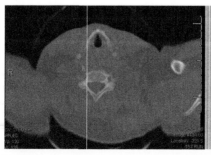
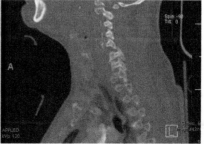

Fig. 1. CT, axial (*left*) and sagittal (*right*) reconstructions showing a subaxial cervical spine subluxation resulting from a flexion-distraction mechanism in a patient following motor vehicle collision.

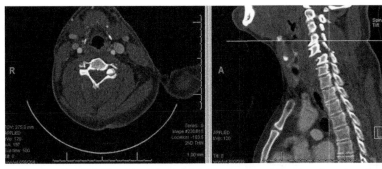

Fig. 2. CT angiography, axial (*left*) and sagittal (*right*) reconstructions showing the absence of flow-related enhancement in either vertebral artery.

with SCI and associated AS have an increased risk of poor functional outcomes, but patients with AS also have an increased incidence of other underlying comorbidities, which further complicates their postinjury care and recovery; patients with AS have been quoted as having a medical comorbidity rate as high as 80%.[31] Underlying cardiac conduction abnormalities, pulmonary fibrosis or interstitial lung disease, and renal impairment from chronic nonsteroidal antiinflammatory drug use all increase the risk of complication in patients with AS-SCI.[32] Respiratory complications are more common with AS as a result of chest-wall rigidity and reduced thoracic expansion.[31,33] Furthermore, surgical reduction of any fracture and fusion to treat instability carries a higher risk because of increased blood loss and the stiff and rigid spine.[34] When considering all of these compounding issues, it is not surprising that the complication rate in patients with AS and SCI is higher than 80%[31] and mortality is reported between 35% and 40%, compared with from 4% to 16% mortality in the general SCI population.[29,32,35]

MEDICAL COMPLICATIONS

Patients with SCI have an increased risk of developing medical complications as a result of their injuries: almost 50% have at least 2 complications,

with patients with more severe neurologic injuries (ASIA A or B) being associated with a higher chance of complications than less severely injured patients (ASIA C, D, or E).[5,8] Although large data sets have suggested that the annual incidence of SCI has remained fairly stable since the 1990s,[36] the demographics of patients diagnosed with SCI have evolved with a significant increase in the proportion of elderly patients (variably defined as 60–70 years of age).[36,37] This finding is important because older patients are more likely to have underlying medical comorbidities before their injuries and have an increased risk of developing medical complications associated with the acute phase of the injury and subsequent recovery.[38–40] Accordingly, the elderly have a significantly greater rate of mortality following SCI.[36,37] Thus, it is important to be vigilant in the assessment of all patients with SCI, but particularly in those who are older and more severely injured, for the presence of any medical complications that could impede their recovery or, even worse, hasten their demise.

Pulmonary Complications

Pulmonary complications in patients with SCI are the leading cause of mortality[7,11] and significantly increase length of hospital stay.[41] The list of pulmonary complications is extensive and includes acute

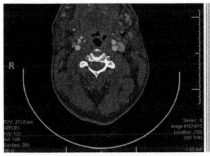
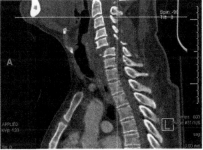

Fig. 3. CT, axial (*left*) and sagittal (*right*) reconstructions showing partial distal reconstitution of the bilateral vertebral arteries.

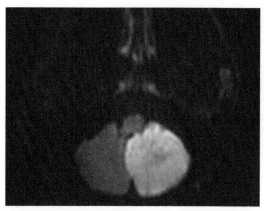

Fig. 4. MR axial sequence of the brain, diffusion-weighted imaging through the cerebellum, showing a symptomatic left cerebellar infarct 2 days postinjury. The patient ultimately required surgical decompression via a suboccipital craniectomy.

lung injury, acute respiratory distress syndrome, respiratory failure, pulmonary embolus, pleural effusion, lobar collapse, mucous plug, pneumonia, aspiration, pneumothorax, and hemothorax (**Box 1**).[5] From 10% to 60% of patients with SCI have some form of pulmonary complication,[2,5] but pneumonia is the most deadly.[42] In addition to any primary lung injury attributed to the initial event that precipitated SCI, mechanisms underlying compromised pulmonary function include decreased or absent innervation of the diaphragm and intercostal muscles, which can impair respiratory effort and inspiratory capacity; loss of sympathetic tone leading to bronchial constriction; and weak or paralyzed abdominal muscles, which prevents an effective cough and impairs the ability to clear secretions. Patients with complete SCIs are significantly more prone to pulmonary complications and have an increased risk with a more rostral

level of injury: patients with a complete cervical SCI have a 60% to 70% risk of pneumonia compared with a 20% to 30% risk in patients with incomplete SCI.[41,42] Early tracheostomy placement (within 7 days) can reduce the risk of ventilator-associated pneumonia and aspiration.[43] It also reduces the duration of mechanical ventilation and intensive care unit stay, and decreases the rate of orotracheal intubation-associated complications such as tracheal granuloma formation and stenosis.[44] Recent research has suggested that patients with diaphragm paralysis may benefit from placement of a diaphragm pacer because it can reduce dependence on positive-pressure ventilation and may even aid neuroplasticity with the development of alternative diaphragm innervation.[45]

Hematologic Complications

Potential hematologic complications encountered in SCI most commonly include, but are not limited to, deep venous thrombosis (DVT), anemia, thrombocytopenia, and coagulopathy (**Box 2**).[5] DVT is the most common of these; although older studies quote an incidence as high as 50%,[46] more recent reviews of acute SCI found it to be much lower, at approximately 3% to 4%.[36,47] This reduction is most likely caused by aggressive use of mechanical and chemoprophylactic agents. Note that location of SCI may play a role in risk for venous thromboembolism (VTE) because patients with thoracic SCI have been found to have a higher rate for VTE than patients with either cervical or lumbar injury (6% vs 3%).[47] In addition to venous stasis and endothelial injury, other factors may be at play in the development of DVT. Patients with SCI who develop DVT have been found to have higher blood concentrations of fibrinopeptide A, thrombin-antithrombin III, D-dimer, factor VIII antigen, and ristocetin cofactor.[48,49]

The biggest concern in a patient with a DVT is the subsequent risk of pulmonary embolism (PE). Although the rate of SCI-associated PE is approximately 1.5%,[36] all patients with SCI should be managed with a combination of mechanical and pharmacologic prophylaxis beginning within 72 hours of injury and continuing for at least 3 months.[50] Research has shown that there exists

---

Box 1
Pulmonary complications

- Acute lung injury
- Acute respiratory distress syndrome
- Respiratory failure
- Pulmonary embolus
- Aspiration
- Pneumonia
- Pleural effusion
- Lobar collapse
- Mucous plug
- Pneumothorax
- Hemothorax

Box 2
Hematologic complications

- Deep venous thrombosis
- Pulmonary embolus
- Thrombocytopenia
- Coagulopathy

a synergistic effect when both techniques are used concurrently.[51] An inferior vena cava filter is not recommended as a first-line agent given the risk profile and absence of mortality benefit,[52] but can be considered if a patient has failed first-line therapy or there is a contraindication to anticoagulation therapy.[50]

Cardiac Complications

The severity of cardiac dysfunction following SCI is correlated with the anatomic level and degree of SCI.[53,54] Patients with injuries in the cervical or upper thoracic spine to the level of T6 have the highest risk of cardiovascular dysfunction from impairment or loss of sympathetic vascular control, which subsequently allows unopposed parasympathetic input from the vagus nerve[55]; cardiac complications are also more common in patients with more severe neurologic injury (ASIA A and B) and are the second leading cause of death after pulmonary complications.[7,56,57] Common cardiac complications following SCI include arrhythmia, bradycardia, cardiac arrest, myocardial infarction (MI), shock (defined as systolic blood pressure <80 mm Hg), congestive heart failure, and cardiogenic pulmonary edema (**Box 3**).[5] In the acute setting, traumatic SCI requiring emergency surgery is associated with an increased risk of perioperative MI.[58] Loss of central sympathetic regulation of peripheral vascular tone can cause orthostatic hypotension, lower resting blood pressure, and in severe cases neurogenic shock when combined with persistent bradycardia.[59]

Prompt identification and management of cardiac irregularities is critical to improving long-term patient outcomes. Evidence suggests that hypotension (systolic blood pressure <90 mm Hg) in the acute setting following traumatic SCI is associated with worse neurologic outcomes and can perpetuate the development of secondary neurologic injury.[35,60–63] Blood pressure should be supported with fluid resuscitation to the extent that there is adequate intravascular volume repletion, at which point pressor agents may be used[64] with a goal mean arterial pressure between 85 and 90 mm Hg for the first 7 days after injury, based on the most recent guidelines.[65] The risks of aggressive fluid resuscitation should be assessed on a patient-by-patient basis, depending on patient cardiopulmonary status and age. In the setting of trauma, it is important to rule out hypovolemic shock attributable to a hemorrhagic cause before diagnosing a patient with hypotension from neurogenic shock.

Skin Complications

The incidence of pressure ulcers is varied based on the severity of the patient's injury and the point along the recovery pathway, but can be as high as 30% to 40%.[66,67] They are most commonly found in areas that rest on another surface, such as the heels, trochanters, sacrum, scapulae, and occiput. Multidisciplinary focus on prevention and identification of pressure ulcers has led to a decrease in their incidence over time from almost 70% in the early 1980s.[67] Current strategies include early mobilization, frequent turns and repositioning, nutritional support, specialty beds, and targeted care for areas that show early signs of breakdown.

Compared with elective spine patients, patients with SCI requiring emergent surgery have a significantly higher risk of surgical site infection (SSI) and wound dehiscence.[4,5] The rate of postoperative SSI following surgery for spine trauma is between 3% and 5% in the first 3 months after surgery.[68,69] Surgery occurring more than 3 days after the inciting event, significant bleeding (>600 mL), fusion of more than 3 levels, and severity of neurologic injury have been shown to correlate with increased risk of SSI.[68]

Gastrointestinal Complications

Similar to SCI-associated cardiac complications, many gastrointestinal (GI) complications are thought to be the result of unopposed parasympathetic activity. Increased gastric and pancreatic secretions increase the risk of GI hemorrhage and pancreatitis, whereas autonomic imbalance and impaired gut motility increase the risk of ileus (**Box 4**).[70] Delayed transit of gastric contents through the GI system has been found to increase the risk of aspiration in patients with cervical spine immobilization who are receiving nutrition via tube feeds.[71] Note that metabolic demands are decreased following acute SCI, often continuing into the chronic phase, leading to a delayed risk of obesity.[72] Patients with SCI have also been

---

Box 3
Cardiac complications

- Arrhythmia
- Bradycardia
- Cardiac arrest
- Myocardial infarction
- Shock
- Congestive heart failure
- Cardiogenic pulmonary edema
- Orthostatic hypotension

Box 4
GI complications

- GI hemorrhage
- Ileus
- Obesity
- Pancreatitis
- Dysphagia
- Constipation

found to have impaired glucose tolerance and insulin resistance attributed to skeletal muscle atrophy and decreased physical activity.[73,74]

Renal Complications

Hematuria, acute renal failure, urinary incontinence, and urinary tract infection are the renal issues that most commonly occur in patients with SCI.[5] The risk of urinary tract infection is greater than 10% and this is one of the most common complications associated with SCI.[69] Although it remains controversial, sterile intermittent catheterization has been associated with a lower rate of urologic complications compared with chronic indwelling catheters.[75] Improved outcomes have been shown with a longer course (14 days instead of 3 days) of antibiotics for the treatment of acute urinary tract infections, but prophylactic antibiotic use is not supported for all patients with SCI.[76,77]

Neuropsychiatric Complications

SCI has been shown to confer an increased risk of depression, cognitive changes, anxiety, and substance abuse.[5,78] It is important to screen patients with SCI for symptoms suggestive of any psychological disorder and manage them accordingly in order to optimize chances for recovery.

Infectious Complications

Approximately 36% of patients develop some form of infection associated with the care and recovery from SCI.[5] Specific details regarding the most frequent and significant infectious complications in various systems are discussed earlier. Surgeons should have an increased awareness for infectious complications given that SSIs are at a higher risk in patients who undergo spinal decompression and fusion for traumatic SCI.

THERAPEUTIC COMPLICATIONS

The risk of neurologic loss of function in patients with SCI is not temporally limited to the precipitating event. Delayed deterioration may occur in

5% of patients and can be attributed to therapeutic intervention, impaired spinal cord perfusion from cardiac dysfunction, and other causes.[35,63,79] Causes of deterioration include application of a traction device, patient repositioning, halo vest placement, and surgical intervention intended to address instability and/or spinal cord compression.[79] Early studies of the timing of surgery in SCI populations suggested that surgery performed within 5 days of injury may increase the risk of neurologic deterioration,[79,80] but recent research has shown a significant benefit of early surgery (within 24 hours) for cervical spine injuries, with improved functional outcome.[81] In addition, early surgery has also been shown to decrease the rate of adverse events such as pneumonia, pressure ulcers, DVT, PE, and mortality.[4,82] However, before committing any patient with SCI to surgery, it is important to remember that traumatic SCI requiring emergency surgery is associated with a potential increased risk of perioperative MI[58] and that median transfusion requirement for spinal trauma is 4 units of red blood cells; more extensive injuries are more likely to require transfusion.[83]

Debate continues regarding the use of methylprednisolone (MP) in the setting of patients with traumatic nonpenetrating SCI. Three randomized trials have been implemented within the North American Spinal Cord Injury Study (NASCIS) study to evaluate the efficacy of MP. Analysis of the second and third studies with steroid administration within 8 hours of injury showed an improvement in neurologic recovery.[84,85] However, there are potential adverse effect with the use of MP, including an association with an increased rate of wound breakdown, hyperglycemia, GI hemorrhage, and death.[86–88] Use of MP has also been evaluated in the acute setting and the acute plus surgery setting. The investigators found a significantly higher rate of complication and greater severity of complication in patients who received a second loading dose of MP during surgery.[89] Thus, the most recent American Association of Neurological Surgeons/Congress of Neurological Surgeons guidelines recommend against the use of MP in the treatment of SCI[90]; however, further reviews on this topic are in progress.

REFERENCES

1. National Spinal Cord Injury Statistical Center. Facts and figures at a glance. Birmingham (AL): University of Alabama at Birmingham; 2015.
2. Street J, Lenehan B, DiPaola C, et al. Morbidity and mortality of major adult spinal surgery. A prospective cohort analysis of 942 consecutive patients. Spine J 2012;12:22–34.

3. Karstensen S, Bari T, Gehrchen M, et al. Morbidity and mortality of complex spine surgery: a prospective cohort study in 679 patients validating the Spine AdVerse Event Severity (SAVES) system in a European population. Spine J 2016;16:146–53.

4. Kukreja S, Ambekar S, Ahmed O, et al. Impact of elective versus emergent admission on perioperative complications and resource utilization in lumbar fusion. Clin Neurol Neurosurg 2015;136:52–60.

5. Grossman R, Frankowski R, Burau K, et al. Incidence and severity of acute complications after spinal cord injury. J Neurosurg Spine 2012;17(1 Suppl): 119–28.

6. Wilson J, Arnold P, Singh A, et al. Clinical prediction model for acute inpatient complications after traumatic cervical spinal cord injury: a subanalysis from the Surgical Timing in Acute Spinal Cord Injury Study. J Neurosurg Spine 2012;17(1 Suppl):46–51.

7. DeVivo M, Krause J, Lammertse D. Recent trends in mortality and causes of death among persons with spinal cord injury. Arch Phys Med Rehabil 1999;80: 1411–9.

8. Silva Santos E, Santos Filho W, Possatti L, et al. Clinical complications in patients with severe cervical spine trauma: a ten year prospective study. Arq Neuropsiquiatr 2012;70(7):524–8.

9. Chikuda H, Ohya J, Horiguchi H, et al. Ischemic stroke after cervical spine injury: analysis of 11,005 patients using the Japanese Diagnosis Procedure Combination database. Spine J 2014;14:2275–80.

10. Fletcher D, Taddonio R, Byrne D, et al. Incidence of acute care complications in vertebral column fracture patients with and without spinal cord injury. Spine (Phila Pa 1976) 1995;20(10):1136–46.

11. Weaver F, Smith B, Evans C. Outcomes of outpatient visits for acute respiratory illness in veterans with spinal cord injuries and disorders. Am J Phys Med Rehabil 2006;85(9):718–26.

12. Mueller F, Fuechtmeier B, Kinner B, et al. Occipital condyle fractures. Prospective follow-up of 31 cases within 5 years at a level 1 trauma centre. Eur Spine J 2012;21:289–94.

13. Leone A, Cerase A, Colosimo C, et al. Occipital condylar fractures: a review. Radiology 2000;216(3): 635–44.

14. Singh A, Tetreault L, Kalsi-Ryan S, et al. Global prevalence and incidence of traumatic spinal cord injury. Clin Epidemiol 2014;6:309–31.

15. Mueller C, Peters I, Podlogar M, et al. Vertebral artery injuries following cervical spine trauma: a prospective observational study. Eur Spine J 2011; 20(12):2202–9.

16. Munera F, Cohn S, Rivas L. Penetrating injuries of the neck: use of helical computed tomographic angiography. J Trauma 2005;58:413–8.

17. Asensio J, Valenziano C, Falcone R, et al. Management of penetrating neck injuries: the controversy surrounding zone II injuries. Surg Clin North Am 1991;71:267–96.

18. Cothren C, Moore E, Biffl W, et al. Cervical spine fracture patterns predictive in blunt cervical vascular injury. J Trauma 2003;55:811–3.

19. Vilela M, Kim L, Bellabarba C, et al. Blunt cerebrovascular injuries in association with craniocervical distraction injuries: a retrospective review of consecutive cases. Spine J 2015;15:499–505.

20. Eastman A, Muraliraj V, Sperry J, et al. CTA-based screening reduces time to diagnosis and stroke rate in blunt cervical vascular injury. J Trauma 2009;67:551–6.

21. Aydinli U, Karaeminogullari O, Tiskaya K, et al. Dural tears in lumbar burst fractures with greenstick lamina fractures. Spine (Phila Pa 1976) 2001;26:E410–5.

22. Silvestro C, Francaviglia N, Bragazzi R, et al. On the predictive value of radiological signs for the presence of dural lacerations related to fractures of the lower thoracic or lumbar spine. J Spinal Disord 1991;4:49–53.

23. Lee S, Chung C, Jahng T, et al. Dural tear and resultant cerebrospinal fluid leak after cervical spinal trauma. Eur Spine J 2014;23:1772–6.

24. Luszczyk M, Blaisdell G, Wiater B, et al. Traumatic dural tears: what do we know and are they a problem? Spine J 2014;14:49–56.

25. Miller C, Dewey R, Hunt W. Impaction fracture of the lumbar vertebra with dural tear. J Neurosurg 1980; 53:765–71.

26. Cammisa FJ, Eismont F, Green B. Dural laceration occurring with burst fractures and associated laminar fractures. J Bone Joint Surg Am 1989;71: 1044–52.

27. Pickett J, Blumenkopf B. Dural lacerations and thoracolumbar fractures. J Spinal Disord 1989;2:99–103.

28. Kreinest M, Ludes L, Biglari B, et al. Influence of previous comorbidities and common complications on motor function after early surgical treatment of patients with traumatic spinal cord injury. J Neurotrauma 2016. [Epub ahead of print].

29. Tico N, Ramon S, Garcia-Ortun F, et al. Traumatic spinal cord injury complicating ankylosing spondylitis. Spinal Cord 1998;36:349–52.

30. Alaranta H, Luoto S, Konttinen Y. Traumatic spinal cord injury as a complication to ankylosing spondylitis. An extended report. Clin Exp Rheumatol 2002; 20:66–8.

31. Caron T, Bransford R, Nguyen Q. Spine fractures in patients with ankylosing spinal disorders. Spine (Phila Pa 1976) 2005;35:E458–64.

32. Jacobs W, Fehlings M. Ankylosing spondylitis and spinal cord injury: origin, incidence, management, and avoidance. Neurosurg Focus 2008;24(1):E12.

33. Ragnarsdottir M, Geirsson A, Gudbjornsson B. Rib cage motion in ankylosing spondylitis patients: a pilot study. Spine J 2008;8:505–9.

34. Tetzlaff J, Yoon H, Bell G. Massive bleeding during spine surgery in a patient with ankylosing spondylitis. Can J Anaesth 1998;45:903–6.

35. Sekhon L, Felings M. Epidemiology, demographics, and pathophysiology of acute spinal cord injury. Spine 2001;26:S2–12.

36. Jain N, Ayers G, Peterson E, et al. Traumatic spinal cord injury in the United States, 1993-2012. JAMA 2015;313(22):2236–43.

37. Fassett D, Harrop J, Maltenfort M, et al. Mortality rates in geriatric patients with spinal cord injuries. J Neurosurg Spine 2007;7:277–81.

38. Krassioukov A, Furlan J, Fehlings M. Medical comorbidities, secondary complications, and mortality in elderly with acute spinal cord injury. J Neurotrauma 2003;20(4):391–9.

39. Ahn H, Bailey C, Rivers C, et al. Effect of older age on treatment decisions and outcomes among patients with traumatic spinal cord injury. CMAJ 2015; 187(12):873–80.

40. Boakye M, Arrigo R, Kalanithi P, et al. Impact of age, injury severity score, and medical comorbidities on early complications after fusion and halo-vest immobilization for C2 fractures in older adults. Spine (Phila Pa 1976) 2012;37(10):854–9.

41. Aarabi B, Harrop J, Tator C, et al. Predictors of pulmonary complications in blunt traumatic spinal cord injury. J Neurosurg Spine 2012;17(1 Suppl):38–45.

42. Berney S, Bragge P, Granger C, et al. The acute respiratory management of cervical spinal cord injury in the first 6 weeks after injury: a systemic review. Spinal Cord 2011;49(1):17–29.

43. Jaeger J, Littlewood K, Durbin C. The role of tracheostomy in weaning from mechanical ventilation. Respir Care 2002;47(4):469–80.

44. Romero J, Vari A, Gambarrutta C, et al. Tracheostomy timing in traumatic spinal cord injury. Eur Spine J 2009;18(10):1452–7.

45. Onders R, Khansarinia S, Weiser T. Multicenter analysis of diaphragm pacing in tetraplegics with cardiac pacemakers: positive implications for ventilator weaning in intensive care units. Surgery 2010;148(4):893–7.

46. Gunduz S, Ogur E, Mohur H, et al. Deep vein thrombosis in spinal cord injured patients. Paraplegia 1993;31(9):606–10.

47. Maung A, Schuster K, Kaplan L, et al. Risk of venous thromboembolism after spinal cord injury: not all levels are the same. J Trauma 2011;71:1241–5.

48. Rossi E, Green D, Rosen J. Sequential changes in factor VIII and platelets preceding deep vein thrombosis in patients with spinal cord injury. Br J Haematol 1980;45:143–51.

49. Fujii Y, Mammen E, Farag A. Thrombosis in spinal cord injury. Thromb Res 1992;68:357–68.

50. Dhall S, Hadley M, Aarabi B, et al. Deep venous thrombosis and thromboembolism in patients with cervical spinal cord injuries. Neurosurgery 2013; 72:244–54.

51. Merli G, Crabbe S, Doyle L, et al. Mechanical plus pharmacological prophylaxis for deep vein thrombosis in acute spinal cord injury. Paraplegia 1992; 30(8):558–62.

52. Khansarinia S, Dennis J, Veldenz H, et al. Prophylactic greenfield filter placement in selected high-risk trauma patients. J Vasc Surg 1995;22(3):231–5.

53. Furlan J, Fehlings M, Shannon P. Descending vasomotor pathways in humans: correlation between axonal preservation and cardiovascular dysfunction after spinal cord injury. J Neurotrauma 2003;20: 1351–63.

54. Krassioukov A, Furlan J, Fehlings M. Autonomic dysreflexia in acute spinal cord injury: an underrecognized clinical entity. J Neurotrauma 2003;20: 707–16.

55. Garstang S, Miller-Smith S. Autonomic nervous system dysfunction after spinal cord injury. Phys Med Rehabil Clin North Am 2007;18:275–96.

56. Popa C, Popa F, Grigorean V. Vascular dysfunctions following spinal cord injury. J Med Life 2010;3:275–85.

57. Krassioukov A, Claydon V. The clinical problems in cardiovascular control following spinal cord injury: an overview. Prog Brain Res 2006;152:223–9.

58. Wang T, Martin J, Loriaux D, et al. Risk assessment and characterization of 30-day perioperative myocardial infarction following spine surgery: a retrospective analysis of 1346 consecutive adult patients. Spine (Phila Pa 1976) 2016;41(5):438–44.

59. Atkinson P, Atkinson J. Spinal shock. Mayo Clin Proc 1996;71:384–9.

60. Vale F, Burns J, Jackson A, et al. Combined medical and surgical treatment after acute spinal cord injury: results of a prospective pilot study to assess the merits of aggressive medical resuscitation and blood pressure management. J Neurosurg 1997; 87:239–46.

61. Levi L, Wolf A, Belzberg H. Hemodynamic parameters in patients with acute cervical cord trauma: description, intervention, and prediction of outcome. Neurosurgery 1993;33:1007–17.

62. Dumont R, Okonkwo D, Verma S. Acute spinal cord injury, part I: pathophysiologic mechanisms. Clin Neuropharmacol 2001;24(5):254–64.

63. Dyson-Hudson T, Stein A. Acute management of traumatic cervical spinal cord injuries. Mt Sinai J Med 1999;66:170–8.

64. Stevens R, Bhardwaj A, Kirsch J. Critical care and perioperative management in traumatic spinal cord injury. J Neurosurg Anesthesiol 2003;15:215–29.

65. Ryken T, Hurlbert R, Hadley M, et al. The acute cardiopulmonary management of patients with cervical spinal cord injuries. Neurosurgery 2013;77:84–92.

66. Chen D, Apple D, Hudson L, et al. Medical complications during acute rehabilitation following

spinal cord injury–current experience of the Model Systems. Arch Phys Med Rehabil 1999;80(11): 1397–401.

67. Scheel-Sailer A, Wyss A, Boldt C, et al. Prevalence, location, grade of pressure ulcers and association with specific patient characteristics in adult spinal cord injury patients during the hospital stay: a prospective cohort study. Spinal Cord 2013;51:828–33.

68. Lonjon G, Dauzac C, Fourniols E, et al. Early surgical site infections in adult spinal trauma: a prospective, multicentre study of infection rates and risk factors. Orthop Traumatol Surg Res 2012;98:788–94.

69. Dimar J, Fisher C, Vaccaro A, et al. Predictors of complications after spinal stabilization of thoracolumbar spine injuries. J Trauma 2010;69:1497–500.

70. Albert T, Levine M, Balderston R, et al. Gastrointestinal complications in spinal cord injury. Spine (Phila Pa 1976) 1991;16(Suppl 10):S522–5.

71. Dvorak M, Noonan V, Belanger L. Early versus late enteral feeding in patients with acute cervical spinal cord injury: a pilot study. Spine (Phila Pa 1976) 2004; 29(9):E175–80.

72. Buchholz A, Pencharz P. Energy expenditure in chronic spinal cord injury. Curr Opin Clin Nutr Metab Care 2004;7(6):635–9.

73. Jia X, Kowalski R, Sciubba D, et al. Critical care of traumatic spinal cord injury. J Intensive Care Med 2013;28(1):12–23.

74. Raymond J, Harmer A, Temesi J, et al. Glucose tolerance and physical activity level in people with spinal cord injury. Spinal Cord 2010;48(8):591–6.

75. Weld K, Dmochowski R. Effect of bladder management on urological complications in spinal cord injured patients. J Urol 2000;163(3):768–72.

76. Dow G, Rao P, Harding G. A prospective, randomized trial of 3 or 14 days of ciprofloxacin treatment for acute urinary tract infection in patients with spinal cord injury. Clin Infect Dis 2004;39(5):658–64.

77. Morton S, Shekelle P, Adams J. Antimicrobial prophylaxis for urinary tract infection in persons with spinal cord dysfunction. Arch Phys Med Rehabil 2002;83(1):129–38.

78. Craig A, Nicholson Perry K, Guest R, et al. Prospective study of the occurrence of psychological disorders and comorbidities after spinal cord injury. Arch Phys Med Rehabil 2015;96:1426–34.

79. Marshall L, Knowlton S, Garfin S, et al. Deterioration following spinal cord injury. J Neurosurg 1987;66: 400–4.

80. Heiden J, Weiss M, Rosenberg A. Management of cervical spinal cord trauma in Southern California. J Neurosurg 1975;43:732–6.

81. Fehlings M, Vaccaro A, Wilson J, et al. Early versus delayed decompression for traumatic cervical spinal cord injury: results of the Surgical Timing in Acute Spinal Cord Injury Study (STASCIS). PLoS One 2012;7(2):1–8.

82. Bourassa-Moreau E, Mac-Thiong J, Ehrmann Feldman D, et al. Complications in acute phase hospitalization of traumatic spinal cord injury: does surgical timing matter? J Trauma Acute Care Surg 2013;74(3):849–54.

83. Butler J, Burke J, Dolan R, et al. Risk analysis of blood transfusion requirements in emergency and elective spinal surgery. Eur Spine J 2011;20:753–8.

84. Bracken M, Shepard M, Collins W. A randomized, controlled trial of methylprednisolone or naloxone in the treatment of acute spinal-cord injury: results of the Second National Acute Spinal Cord Injury Study. N Engl J Med 1990;322:1405–11.

85. Bracken M, Shepard M, Holford T. Administration of methylprednisolone for 24 or 48 hours or tirilazad mesylate for 48 hours in the treatment of acute spinal cord injury: results of the third national acute spinal cord injury randomized controlled trial. National Acute Spinal Cord Injury Study. JAMA 1997;277: 1597–604.

86. Edwards P, Arango M, Balica L. Final results of MRC CRASH, a randomised placebo-controlled trial of intravenous corticosteroid in adults with head injury-outcomes at 6 months. Lancet 2005;365: 1957–9.

87. Pointillart V, Petitjean M, Wiart L. Pharmacological therapy of spinal cord injury during the acute phase. Spinal Cord 2000;38(2):71–6.

88. Matsumoto T, Tamaki T, Kawakami M, et al. Early complications of high-dose methylprednisolone sodium succinate treatment in the follow-up of acute cervical spinal cord injury. Spine (Phila Pa 1976) 2001;26(4):426–30.

89. Del Rosario Molano M, Broton J, Bean J, et al. Complications associated with the prophylactic use of methylprednisolone during surgical stabilization after spinal cord injury. J Neurosurg Spine 2002;96: 267–72.

90. Hurlbert R, Hadley M, Walters B, et al. Pharmacological therapy for acute spinal cord injury. Neurosurgery 2013;72:93–105.

Minimally Invasive Treatment of Spine Trauma

Jason E. McGowan, MD[a], Christian B. Ricks, MD[b],
Adam S. Kanter, MD[c],*

KEYWORDS

- MIS • Minimally invasive • Spine trauma • Percutaneous

KEY POINTS

- In the setting of trauma where patients can be structurally unstable and hemodynamically labile, operative techniques that minimize morbidity without compromising clinical efficacy have significant value.
- Minimally invasive surgery (MIS) techniques have been associated with decreased intraoperative blood loss, operative time, and morbidity, while providing patients with comparable outcomes when compared with conventional open procedures.
- MIS interventions enable earlier mobilization, decreased hospital stay, decreased pain, and an earlier return to baseline function when compared with traditional techniques.
- MIS techniques designed to reestablish anterior column support include percutaneous vertebral body augmentation procedures and mini-open lateral corpectomy.
- MIS posterior stabilization largely consists of percutaneous fixation techniques that minimize the surgical access footprint and adjacent tissue injury.

INTRODUCTION

Traumatic spine fractures represent 75% of all spinal injuries, thus accounting for 160,000 annually,[1] most of which occur at the thoracolumbar junction (T10–L2) due to the transition from the mobile lumbar spine to the rigid thoracic spine. These fractures are typically caused by high-impact injuries, such as motor vehicle accidents and falls, and can result in persistent pain and disability even without neurologic compromise.[2] Early surgical management can potentially prevent, and sometimes reverse, neurologic injury; this may involve decompression, reduction, anterior column support, and/or restoration of the posterior tension band.[3] Operative stabilization with pedicle screw instrumentation via a posterior approach for reduction and fixation of fractures has traditionally demonstrated good clinical and radiographic outcomes and remains the prevalent treatment for most fractures.[4,5] However, open surgical approaches have been associated with a mixed array of perioperative complications, including infection, significant blood loss, and extended hospitalizations.[6]

Minimally invasive surgery (MIS) has been increasingly used in the treatment of degenerative spinal pathology; however, its utilization in traumatic injury was not reported until 2004 and

Disclosure: The authors have no commercial or financial conflicts of interest to disclose as it relates to this article.
[a] Georgetown University, Washington, DC, USA; [b] University of Pittsburgh Medical Center, Pittsburgh, PA, USA; [c] Neurological Surgery Spine Services, University of Pittsburgh Medical Center, UMPC – Presbyterian, Suite B400, 200 Lothrop Street, Pittsburgh, PA 15213, USA
* Corresponding author.
E-mail address: kanteras@upmc.edu

indications for its usage remained controversial. Due to evolving advancements in MIS technology and practice over the past decade, spine surgeons have established 360° MIS access to the vertebral column enabling anterior, lateral, and posterior less-invasive surgical approaches. Select examples of MIS procedures include percutaneous segmental fixation, vertebroplasty/kyphoplasty, and mini-open lateral access corpectomy/fusion, enabling a less destructive method of fixation and stabilization with limited adjacent tissue destruction. Moreover, proper use of these techniques has been shown to shorten hospital and recovery times, as well as reduce blood loss and perioperative complications.[7–22] Here we summarize the techniques, controversy, and indications for the use of minimally invasive procedures in traumatic spine injuries.

Preoperative Considerations and Indications

The goals of spinal surgery in the setting of trauma remain consistent with those associated with all forms of spinal pathology, and irrespective of surgical invasiveness: decompression of neural elements, and realignment and stabilization of the vertebral column. The maintenance of adequate spinal perfusion remains critical before, during, and even after decompression of neural elements is achieved. Any injury that results in compression or spinal cord swelling can interrupt the blood supply to the spinal cord; it is thus recommended to elevate Mean Arterial Pressure (MAP) to greater than 90 mm Hg to mitigate hypoperfusion ischemic injury. If intravenous fluids alone cannot achieve target MAP, the use of vasopressors can be initiated to augment spinal perfusion.

The role of intraoperative neurophysiologic monitoring has expanded considerably with the advancements in MIS techniques, as direct visualization of neural structures is limited or absent. The use of electromyography (EMG), motor evoked potentials, and somatosensory evoked potentials (SSEPs) enables the detection of alterations in spinal cord and peripheral nerve function secondary to mechanical or ischemic events.

Patients with minor stable injuries are routinely managed nonoperatively. Those with unstable spinal injuries requiring surgical intervention can largely be divided into 2 groups: those requiring anterior column reconstruction and those requiring posterior segmental stabilization. MIS techniques designed to reestablish anterior column support include percutaneous vertebral body augmentation procedures and mini-open lateral corpectomy. Posterior stabilization largely consists of percutaneous fixation techniques that minimize

access footprint and adjacent tissue injury. The following select techniques represent the preponderance of trauma-related MIS procedures in modern day spine practice:

- *Vertebroplasty*: indicated in patients with focal back pain without evidence of cord compression, minimal loss of vertebral body height (<50%), absence of abnormal angulation (<20°), and no evidence of posterior wall involvement.
- *Kyphoplasty*: indicated in patients with focal back pain, significant loss of vertebral body height (>50%), and/or kyphotic angulation (>20°) without evidence of canal compromise or posterior wall involvement.
- *Lateral Mini-Open Corpectomy*: indicated in patients with canal stenosis secondary to comminuted or "burst" fracture patterns, kyphotic angulation, and a greater degree of instability (ie, disco-ligamentous involvement) seen on static or dynamic imaging.
- *Percutaneous Posterior Segmental Fixation*: indicated in patients with comminuted or "burst" fracture patterns with canal compromise, but with evidence of an intact posterior longitudinal ligament (PLL). Instrumentation serves as a form of "internal brace" to stabilize the segment while fracture healing occurs.

Vertebral Body Augmentation

Vertebral compression fractures commonly occur in the aging osteoporotic population and account for more than $1 billion annual medical expenditures in the United States. MIS treatments are ideal for this population due to their numerous medical comorbidities and risk of perioperative complications, particularly in those suffering and deemed unsuitable for operative intervention. Vertebral body fracture treatment considerations include evaluation of spinal stability, focal kyphotic angulation, presence of canal retropulsion, and involvement of the posterior vertebral wall and ligament. These procedures have historically low operative morbidity and high patient satisfaction rates, and remain an excellent option for elderly patients and those with multiple medical comorbidities in whom greater interventions could not be tolerated. In osteoporotic patients, some institutions advocate prophylactic cement augmentation adjacent to the index fracture level to fortify neighboring vertebral bodies. Rates of new vertebral body fractures in osteoporotic patients following initial vertebral body augmentation have been reported in the literature at rates ranging from 5% to 18%.

Percutaneous vertebroplasty

Patients with focal back pain secondary to a vertebral compression fracture with the posterior wall intact are candidates for vertebral body augmentation. In patients in whom the vertebral body height is grossly maintained (<50% loss), with kyphotic angulation <20°, MIS techniques can be used to perform percutaneous vertebroplasty in which the injured vertebral level is augmented with polymethylmethacrylate (PMMA) to diminish pain by eliminating micro-motion within the fracture. The procedure involves bipedicular cannulation to access the injured vertebral body. The patient is placed in the prone position on the operating table. Anesthesia is delivered via intravenous conscious sedation or alternatively endotracheal intubation. Fluoroscopy is used to identify the target level. The skin is prepped and local anesthetic injected. The needle is carefully introduced under fluoroscopic guidance in a lateral to medial trajectory. The ideal docking site is mid-pedicle on lateral fluoroscopy, and the lateral border of the pedicle on anteroposterior (AP) projection. Tactile resistance of intrapedicular cancellous bone and fluoroscopic confirmation are used to confirm intrapedicular position. PMMA is injected under live fluoroscopy to verify injection site and lack of cement extravasation in real-time. If cement extravasation is detected, the needle can be carefully repositioned to fill the remaining portion of the vertebral body.

Percutaneous kyphoplasty

In the setting of significant vertebral body collapse (>50%) or kyphotic angulation (>20°), kyphoplasty offers a viable option to restore vertebral body height and fortify the effected vertebral body. Kyphoplasty uses the same positioning and approach required to perform a vertebroplasty; however, before cement augmentation, a balloon is introduced into the vertebral body and expanded under live fluoroscopy to reestablish vertebral body height and reduce focal kyphotic angulation. Similarly, PMMA is injected into the vertebral body to provide permanent stability within the fracture.

A systematic review found that vertebroplasty and kyphoplasty provided significant pain relief in 87% and 92% of patients, respectively. However, cement extravasation was seen in up to 41% of patients with vertebroplasty and 9% with kyphoplasty. Postprocedural rates of adjacent level vertebral body fractures after vertebral body augmentation in the vertebroplasty group was approximately 7.4% and 6.5% in kyphoplasty. This is thought to be due to alteration of forces distributed across adjacent levels secondary to increased stiffness at the treated segment. Other factors that contribute to an increased rate of adjacent level vertebral body fractures are decreased bone mineral density, and postprocedure kyphotic angulation (>9°). Remotely, there have been rare case reports of pulmonary embolus secondary to hematogenous spread of bone cement via the epidural venous plexus.

Anterior Approach

In cases in which trauma to the spine results in injury to the anterior and middle columns, it is important to determine if surgical intervention needs to include anterior column support and stabilization. The thoracolumbar junction is particularly prone to injury given the unique biomechanical properties of the region. Angulated 2-column fractures, 3-column fractures, and fractures with evidence of disco-ligamentous involvement represent injury patterns that are traditionally treated with anterior column repair techniques, as it enables direct visualization of the anterior spinal elements and thecal sac.

Mini-open corpectomy

Patients are placed in the true lateral position. After padding of all pressure points, including the brachial plexus with an axillary roll, proper patient positioning is confirmed with fluoroscopy using both AP and lateral projections. On AP fluoroscopy, it is important to eliminate endplate parallax at each level of interest and confirm the spinous process bisects the pedicles. On lateral imaging, endplate parallax also should be eliminated and the pedicles well-defined. For lower lumbar levels, it is important to assess the superior aspect of the iliac crest, as a high-riding crest can present a relative contraindication to the mini-open approach. Similarly, the ribs may impede direct access to the rostral lumbar levels. Manipulation of the table can be used to enhance access to the spinal column; however, recent evidence suggests that the latter maneuver increases the risk of postoperative iliopsoas weakness.

An oblique incision is fashioned directly above the fractured vertebral body and careful dissection is performed through the muscle layers of the abdominal wall (external oblique, internal oblique, and transversus abdominis) and fascia into the retroperitoneal space. The transverse process is palpated and the finger turned to sweep the peritoneal contents anteriorly away from the psoas. Lateral fluoroscopy is used to confirm the level before introducing a dilator and Kirschner wire (K-wire) into the target disc space above or below the fractured vertebrae. Serial dilators are then advanced using continuous EMG neuromonitoring to safely advance the retractor while minimizing injury to the traversing lumbar plexus. Complete discectomy and annulotomy is performed above and below the fractured body. The intervening bone is then removed with the drill and rongeurs being mindful not to disrupt the anterior longitudinal ligament. The PLL can then be carefully taken to complete the decompression and expose retropulsed fragments in the canal. Once complete, an appropriately sized and angled cage is deployed in the intervertebral space. Supplemental stabilization can be achieved with lateral plating or percutaneous segmental pedicle screw and rod instrumentation.

When performing the lateral approach to the thoracic spine, the incision is fashioned along the superior aspect of the inferior adjacent rib. A right-sided approach is favorable for patients with fractures from above, and a left-sided approach is preferred for lower thoracic fractures to avoid retraction on the liver and injury to the inferior vena cava. Careful dissection of the rib from the underlying pleura is performed while mindful of the neurovascular bundle traversing the caudal border of the superior rib. The corridor can be created between the ribs or a small section of rib overlying the index vertebrae can be removed, which later can be used to provide autograph for fusion. The dilators are advanced along the posterior rib wall and gently swept forward to land atop the lateral edge of the spine. The lung is protected by using a spatula retractor as the surgical access corridor is widened. The crus of the diaphragm can be lifted or incised if it presents an obstruction to docking. Once positioned and the level is confirmed, the corpectomy is carried out similar to what was described previously, from discectomies to removal of the intervening bone including the medial rib heads depending on the necessity for canal exploration. Inadvertent injury to the pleura during the approach may necessitate a chest tube that can either be pulled as the chest wall is sealed via purse string suture under positive pressure ventilation, or after a postoperative chest radiograph rules out pneumothorax.

Reported fusion rates in patients with lateral mini-open corpectomies and minimum 1-year follow-up range from 85% to 93%, with significant improvements on Short Form-12 and Oswestry Disability Index patient satisfaction surveys. Hardware subsidence was reported in 8.1% with an overall complication rate of approximately 12%.

Posterior Approach

Posterior approaches to the spine remain the surgical workhorse in both open and MIS techniques when treating patients with destabilizing traumatic spinal injuries. MIS options aim to decrease disruption of the overlying paraspinal musculature, thus minimizing blood loss and hospitalization as these adjacent tissues contribute extensively to spinal recovery and rehabilitation. Patients with burst fractures with an intact PLL are often suitable candidates for percutaneous pedicle screw fixation and ligamentotaxy to reduce the retropulsed fracture fragments. This is represented numerically in patients with a Thoracolumbar Injury Classification and Severity score of less than 5 or Magerl type A fractures. Fractures with resultant neural deficits almost always require open decompression, in addition to those with significant rotational deformity, pedicle fractures, and adjacent vertebral body fractures, particularly when occurring over multiple levels.

Percutaneous pedicle screw placement

The patient is placed on an open Jackson radiolucent table in the prone position. Intraoperative fluoroscopy is used to confirm proper anatomic alignment and surgical level. Pedicle cannulation is performed similarly as described in the vertebral body augmentation procedures; however, the initial incision must take into account the distance to be traveled from the skin to the lateral facet/transverse process junction. Jamshidi needles are inserted and fluoroscopy is used to a confirm a mid-pedicular starting point on the AP projection. The needle is advanced approximately 1 cm to the AP midpoint of the pedicle, after which a lateral projection is then performed to confirm traversal into the pedicle and lack of any medial breach. Pedicular cannulation is completed and the K-wire is passed, followed by removal of the Jamshidi, and advancement of tissue dilators, and the pedicle screw itself. Serial fluoroscopy is used to confirm screw depth and position. This is typically accomplished either 1 or 2 levels above and below the index fracture, depending on the fracture severity and stabilization required, as well as the fracture site itself. The rods are then introduced and secured and reduction techniques performed via distractive instrumentation. Ease of rod passing is facilitated by a properly sized and bent rod inserted from where the screws are most superficial to where they are deepest, typically in a cranial to caudal direction. Final cap placement and tightening is completed and imaging obtained to verify spinal alignment and hardware placement.

For young healthy patients with pure bone injuries, short-segment fusions can be used as internal bracing to provide ample rigid fixation for fracture healing. For segments with kyphotic angulation, or those that cross the thoraco-lumbar junction, increased construct lengths are often necessary. It is important to note that this is *not* a fusion procedure, as no arthrodesis is performed. Controversy remains regarding the necessity to remove the hardware after adequate time for fracture healing has occurred, but sufficient data to support hardware removal are currently lacking.

A meta-analysis of 12 studies identifying 279 patients with percutaneous fixation compared with 340 open fixation procedures found statistically significant shorter operative duration ($P = .0002$), shorter hospital stay ($P = .0007$), reduced infection rates ($P = .05$), and improved visual analog scale clinical outcomes ($P = .001$). There was no difference noted in screw malpositioning ($P = .56$), postoperative Cobb angles ($P = .22$), body angles ($P = .66$), or anterior body height ($P = .19$). These differences are particularly important in the trauma population where comorbidities and physiologic demands increase the propensity for intraoperative blood loss and perioperative complications, such as infection.

POSTOPERATIVE MANAGEMENT

Postoperative intensive care unit monitoring may be necessary in some patients requiring maintenance of elevated blood pressure in the perioperative period to ensure adequate spinal cord perfusion. At the author's (Kanter AS) institution, target MAP is greater than 85 mm Hg for the first 24 hours postoperatively. Subsequent relaxation of MAP goals is titrated per the patient's examination status. Sequential compression devices are worn until patients are ambulatory to minimize the risk of venous thrombosis, and subcutaneous heparin is routinely started on postoperative day 1. In cases of severe fractures, patients can additionally use an external back brace to provide comfort and support as the fracture heals. Controversy remains as it relates to using a brace to minimize the incidence of hardware failure secondary to excessive flexion, extension, or lateral bending. Early mobilization marks one of the primary benefits of MIS techniques when compared with open conventional techniques. Reduction in postoperative pain, and decreased paraspinal musculature morbidity (ischemia, denervation) promote early patient mobilization, which also decreases the risk of postoperative complications, including atelectasis and deep venous thrombosis/pulmonary embolism.

SUMMARY

Minimally invasive techniques provide viable options for patients who have suffered traumatic injury to the spinal column. The goals of surgical intervention remain the same as those used when performing open procedures; however, doing so with lessened perioperative morbidity to enable early postoperative mobilization and rehabilitation. A variety of techniques have been developed as the realm of minimally invasive spinal instrumentation has evolved. Prospective randomized studies remain scarce as it relates to the spine-injured trauma population due to the historic follow-up difficulties inherent in this group. Surgeon-driven scrutiny and long-term assessment will continue to advance the implications and applications of MIS techniques in the treatment of the spine-injured patient population.

REFERENCES

1. Ozgur BM, Aryan HE, Pimenta L, et al. Extreme lateral interbody fusion (XLIF): a novel surgical technique for anterior lumbar interbody fusion. Spine J 2006;6:435–43.
2. Evans AJ, Jensen ME, Kip KE, et al. Vertebral compression fractures: pain reduction and improvement in functional mobility after percutaneous methylmethacrylate vertebroplasty in the treatment of osteoporotic vertebral body compression fractures: technical aspects. Am J Neuroradiol 1997;18:1897–904.
3. Ledlie JT, Renfro M. Balloon kyphoplasty: one-year outcomes in vertebral body height restoration, chronic pain, and activity levels. J Neurosurg 2003;98(1 Suppl):36–42.
4. Mayer MH. A new microsurgical technique for minimally invasive anterior lumbar interbody fusion. Spine 1997;22:691–9.
5. McAffe PC, Regan JJ, Geis PW, et al. Minimally invasive anterior retrperitoneal approach to the lumbar spine: emphasis on the lateral BAK. Spine 1998;23:1476–84.
6. Sandhu FA, Voyadzis JM, Fessler RG. Decision making for minimally invasive spine surgery. New York: Thieme; 2011.
7. Smith WD, Dakwar E, Tien V, et al. Minimally invasive surgery for traumatic spinal pathologies: a mini-open, lateral approach in the thoracic and lumbar spine. Spine 2010;35:338–46.
8. Uribe J, Vale FL, Dakwar E. Electromyographic monitoring and its anatomical implications in minimally invasive spine surgery. Spine (Phila Pa 1976) 2010;35:S368–74.
9. Oskouian RJ, Schaffrey CI, Kanter AS, et al. Anterior stabilization of three-column thoracolumbar spinal trauma. J Neurosurg Spine 2006;5:18–25.
10. Tempel ZJ, Gandhoke GS, Bonfield CM, et al. Radiographic and clinical outcomes following combined lateral lumbar interbody fusion and posterior

segmental stabilization in patients with adult degenerative scoliosis. Neurosurg Focus 2014;36:E11.

11. Ry Rampersaud, Annand N, Dekutoski MB. Use of minimally invasive surgical techniques in the management of thoracolumbar trauma. Spine 2006;3: S96–102.

12. Seng C, Siddiqui MA, Wong KPL, et al. Five-year outcomes of minimally invasive versus open transforaminal lumbar interbody fusion: a matched-pair comparison study. Spine 2013;38:2049–55.

13. Ahmadian A, Deukmedjian AR, Abel N, et al. Analysis of lumbar plexopathies and nerve injury after lateral retroperitoneal transpsoas approach: diagnostic standardization. J Neurosurg Spine 2013;18: 289–97.

14. Park DK, Lee MJ, Lin EL, et al. The relationship of intrapsoas nerves during a transpsoas approach to the lumbar spine: anatomic study. J Spinal Disord Tech 2010;23:223–8.

15. Watkins RG, Hanna RS, Chang D, et al. Sagittal alignment after lumbar interbody fusion: comparing anterior, lateral, and transforaminal approaches. J Spinal Disord Tech 2014;27:253–6.

16. Wiesel SW, Bolden SD. Semin Spine Surg 2015;27.

17. Schroeder GD, Kepler CK, Millhouse PW, et al. L5/S1 fusion rates in degenerative spine surgery: a systemic review comparing ALIF, TLIF, and axial interbody arthrodesis. Clin Spine Surg 2016;29(4):150–5.

18. Petteys RJ, Sandhu FA. Minimally invasive lateral retroperitoneal corpectomy for treatment of focal thoracolumbar kyphotic deformity: case report and review of literature. J Neurol Surg A Cent Eur Neurosurg 2014;75:305–9.

19. Cox JB, Yang M, Jacob RB, et al. Temporary percutaneous pedicle fixation for treatment of thoracolumbar injuries in young adults. J Neurol Surg A Cent Eur Neurosurg 2013;74:7–11.

20. Widi GA, Williams SK, Levi AD. Minimally invasive direct repair of bilateral lumbar spine pars defects in athletes. Case Rep Med 2013;1:5–6.

21. Amoretti N, Huwart L, Hauger O, et al. Computed tomography- and fluoroscopy-guided percutaneous screw fixation of low-grade isthmic spondylolisthesis in adults: a new technique. Eur Radiol 2012;22: 2841–7.

22. Molinares DM, Davis TT, Fung DA, et al. Is the lateral jack-knife position responsible for cases of transient neurapraxia? J Neurosurg Spine 2016;24:189–96.

Return to Play for Athletes

Brett D. Rosenthal, MD*, Barrett S. Boody, MD, Wellington K. Hsu, MD

KEYWORDS

- Return to play • Athlete • Stinger • Sports-related trauma • Cervical cord neurapraxia

KEY POINTS

- Sports-related trauma can cause a variety of spinal injuries.
- Each type of sports-related spine injury has unique clinical characteristics that should be considered before allowing an athlete to return to play.
- In general, athletes should be neurologically intact, pain free, at full strength, and have full range of motion before returning to full, unrestricted athletic activity.

INTRODUCTION

Spinal cord injuries have an estimated annual incidence of 40 cases per 1 million Americans, with the fourth most common cause of spinal cord injury being sports-related trauma (8.2%).[1] The incidence of sports-related spinal cord injury has decreased since the 1970s (about 14%),[2] which many attribute to injury prevention initiatives and advancements in personal protective equipment.[3] Although spinal cord injury is the most severe form of spine trauma sustained during athletics, lower impact traumas that may result in strains, stingers, disc herniations, or other forms of neural compression are far more common. The spine surgeon is often under substantial extrinsic pressures to determine an athlete's readiness to return to play, so it is critical to base this decision on reproducible metrics.

Most experts agree that, at the very least, an athlete should be neurologically intact, be pain free, be at full strength, and have full range of motion before returning to competitive athletic activities after a sports-related spine injury.[4] However, because of the variety of spine conditions associated with athletes, a single algorithm for determining an athlete's readiness for sport will likely never exist. As of yet, no major sporting organization has adopted a singular return-to-play guideline or algorithm, which reflects the complexity of the treatment of these patients. Guidelines to determine an athlete's ability to return to play are likely better described based on patient-specific factors. The most common spine conditions sustained during sport activity are described in greater detail in the sections that follow.

CERVICAL TRAUMA

Cervical spine sport injuries range from minor and transient muscle strains to catastrophic spinal cord injury. During contact sports, the most frequent mechanism responsible for catastrophic spinal cord injury involves an axial load applied to the cervical spine.[5] After spear tackling (head-first tackling) was banned from high school football in the late 1970s, the rate of cervical injuries and traumatic quadriplegia decreased by more than 70% within the first 12 years.[5] Nonetheless, cervical spine injuries accounted for 44.7% of all spinal injuries sustained by National Football League (NFL) athletes during the 2000 to 2010 seasons.[6] These conditions result in a career mean of 23.4 practices and 4.1 games missed among NFL

Disclosure: See last page of article.
Department of Orthopaedic Surgery, Northwestern University, 676 North Saint Clair Street, Suite 1350, Chicago, IL 60611, USA
* Corresponding author. Department of Orthopaedic Surgery, Northwestern University, 676 North Saint Clair Street, Suite 1350, Chicago, IL 60611.
E-mail address: brett.david.rosenthal@gmail.com

athletes per injury,[6] and the presence of a cervical spine diagnosis reduces an athlete's likelihood to be drafted despite the absence of differences in career performance.[7]

Cervical Strain/Sprains

Cervical spine injuries that are predominantly muscular or ligamentous are considered cervical strains or sprains, respectively. Cervical strains and sprains accounted for 21.7% and 15.5% of cervical spine injuries in NFL athletes and were responsible for a career mean of 6.0 and 9.6 days of activity lost per injury, respectively, from 2000 to 2010.[6] Most of these injuries are self-limited, however, despite the lack of direct neurologic insult, spinal instability should still be ruled out to avoid delayed injury. In addition to a detailed history and physical examination, dynamic radiographs are critical to the diagnosis of cervical spine instability. Cantu and colleagues[8] recommended that any subluxation noted after a sport-related injury necessitates a hard cervical collar to be worn at all times with follow-up imaging taken at 2 and 4 weeks after injury. Based on cadaveric studies, the definition of a subluxation is reported at greater than 3.5 mm of horizontal displacement of 1 vertebral body relative to the next or angular displacement of greater than 11° between adjacent vertebrae.[9] These investigators also cautioned that adolescent athletes have increased ligamentous laxity of unclear significance, which may account for measurements outside this norm.[8] If repeat imaging shows stability and pain and range of motion have resolved, most experts agree that return to play for these athletes is safe.

Stingers/Burners

A stinger or burner is a temporary episode of unilateral upper extremity dysesthesia, which is estimated to occur at least once during the career of more than 50% of athletes participating in contact/collision sports.[10] Although improvements in shoulder pads have reduced the frequency of stinger injuries,[11,12] nerve injuries without evidence of causal anatomic conditions were still the most common cause of cervical spine injury among NFL athletes between 2000 and 2010.[6] Cervical nerve injuries comprised 45.9% of all cervical spine injuries and resulted in a career mean of 15.3 days of activity lost per injury.[6] Motor weakness may not occur during a stinger but, if present, is most common in the C5 and C6 myotomes. Proposed mechanisms of injury include traction injury to the brachial plexus, nerve root compression at the neural foramina, and direct trauma to the

brachial plexus, most often at Erb's point (where the upper trunk can be compressed against a transverse process).[13]

Typically, symptoms resolve within a few minutes. If symptoms have resolved and it is the athlete's first episode of having a stinger, he or she can return to the sporting event as long as cervical range of motion is maintained and no neurologic deficits are present. After the resolution of an athlete's second episode of stinger, Cantu[10] recommends considering use of high shoulder pads, a soft cervical roll to limit neck flexion and extension, and review of the athlete's blocking and tackling techniques to identify if modifications may decrease the likelihood of recurrent injury. Some experts suggest that the occurrence of 3 or more stingers, especially if in rapid succession, is a relative contraindication to continued sport participation.[10,14] Certain athletes, those with foraminal stenosis, are predisposed to recurrent and chronic stinger injuries.[15] Because the dorsal root ganglion occupies the largest proportion of space within the neural foramen, it often takes the brunt of the injury, which is why purely sensory findings may be the result of a stinger.[8] Although the long-term natural history of athletes who have recurrent stingers is not well described in the scientific literature, some believe that recurrent episodes may lead to long-term proximal arm weakness and persistent pain.[10]

If symptoms persist after a stinger injury, alternative etiologies for the athlete's symptoms should be explored. In that situation, radiographs to rule out fractures or instability and an MRI to rule out disc herniation or other structural abnormalities should be performed. Cantu[10] recommends that electromyography be performed if symptoms persist greater than 2 weeks to accurately assess the extent of injury.[10] Weinstein[16] recommends continued cessation from sport if the athlete has clinical weakness and moderate fibrillation potentials 2 weeks postinjury.[16]

Cervical Stenosis, Cervical Cord Neurapraxia, and Transient Quadriplegia

Cervical stenosis may be present congenitally or caused by degenerative spondylotic changes. One phenomenon, initially described by Torg and colleagues,[17] is that of cervical cord neurapraxia (CCN), wherein an athlete sustains transient bilateral motor or sensory neurologic symptoms that begin after a blow to the head or a whiplash neck injury. One manifestation of this condition is referred to as transient quadriplegia. These clinical entities seem to most often occur in athletes who have cervical stenosis.[17–20] Narrowing of the cervical spinal canal places individuals at increased risk of cord injury during cervical trauma.[21] Most of these injuries occur with a hyperextension and axial load mechanism, because this position further narrows the anteroposterior space available for the cord.[22]

CCN tends to occur in high-velocity, high-impact sports such as football, rugby, and hockey. CCN is estimated to occur in 7.3 per 10,000 football players.[23] In one series, 57% returned to contact activities after their first episode, and 56% of the athletes who returned to play suffered a second episode of CCN.[20] Recurrence of symptoms was associated with radiographic and MRI evidence of progressive cervical stenosis.[20] The diagnostic workup for CCN after determination of a stable cervical spine often includes dynamic plain films to assess for fractures and subtle instability and an MRI to identify sources of ongoing neural impingement.[10]

Screening for cervical stenosis and the risk of CCN is far more controversial. Athletes may be exposed to repetitive loads or collisions that the general population are typically spared. Evidence suggests that long-term athletic participation increases the risk of radiographic signs of cervical spondylosis.[24] Additionally, some individuals with morphologic abnormalities of the posterior elements (eg, shorter lamina length) may have congenital cervical stenosis.[25] Although an athlete may be asymptomatic outside of sporting activity, his or her functional reserve may be compromised to a critical point, increasing the risk of sustaining spinal cord injury during participation in contact/collision sports. Radiographic assessment of the Pavlov/Torg ratio may be used as an adjunct to an athlete's assessment. The Pavlov/Torg ratio is the distance from the midpoint of the posterior aspect of a vertebral body to its corresponding spinolaminar line divided by the anteroposterior diameter of the same vertebral body, as measured on a lateral radiograph. A normal ratio is 1, and a ratio less than 0.8 indicates spinal stenosis.[26] Torg and colleagues[27] identified that a ratio of less than 0.8 was highly sensitive for athletes who had sustained an episode of transient neurapraxias, but the ratio had a low specificity (about 58%) and low positive predictive value (0.2%), which diminish its utility as a screening tool for determining an athlete's ability to participate in contact/collision sports. Additionally, Herzog and colleagues[28] identified that athletes tended to have larger vertebral bodies, which resulted in 41% of the asymptomatic professional football players having a Pavlov/Torg ratio less than 0.8 in their series.

Alternatively, Cantu[29] posits that a loss of cerebrospinal fluid surrounding the spinal cord or the presence of cord deformation, as measured on axial MRI slices, indicates the presence of a functional stenosis, suggesting a loss of the patient's functional reserve (eg, protective CSF cushion). Cantu and his associates[8,29] considered this a contraindication to participate in contact/collision sports even if the player is asymptomatic because of a theorized increased risk of CCN. However, obtaining an MRI on every athlete who wishes to engage in contact/collision sports is not cost effective and can lead to many incidental diagnoses. A recent systematic review by Dailey and colleagues[30] summarizes the available evidence and puts forth a weak recommendation that patients with transient neurapraxias and evidence of stenosis on MRI should not return to full participation in high-energy contact sports. Additionally, a strong recommendation was made that if no evidence of stenosis is identified on MRI and the CCN symptoms are transient, consideration should be made for full return to sport activities.[30] Torg and Ramsey-Emrhein[31] considered a history of CCN with the presence of a cord lesion on MRI as a relative contraindication to return to play. The persistence of symptoms for greater than 36 hours, recurrence of CCN, or evidence of ligamentous instability are also considered absolute contraindications to return to play.[31]

Cervical Disc Herniation

Contact sport athletes have higher rates of cervical disc herniations (CDH) than the general population[32]; whereas, noncontact athletics may provide a slight protective effect because of dynamic muscular support of the cervical spine.[33] An asymptomatic cervical disc condition that is incidentally identified necessitates a thorough history and physical of the athlete. In the absence of pain, limited range of neck motion, neurologic deficits, or signs of myelopathy, it is appropriate to allow the player to continue his participation in sport.[34] Of patients younger than 40 years, 10% of asymptomatic individuals have a herniated nucleus pulposus of the cervical spine identifiable on MRI.[35] The presence of symptoms, myelopathic signs, deficits of strength, or diminished range of motion are contraindications to the participation in athletics because the concern remains that sport-related activities could exacerbate current signs and symptoms of neurologic compression.[34] CDHs accounted for 5.8% of cervical spine injuries to NFL athletes between 2000 and 2010 and were responsible for a career mean of 84.8 days of activity lost per injury.[6] In a retrospective review, Hsu[36] identified CDH as a potentially career-ending injury, with 28% of operatively treated and 54% of nonoperatively treated NFL athletes never returning to professional play. Despite the potential severity of the condition, many athletes return to professional sport and perform well after CDH.[36,37] Athletes show no significant differences in sport performance whether operative or nonoperative treatment was selected; however, operatively treated CDH athletes had higher rates of return to play, played more games after their return, and had longer careers posttreatment.[36]

After failure of conservative measures, surgical treatment options that may be considered include posterior foraminotomy/decompression and anterior cervical discectomy and fusion (ACDF). Current guidelines are based on expert opinions and are experiential in nature. The general consensus is that posterior foraminotomy poses minimal change to the cervical spine's structural integrity; therefore, return to play with full contact is possible.[38] Burnett and Sonntag[38] cautioned that if a 2-level or more cervical laminectomy was required for adequate decompression, return to full-contact play would not be admissible regardless of whether posterolateral fusion was performed.

Single-level ACDFs less than C3 are generally deemed safe for return to play if range of motion is preserved, neurologic deficits resolve, and a solid fusion occurs.[13,31,37] Although some caution that a 2-level ACDF is a relative contraindication to return to play,[34] other surgeons suggest that this procedure should not preclude a collision athlete from returning to play.[37,39] Most experts agree that a 3-level ACDF is a contraindication to return to contact sports.[34,37]

Fractures

A broad range of cervical fractures may be sustained during athletic performance. The fracture morphology, location, and extent of neurovascular involvement all contribute to determining a player's prognosis. Return-to-play criteria are based on multiple factors because of the breadth of potential injuries. Cervical fractures are the least frequently sustained cervical injury among NFL athletes (1.8%), but they result in the greatest career mean number of days of activity lost per injury (119.7 days).[6]

Spinous process fractures typically occur in the lower cervical spine and may occur secondary to avulsion, direct blow, or hyperflexion.[40] Historically, these injuries were identified in manual laborers, which is why they are also referred to as clay-shoveler's fractures.[41] More recently, spinous process avulsion fractures have been reported in dance,[42] golf,[43] weight lifting,[44] and volleyball.[45] Their clinical

course is generally benign, and return to play can occur as soon as osseous healing has completed, pain has resolved, and range of motion is restored. Rarely have nonunions been reported that required excision of the nonunited fragment.[46]

Axial loads have been implicated in many football-induced cervical spine traumas,[5] which is a common mechanism to sustain burst or compression fractures of the cervical spine. Unstable Jefferson fractures require C1 to C2 fusion or occipitocervical fusion. Among the fragility of C1, the importance of the transverse and alar odontoid ligaments, and the functional limitations incurred from upper cervical arthrodesis, fusion of the upper cervical spine is an absolute contraindication for return to play.[31] Subaxial cervical spine fractures also may require fusion procedures. As discussed previously, ACDF is not an absolute contraindication to return to play. Range of motion, neurologic deficits, pain, and strength must all be improved before returning to full athletic activities. In the setting of prior fracture, it is of utmost importance to assess for residual instability on follow-up radiographs before allowing an athlete to return to sport activities. Additionally, in athletes who use a head-first tackle technique, also known as spearing, the cervical spine may progressively kyphose because of cumulative trauma and residual deformity from prior vertebral injuries. This clinical entity, known as spear tackler's spine, is regarded an absolute contraindication to return to contact/collision sports.[40]

THORACIC TRAUMA

Thoracic spine injuries are uncommon during sports activities and, as such, have limited published evidence regarding the appropriateness for return to play. The rarity of thoracic spine injuries is in part owing to the added stability provided by the thoracic cage anteriorly. This added rigidity may, however, be the reason for the most common sport-related injuries—compression and transverse process fractures.[47] The thoracic region was the least frequently injured by professional NFL athletes between 2000 and 2010.[6] Of the NFL thoracic spine injuries, the greatest number of days lost was for disc herniations, which had a mean of 189 days (n = 4). Thoracic spine fractures had a mean of 33.5 days of activity lost (n = 10).[6]

Stress fractures of the spinous or transverse processes may occur because of overuse activities and are usually managed nonoperatively. Similarly, thoracic vertebral compression fractures rarely require operative management, as they do not create instability. Thoracic fractures with evidence of instability are absolute contraindications to return to play in contact sports. Disc herniations, although uncommon in the thoracic spine, may result in axial pain, radiculopathy, or myelopathy. Barring the signs of myelopathy, a trial of nonoperative management is usually the appropriate starting treatment.

Once symptoms resolve, as long as the athlete remains neurologically intact and has unimpaired range of motion and strength, return to play is usually appropriate.[47]

LUMBAR TRAUMA

Lumbar spine trauma is the second most common region for spine trauma among NFL athletes,[6] and injuries sustained vary from minor to severe. In one series of college athletes from all sports, back injuries were most often acute (59%), whereas overuse (12%) and injuries associated with pre-existing conditions (29%) were less common.[48]

Lumbar Strain

The most frequent lumbar spine conditions encountered during athletic activity are strains of the lumbar paraspinal muscles. One series of college athletes from 17 varsity sports (football, basketball, track and field, cross country, ice hockey, gymnastics, crew, swimming, soccer, tennis, badminton, volleyball, wrestling, baseball, golf, fencing, and field hockey) identified 59% of strains as acute and 41% as chronic in nature.[48] In the acute setting, the disruption of muscle fibers results in pain that is typically worst within 48 hours of initial injury and may subsequently localize to a trigger point. The published prevalence of lumbago among athletes is widely variable, from 1% to greater than 30%, and depends on sport, sex, training intensity, and training frequency.[49] Nonoperative treatment with physical therapy and anti-inflammatory medications is the gold standard for initial management. Once athletes are pain free and have restoration of athletic function, return to play at their previous level of competition is appropriate. Among professional NFL athletes, lumbar strain was the cause of 41.9% of lumbar spine injuries and resulted in a career mean of 7 days of activity lost per injury.[6]

Lumbar Disc Herniation

Disc herniations are another common lumbar spine condition found in athletes. Among professional NFL players, lumbar disc herniations (LDHs) were the second most common lumbar spine condition, representing 28% of lumbar spine injuries and resulting in a mean of 51.7 days of activity lost.[6] Asymptomatic LDHs are common, with an estimated prevalence of 27% in asymptomatic adults and, therefore, do not require athletic restrictions or treatment.[50] Symptomatic LDHs, however, are a potentially career-ending injury for elite athletes. One multisport meta-analysis did not identify a significant difference in return-to-play rates between elite athletes who underwent single-level lumbar microdiscectomy or nonoperative management.[51] A large retrospective cohort study of National Basketball Association, National Hockey League (NHL), Major League Baseball (MLB), and NFL players identified MLB athletes as having a significantly greater return to play regardless of treatment modality than athletes in other sports (96% operative, 97% nonoperative); conversely, NFL athletes had a lower return-to-play rate than players of other sports (78% operative, 59% nonoperative).[52] Sport-specific analyses failed to identify differences in return-to-play rates among NHL,[53] National Basketball Association,[54,55] and MLB[56] athletes regardless of whether surgical or nonoperative management was chosen. In one series, operatively treated NFL lineman showed a significantly greater rate of return to play (42 of 52; 80.8%) than those treated nonoperatively (4 of 14; 28.6%; P<.05).[57] It is currently unclear whether the differences identified among NFL lineman are owing to sport-specific differences in the demands required to play at an elite level. In a systematic review, Nair and colleagues[58] identified postoperative athletic performance as variable, depending on the sport. Postoperative performance ranged from 64.4% (NHL athletes) to 103.6% (NFL athletes) of baseline.

Most guidelines for return-to-play criteria in the setting of LDH are experiential in nature. With appropriate physical therapy and rehabilitation, most experts believe athletes can return to contact/collision sports regardless of whether nonoperative or operative treatment is conducted.[38,59] Return to play should be considered once the athlete has resolution of pain, full strength, and full range of motion. As a point of reference, based on surveys of North American Spine Society members, the most frequently recommended time before return to golf activities was 4 to 8 weeks after lumbar microdiscectomy. Shorter durations were more commonly recommended if the patient was a professional or college golfer.[60] Contact sports may require 2 to 6 months of postoperative rehabilitation before return to play.[61]

Spondylolysis and Spondylolisthesis

Spondylolysis is the condition in which there is a defect of the posterior portion of the neural arch, most commonly at the pars interarticularis. This condition is believed to be the result of a stress fracture,[62] and most cases are asymptomatic. Within the general population, spondylolysis has an estimated prevalence of 3% to 6%, and roughly a quarter of symptomatic cases have associated spondylolisthesis.[49] In one series of adolescent athletes complaining of low back pain, 47% were ultimately found to have spondylolysis in the lumbar spine.[63] Repetitive trunk movements, particularly hyperextension and rotation, increase stress within the pars interarticularis and likely contribute to the formation of spondylolysis, so it is not surprising that certain sports (eg, gymnastics, American football, and baseball) have been associated with increased risk of spondylolysis development.[64,65]

The diagnosis of spondylolysis can be made on plain radiographs, but computed tomography scans improve sensitivity of identifying the lesion. Single photon emission computed tomography scans can identify active lesions, which is especially useful if it is not apparent on plain radiographs. Unilateral lesions are not associated with spondylolisthesis or disability.[66]

Asymptomatic spondylolysis and low-grade spondylolisthesis have a benign clinical course over the first 50 years of life and, therefore, do not require any restrictions from competitive sports.[66] The goals of treatment for symptomatic spondylolysis are to minimize pain, restore function, and restore motion. Nonoperative treatment, including activity modification, cessation of competitive play, and bracing, is the mainstay of first-line therapy. With early diagnosis (single photon emission computed tomography findings but not plain radiographs), the prognosis with nonoperative management is excellent; more than 90% of patients will have good or excellent outcomes with 11-year follow-up.[67] Much like a stress fracture of a long bone, activity cessation, regardless of brace compliance, was found to result in better self-reported outcomes and is, therefore, a critical element of conservative treatment.[68] Unilateral defects are more likely to undergo bony union, whereas bilateral defects often undergo further degeneration over time.[67,69] Nonunion does not seem to be detrimental to outcome or ability to return to play.[69]

Indications for surgery include persistent symptoms after 6 months of failed nonoperative treatment, progression of spondylolisthesis, high-grade (Meyerding grade III or IV) slip at initial presentation, or neurologic deficit.[49,70] Surgical treatments include either direct pars defect repair or arthrodesis. The theoretic benefit of a pars repair is the maintenance of the vertebral motion segment, which may help athletic performance. In one series of 22 athletes who underwent pars repair, 82% were able to return to their previous sporting activity.[71]

Limited evidence exists with regard to making recommendations for an athlete to return to play after treatment for spondylolysis and spondylolisthesis. A survey of Scoliosis Research Society members had highly variable responses regarding surgeon preference of duration before allowing an athlete to return to play.[72] For noncontact sports (eg, running, tennis), the 2 most common surgeon preferences were for athletes to take 6 months or 1 year of time off postoperatively. Most respondents preferred that athletes abstain from contact sports (eg, basketball, soccer) for 1 year postoperatively before resumption, regardless of slip level. Collision sports (eg, football, hockey) were more controversial. A total of 27% and 36% of respondents allowed return to collision sports 1 year postoperatively for low-grade and high-grade slips, respectively; whereas 49% and 58% of respondents either recommended against or forbade collision sports for low-grade and high-grade slips, respectively.[72] Although resumption of contact or collision sports is controversial,[38,59] most experts agree that all athletes should have relief of pain, normal strength, and normal range of motion before return to athletic activities.[73] Radcliff and colleagues[74] recommended a postoperative rehabilitation protocol that entails 2 weeks of supervised core strengthening, flexibility, and water exercise. Nonimpact aerobic activity could be introduced at postoperative weeks 2 to 4. Gradual increases in impact can be introduced over the first 3 months, but all exercises must be performed with a neutral spine. After 3 months, sport-specific training may commence.

Lumbar Stenosis

Lumbar spinal stenosis is usually the result of structural deformities such as spondylolisthesis, LDH, or scoliosis in the setting of young athletes, unlike degenerative changes (spondylosis) responsible for lumbar spinal stenosis in middle age and older adults. Conservative management with cessation of activity, nonsteroidal anti-inflammatory medications, and progressive therapy are first-line treatments for most patients. Surgical indications include failure of nonoperative management, cauda equina syndrome, substantial neurologic deficits, and vertebral instability.[4] With isolated decompression, expert opinion is highly variable as to the appropriate amount of time before return to play. A survey of North American Spine Society members found the most common recommendation to be 4 to 8 weeks of time off before resumption of golf.[60] Eck and Riley,[59] however, recommended 4 to 6 months with no resumption of contact sports. If fusion is necessary, Eck and Riley[59] recommended 1 year of postoperative time elapse before resumption of noncontact sports.

SACRAL TRAUMA

Sacral injuries are uncommon among athletes; however, sacral stress fractures should be considered a part of the differential diagnosis for athletes with low back pain. This clinical entity is almost exclusively encountered among running athletes. The female athlete triad has been implicated in the development of sacral stress fractures,[75] much like the formation of tibial stress fractures. Standard radiographs often inadequately identify sacral stress fractures because of overlying bowel gas and pelvic geometry, so computed tomography, bone scans, and MRI are often required to assist with determining the diagnosis. Nonoperative treatment with rest and protected or non–weight bearing are the mainstays of management.[49] Athletes typically return to sports activity after 4 to 6 weeks of rest.[76]

SUMMARY

Given the breadth of conditions encountered during athletic activity, there is no standardized algorithm for determining a player's readiness to return to play after spine injury. Regardless of the condition present, an athlete should be pain free, neurologically intact, and without deficits of strength or range of motion before returning to sports.

DISCLOSURES

Dr. B.D. Rosenthal and Dr. B.S. Boody have no disclosures. Dr. W.K. Hsu has the following disclosures. American Academy of Orthopaedic Surgeons: Board or committee member. Arbeitsgemeinschaft für Osteosynthesefragen North America: Paid consultant; Paid presenter or speaker. Bacterin: Paid consultant. Bioventus: Paid consultant. CeramTec: Paid consultant. Cervical Spine Research Society: Board or committee member. Globus: Paid consultant. Graftys: Paid consultant. *Journal of Spinal Disorders and Techniques*: Editorial or governing board. Lifenet: Paid consultant. Lumbar Spine Research Society: Board or committee member. Medtronic: Paid consultant; Research support. North American Spine Society: Board or committee member. Pioneer: Paid consultant. Relievant: Paid consultant. SI Bone: Paid consultant. Stryker Spine: Paid consultant. Synthes: Paid consultant.

REFERENCES

1. National Spinal Cord Injury Statistical Center. Spinal cord injury facts and figures at a glance. J Spinal Cord Med 2013;36(1):1–2.
2. Devivo MJ. Epidemiology of traumatic spinal cord injury: trends and future implications. Spinal Cord 2012;50(5):365–72.
3. Torg JS. Epidemiology, pathomechanics, and prevention of athletic injuries to the cervical spine. Med Sci Sports Exerc 1985;17(3):295–303.
4. Huang P, Anissipour A, McGee W, et al. Injuries: A Comprehensive Review. Sports Health 2016;8(1):19–25.
5. Torg JS, Vegso JJ, O'Neill MJ, et al. The epidemiologic, pathologic, biomechanical, and cinematographic analysis of football-induced cervical spine trauma. Am J Sports Med 1990;18(1):50–7.
6. Mall NA, Buchowski J, Zebala L, et al. Spine and axial skeleton injuries in the National Football League. Am J Sports Med 2012;40(8):1755–61.
7. Schroeder GD, Lynch TS, Gibbs DB, et al. The impact of a cervical spine diagnosis on the careers of National Football League athletes. Spine 2014;39(12):947–52.
8. Cantu RC, Li YM, Abdulhamid M, et al. Return to play after cervical spine injury in sports. Curr Sports Med Rep 2013;12(1):14–7.
9. White AA, Johnson RM, Panjabi MM, et al. Biomechanical analysis of clinical stability in the cervical spine. Clin Orthop 1975;109:85–96.
10. Cantu RC. Stingers, transient quadriplegia, and cervical spinal stenosis: return to play criteria. Med Sci Sports Exerc 1997;29(7 Suppl):S233–5.
11. Markey KL, Di Benedetto M, Curl WW. Upper trunk brachial plexopathy. The stinger syndrome. Am J Sports Med 1993;21(5):650–5.
12. Di Benedetto M, Markey K. Electrodiagnostic localization of traumatic upper trunk brachial plexopathy. Arch Phys Med Rehabil 1984;65(1):15–7.
13. Vaccaro AR, Klein GR, Ciccoti M, et al. Return to play criteria for the athlete with cervical spine injuries resulting in stinger and transient quadriplegia/paresis. Spine J 2002;2(5):351–6.
14. Vaccaro AR, Watkins B, Albert TJ, et al. Cervical spine injuries in athletes: current return-to-play criteria. Orthopedics 2001;24(7):699–703 [quiz: 704–5].
15. Levitz CL, Reilly PJ, Torg JS. The pathomechanics of chronic, recurrent cervical nerve root neurapraxia. The chronic burner syndrome. Am J Sports Med 1997;25(1):73–6.
16. Weinstein SM. Assessment and rehabilitation of the athlete with a "stinger". a model for the management

of noncatastrophic athletic cervical spine injury. Clin Sports Med 1998;17(1):127–35.

17. Torg JS, Pavlov H, Genuario SE, et al. Neurapraxia of the cervical spinal cord with transient quadriplegia. J Bone Joint Surg Am 1986;68(9):1354–70.

18. Grant TT, Puffer J. Cervical stenosis: a developmental anomaly with quadriparesis during football. Am J Sports Med 1976;4(5):219–21.

19. Ladd AL, Scranton PE. Congenital cervical stenosis presenting as transient quadriplegia in athletes. Report of two cases. J Bone Joint Surg Am 1986;68(9):1371–4.

20. Torg JS, Corcoran TA, Thibault LE, et al. Cervical cord neurapraxia: classification, pathomechanics, morbidity, and management guidelines. J Neurosurg 1997;87(6):843–50.

21. Eismont FJ, Clifford S, Goldberg M, et al. Cervical sagittal spinal canal size in spine injury. Spine 1984;9(7):663–6.

22. Penning L. Some aspects of plain radiography of the cervical spine in chronic myelopathy. Neurology 1962;12:513–9.

23. Torg JS, Pavlov H. Cervical spinal stenosis with cord neurapraxia and transient quadriplegia. Clin Sports Med 1987;6(1):115–33.

24. Triantafillou KM, Lauerman W, Kalantar SB. Degenerative disease of the cervical spine and its relationship to athletes. Clin Sports Med 2012;31(3):509–20.

25. Jenkins TJ, Mai HT, Burgmeier RJ, et al. The triangle model of congenital cervical stenosis. Spine 2016;41(5):E242–7.

26. Pavlov H, Torg JS, Robie B, et al. Cervical spinal stenosis: determination with vertebral body ratio method. Radiology 1987;164(3):771–5.

27. Torg JS, Naranja RJ Jr, Pavlov H, et al. The relationship of developmental narrowing of the cervical spinal canal to reversible and irreversible injury of the cervical spinal cord in football players. J Bone Joint Surg Am 1996;78(9):1308–14.

28. Herzog RJ, Wiens JJ, Dillingham MF, et al. Normal cervical spine morphometry and cervical spinal stenosis in asymptomatic professional football players. Plain film radiography, multiplanar computed tomography, and magnetic resonance imaging. Spine 1991;16(6 Suppl):S178–86.

29. Cantu RC. Functional cervical spinal stenosis: a contraindication to participation in contact sports. Med Sci Sports Exerc 1993;25(3):316–7.

30. Dailey A, Harrop JS, France JC. High-energy contact sports and cervical spine neuropraxia injuries: what are the criteria for return to participation? Spine 2010;35(21 Suppl):S193–201.

31. Torg JS, Ramsey-Emrhein JA. Management guidelines for participation in collision activities with congenital, developmental, or postinjury lesions involving the cervical spine. Clin J Sport Med 1997;7(4):273–91.

32. Zmurko MG, Tannoury TY, Tannoury CA, et al. Cervical sprains, disc herniations, minor fractures, and other cervical injuries in the athlete. Clin Sports Med 2003;22(3):513–21.

33. Mundt DJ, Kelsey JL, Golden AL, et al. An epidemiologic study of sports and weight lifting as possible risk factors for herniated lumbar and cervical discs. the northeast collaborative group on low back pain. Am J Sports Med 1993;21(6):854–60.

34. Kepler CK, Vaccaro AR. Injuries and abnormalities of the cervical spine and return to play criteria. Clin Sports Med 2012;31(3):499–508.

35. Boden SD, McCowin PR, Davis DO, et al. Abnormal magnetic-resonance scans of the cervical spine in asymptomatic subjects. A prospective investigation. J Bone Joint Surg Am 1990;72(8):1178–84.

36. Hsu WK. Outcomes following nonoperative and operative treatment for cervical disc herniations in National Football League athletes. Spine 2011;36(10):800–5.

37. Maroon JC, Bost JW, Petraglia AL, et al. Outcomes after anterior cervical discectomy and fusion in professional athletes. Neurosurgery 2013;73(1):103–12 [discussion: 112].

38. Burnett MG, Sonntag VKH. Return to contact sports after spinal surgery. Neurosurg Focus 2006;21(4):E5.

39. Hecht AC, Vaccaro A, Hsu WK, et al. Cervical spine and sports: a roundtable. Rosemont (IL): AAOS Now; 2015.

40. Paulus S, Kennedy DJ. Return to play considerations for cervical spine injuries in athletes. Phys Med Rehabil Clin N Am 2014;25(4):723–33.

41. Hall RDM. Clay-shoveler's fracture. J Bone Jt Surg Am 1940;22(1):63–75.

42. Thomson LP, Stein LA, Fish WW. Lambada fracture. N Engl J Med 1991;324(12):852.

43. Kang D-H, Lee S-H. Multiple spinous process fractures of the thoracic vertebrae (Clay-Shoveler's Fracture) in a beginning Golfer: a case report. Spine 2009;34(15):E534–7.

44. Herrick RT. Clay-shoveler's fracture in power-lifting. a case report. Am J Sports Med 1981;9(1):29–30.

45. Hetsroni I, Mann G, Dolev E, et al. Clay shoveler's fracture in a volleyball player. Phys Sportsmed 2005;33(7):38–42.

46. Murphy RF, Hedequist D. Excision of symptomatic spinous process nonunion in adolescent athletes. Am J Orthop (Belle Mead NJ) 2015;44(11):515–7.

47. Menzer H, Gill GK, Paterson A. Thoracic spine sports-related injuries. Curr Sports Med Rep 2015;14(1):34–40.

48. Keene JS, Albert MJ, Springer SL, et al. Back injuries in college athletes. J Spinal Disord 1989;2(3):190–5.

49. Bono CM. Low-back pain in athletes. J Bone Joint Surg Am 2004;86-A(2):382–96.

50. Jensen MC, Brant-Zawadzki MN, Obuchowski N, et al. Magnetic resonance imaging of the lumbar spine in people without back pain. N Engl J Med 1994;331(2):69–73.

51. Overley SC, McAnany SJ, Andelman S, et al. Return to play in elite athletes after lumbar microdiscectomy: a meta-analysis. Spine (Phila Pa 1976) 2016; 41(8):713–8.

52. Hsu WK, McCarthy KJ, Savage JW, et al. The professional athlete spine initiative: outcomes after lumbar disc herniation in 342 elite professional athletes. Spine J 2011;11(3):180–6.

53. Schroeder GD, McCarthy KJ, Micev AJ, et al. Performance-based outcomes after nonoperative treatment, discectomy, and/or fusion for a lumbar disc herniation in National Hockey League athletes. Am J Sports Med 2013;41(11):2604–8.

54. Anakwenze OA, Namdari S, Auerbach JD, et al. Athletic performance outcomes following lumbar discectomy in professional basketball players. Spine 2010;35(7):825–8.

55. Minhas SV, Kester BS, Hsu WK. Outcomes after lumbar disc herniation in the national basketball association. Sports Health 2016;8(1):43–9.

56. Earhart JS, Roberts D, Roc G, et al. Effects of lumbar disk herniation on the careers of professional baseball players. Orthopedics 2012;35(1):43–9.

57. Weistroffer JK, Hsu WK. Return-to-play rates in National Football League linemen after treatment for lumbar disk herniation. Am J Sports Med 2011; 39(3):632–6.

58. Nair R, Kahlenberg CA, Hsu WK. Outcomes of lumbar discectomy in elite athletes: the need for high-level evidence. Clin Orthop 2015;473(6):1971–7.

59. Eck JC, Riley LH. Return to play after lumbar spine conditions and surgeries. Clin Sports Med 2004; 23(3):367–79, viii.

60. Abla AA, Maroon JC, Lochhead R, et al. Return to golf after spine surgery. J Neurosurg Spine 2011; 14(1):23–30.

61. Li Y, Hresko MT. Lumbar spine surgery in athletes:: outcomes and return-to-play criteria. Clin Sports Med 2012;31(3):487–98.

62. Wiltse LL, Widell EH, Jackson DW. Fatigue fracture: the basic lesion is inthmic spondylolisthesis. J Bone Joint Surg Am 1975;57(1):17–22.

63. Micheli LJ, Wood R. Back pain in young athletes. Significant differences from adults in causes and patterns. Arch Pediatr Adolesc Med 1995;149(1): 15–8.

64. Sakai T, Sairyo K, Suzue N, et al. Incidence and etiology of lumbar spondylolysis: review of the literature. J Orthop Sci 2010;15(3):281–8.

65. Jackson DW, Wiltse LL, Cirincoine RJ. Spondylolysis in the female gymnast. Clin Orthop 1976;117:68–73.

66. Beutler WJ, Fredrickson BE, Murtland A, et al. The natural history of spondylolysis and spondylolisthesis: 45-year follow-up evaluation. Spine 2003; 28(10):1027–35 [discussion: 1035].

67. Miller SF, Congeni J, Swanson K. Long-term functional and anatomical follow-up of early detected spondylolysis in young athletes. Am J Sports Med 2004;32(4):928–33.

68. El Rassi G, Takemitsu M, Woratanarat P, et al. Lumbar spondylolysis in pediatric and adolescent soccer players. Am J Sports Med 2005;33(11):1688–93.

69. Sys J, Michielsen J, Bracke P, et al. Nonoperative treatment of active spondylolysis in elite athletes with normal X-ray findings: literature review and results of conservative treatment. Eur Spine J 2001; 10(6):498–504.

70. Blanda J, Bethem D, Moats W, et al. Defects of pars interarticularis in athletes: a protocol for nonoperative treatment. J Spinal Disord 1993;6(5):406–11.

71. Debnath UK, Freeman BJC, Gregory P, et al. Clinical outcome and return to sport after the surgical treatment of spondylolysis in young athletes. J Bone Joint Surg Br 2003;85(2):244–9.

72. Rubery PT, Bradford DS. Athletic activity after spine surgery in children and adolescents: results of a survey. Spine 2002;27(4):423–7.

73. Radcliff KE, Kalantar SB, Reitman CA. Surgical management of spondylolysis and spondylolisthesis in athletes: indications and return to play. Curr Sports Med Rep 2009;8(1):35–40.

74. Radcliff KE, Limthongkul W, Kepler CK, et al. Cervical laminectomy width and spinal cord drift are risk factors for postoperative C5 palsy. J Spinal Disord Tech 2014;27(2):86–92.

75. Nusselt T, Klinger H-M, Schultz W, et al. Fatigue stress fractures of the pelvis: a rare cause of low back pain in female athletes. Acta Orthop Belg 2010;76(6):838–43.

76. Major NM, Helms CA. Sacral stress fractures in long-distance runners. AJR Am J Roentgenol 2000; 174(3):727–9.

Index

Note: Page numbers of article titles are in **boldface** type.

A

Abdominal injuries, in seat belt injury, 106–107
Acidosis, in spinal cord injury, 50
Acute respiratory distress syndrome, with spinal cord injury, 149–150
Allen and Ferguson classification, of cervical spine facet injuries, 126
Allen classification, of cervical spine facet injuries, 126
American Spinal Injury Association Classification Standards/International Standards for Neurological Classification of Spinal Cord Injury, 32–33
American Spinal Injury Association Impairment Scale, 32–33
Anderson and D'Alonza odontoid fracture classification, 116
Anesthesia, for subaxial cervical spine treatment, 99
Ankylosing spondylitis, spinal cord injury with, 148–149
Anterior approach, to cervical spine facet repair, 132–135
Anxiety, with spinal cord injury, 153
AOSpine Thoracolumbar Spine Injury Classification System (2013), 26–28, 126, 128
Apoptosis, in spinal cord injury, 150–151
Arrhythmias, with spinal cord injury, 152
Aspen cervical collar, for odontoid fractures, 117–118
Aspiration, pulmonary, with spinal cord injury, 149–150, 152–153
Athletes, return to play for, **163–171**
ATI-355, for spinal cord injury, 56
Atlantoaxial instability, 79–80
Atlantoaxial rotary fixation, 75–76
Atlantoaxial rotary subluxation, 75–76
Atlantoaxial subluxation, translational, 75
Atlantoaxial techniques, for craniocervical injuries, 85–86
Atlantooccipital dislocation, 74–75

B

Bilateral cervical spine facet dislocation, 128–129
Blood disorders, with spinal cord injury, 150–151
Bone grafts, for subaxial cervical spine injuries, 95, 98–99
Bone marrow stem cells, transplantation of, for spinal cord injury, 65–66
Bone morphogenetic protein, for thoracolumbar trauma, 110–111
Braces
  for odontoid fractures, 117–118
  for thoracolumbar trauma, 105, 110
Bradycardia, with spinal cord injury, 152
Brain computer interfaces, for spinal cord injury, 67–68
Brain injury, with spinal cord injury, 148
Burners, 164
Burst fractures, 24, **103–114**
  of thoracolumbar junction, **139–145**
  of thoracolumbar spine, 105

C

Cage placement, for thoracolumbar junction burst fractures, **139–145**
Car seats, regulation of, 104
Cardiac arrest, with spinal cord injury, 152
Cardiac complications, with spinal cord injury, 151
Cardiogenic pulmonary edema, with spinal cord injury, 152
Carotid artery injury, with spinal cord injury, 148
Cell transplantation, for spinal cord injury, 64–66
Cellular transplantation, for spinal cord injury, 56–58
Central cord syndrome, **41–47**
  anatomy of, 42
  clinical features of, 41
  diagnosis of, 43
  incidence of, 41–42
  mechanism of injury in, 42–43
  natural history of, 43–44
  pathophysiology of, 42
  treatment of, 34–35, 44–46
Cervical collar
  for craniocervical injuries, 81–82
  for odontoid fractures, 117–118
Cervical spine, clearance of, 80
Cervical spine injuries
  facet, **125–137**
  return to play after, 163–166
  strains and sprains, 164
  subaxial, **91–102**
Cervical Spine Injury Severity Score System (CSISS), 93
Cethrin, for spinal cord injury, 53
Chance fractures, 23–24

neurosurgery.theclinics.com

Chondroitin sulfate proteoglycans, in spinal cord injury, 50
Closed reduction
    for cervical spine facet injuries, 131–132
    for subaxial cervical spine injuries, 95
Coagulopathy, with spinal cord injury, 150–151
Cognitive dysfunction, with spinal cord injury, 153
Combined approach, to cervical spine facet repair, 132–135
Compression fractures, of thoracolumbar spine, 104–105
Computed tomography, 3–4
    for cervical spine facet injuries, 128–129
    for craniocervical injuries, 78
    for odontoid fractures, 116
    for subaxial cervical spine injuries, 93
Computer, brain interface with, 67–68
Congestive heart failure, with spinal cord injury, 152
Constipation, with spinal cord injury, 151–152
Cooling, for spinal cord injury, 63–64
Corpectomy
    lateral mini-open, 158, 160
    with thoracolumbar junction burst fractures, **139–145**
Corticosteroids, for spinal cord injury, 54–55
Craniocervical injuries, **73–90**
    biomechanics of, 73–74
    clinical presentation of, 74
    epidemiology of, 73
    patterns of, 74–77
    radiography for, 77–80
    treatment of, 80–87
Cutaneous disorders, with spinal cord injury, 151
Cytokines, in spinal cord injury, 50

D

Decompressive surgery
    for cervical spine facet repair, 132–135
    for disk herniation, 165–166
    for spinal cord injury, timing of, **31–39**
        complications and, 35–36
        factors influencing, 35–36
        initial assessment for, 32–33
        non-neurologic outcome and, 36
        pathophyiologic basis of, 31–32
        recovery and, 33–34
        with central cord syndrome, 34–35
    for thoracolumbar trauma, 105, 110
Deep venous thrombosis, with spinal cord injury, 150–151
Denis classification, of thoracolumbar trauma, 24–25
Dens, fractures of, **115–123**
Depression, with spinal cord injury, 153
Diaphragm paralysis, with spinal cord injury, 150
Disc(s)

herniation of, 165–167
injury of, imaging for, 5–6
Discectomy for cervical spine facet repair, 132–135
Dobutamine, for spinal cord injury, 54
Dopamine, for spinal cord injury, 54
Dorsal fixation, for odontoid fractures, 119–120
Driveway injury, of thoracolumbar spine, 107
Dural injuries, with spinal cord injury, 148
Dysphagia, with spinal cord injury, 151–152

E

Edema, spinal cord, imaging for, 7
Elderly persons, odontoid fractures in, **115–123**
Electrical stimulation, for spinal cord injury, 66–68
Ephrin B3, in spinal cord injury, 50
Epidural stimulation, for spinal cord injury, 67
Epinephrine, for spinal cord injury, 54
External immobilization
    for craniocervical injuries, 81–82
    for odontoid fractures, 118

F

Facet injuries, of cervical spine, **125–137**
Ferguson and Allen classification, of thoracolumbar trauma, 25
Fiber tractography, 13
Fibroblast growth factor, for spinal cord injury, 53, 56
Fluid therapy, for spinal cord injury, 54
Foraminotomy, for disk herniation, 166
Fractures
    cervical spine, 166
    cervical spine facet, **125–137**
    craniocervical, 75, 77, 82–87
    imaging for, 3–4
    minimally invasive treatment of, **157–162**
    odontoid, in elderly persons, **115–123**
    sacral spine, 169
    thoracolumbar junction, **139–145**
    thoracolumbar spine, **103–114**
Functional electrical stimulation, for spinal cord injury, 66–67
Functional MRI, 14–15
Fusion, for thoracolumbar spine fractures, 105

G

Gacyclidine, for spinal cord injury, 51–52
Gait orthosis, for spinal cord injury, 67
Gangliosides, for spinal cord injury, 51, 53
Gastrointestinal complications, with spinal cord injury, 151–152
Gibenclamide, for spinal cord injury, 52
Glial cell transplantation, for spinal cord injury, 64

Glucose intolerance, with spinal cord injury, 153
Glyburide, for spinal cord injury, 52, 55
Granulocyte colony-stimulating factor, for spinal cord
     injury, 53, 56

H

Halo ring and vest
     for craniocervical injuries, 81
     for odontoid fractures, 117–118
     for subaxial cervical spine injuries, 95
Hangman's fractures, 77
Harris classification, of cervical spine facet injuries,
     126
Heart problems, with spinal cord injury, 151
Hematologic complications, with spinal cord injury,
     150–151
Hematuria, with spinal cord injury, 153
Hemorrhage, spinal cord, imaging for, 7
Hemothorax, with spinal cord injury, 149–150
Herniation, disc, 165–167
Holdsworth classification, of thoracolumbar
     trauma, 24
Hypothermia, therapeutic, for spinal cord injury,
     63–64

I

Iatrogenic complications, with spinal cord injury, 152
Ileus, with spinal cord injury, 151–152
Imaging. See Computed tomography; Magnetic
     resonance imaging.
Immobilization
     for craniocervical injuries, 81–82
     for subaxial cervical spine injuries, 95
Immunoglobulin-like receptor B, in spinal cord
     injury, 50
Infections, with spinal cord injury, 152
Inflammation, in spinal cord injury, 50
Instrumentation
     for subaxial cervical spine injuries, 95–99
     for thoracolumbar spine fractures, 105
Insulin resistance, with spinal cord injury, 153
Intracranial injury, with spinal cord injury, 148
Intraspinal microstimulation, for spinal cord injury, 67
Ischemia, in spinal cord injury, 50

J

Jefferson fractures, 75

K

Kelly and Whiteside classification, of thoracolumbar
     trauma, 24
Kidney disorders, with spinal cord injury, 152
Kyphoplasty, 158–159

L

Lateral mass screw, C1, for craniocervical injuries,
     83–84
Ligamentous injury, imaging for, 5
Lobar collapse, with spinal cord injury, 149–150
Locomat device, for spinal cord injury, 67
Lumbar spine injuries, return to play after, 167–169
Lung injury, with spinal cord injury, 149–150

M

McAfee classification, of thoracolumbar trauma, 25
Macrophages, transplantation of, 58
Mageri classification, of thoracolumbar trauma, 25
Magnesium, for spinal cord injury, 52
Magnetic resonance imaging, 1–17
     advanced methods for, 11–16
     for cervical spine facet injuries, 129–131
     for cervical stenosis, 165
     for craniocervical injuries, 78
     for odontoid fractures, 116–117
     for subaxial cervical spine injuries, 93
     for thoracolumbar trauma, 110
     limitations of, 16–17
Magnetic resonance spectroscopy, 14
Mechanical ventilation, 150
Mersilene Polyester Fiber Suture, for subaxial cervical
     spine injuries, 95
Methylprednisolone, 52, 54–55, 64, 152
Miami Project to Cure Paralysis, 64–65
Miami-J collar, for odontoid fractures, 117–118
Minerva brace
     for craniocervical injuries, 81
     for odontoid fractures, 117–118
Minerva orthosis, for subaxial cervical spine
     injuries, 95
Minimally invasive surgery, **157–162**
Miniopen thoracopic-assisted approach, for
     thoracolumbar junction burst fractures,
     139–145
Minocycline, for spinal cord injury, 52, 55, 64
Mitochondrial dysfunction, in spinal cord injury, 50
Monoclonal antibody IN-1, for spinal cord injury, 56
Motor vehicle crashes, thoracolumbar trauma in, 104
Myelin-associated inhibitors, for spinal cord injury, 56
Myelin-associated proteins, in spinal cord injury, 50
Myocardial infarction, with spinal cord injury, 152

N

Naloxone, for spinal cord injury, 53
NASCIS (National Acute Spinal Cord Injury Studies),
     52, 54–55, 152
Netrin, in spinal cord injury, 50
Neural progenitor cells, transplantation of, for spinal
     cord injury, 66

Neural stem cells, transplantation of, for spinal cord injury, 65–66
Neuraxial, cervical, 164–165
Neuroprotective agents, for spinal cord injury, 52–56, 63–64
Neuropsychiatric complications, with spinal cord injury, 152
NEXUS (National Emergency X-Radiography Utilization Study) criteria, 80, 93
Nogo, in spinal cord injury, 50
Norepinephrine, for spinal cord injury, 54

O

Obelisc cage, 142–143
Obesity, with spinal cord injury, 152–153
Occipital condyle-C1 joint, measurement of, 79
Occipital screws, for craniocervical injuries, 84–85
Occipital-cervical techniques, for craniocervical injuries, 82
Odontoid fractures, 77
Odontoid screws, for craniocervical injuries, 86
Olfactory ensheathing cell transplantation, for spinal cord injury, 64–65
Oligodendrocyte myelin glycoprotein, in spinal cord injury, 50
Orthoses
    for odontoid fractures, 117–118
    for subaxial cervical spine injuries, 95
    for thoracolumbar trauma, 105
Orthostatic hypotension, with spinal cord injury, 152
Os odontoideum, 77
Osteotomy, for thoracolumbar junction burst fractures, **139–145**
Oxidative stress, in spinal cord injury, 50

P

Pancreatitis, with spinal cord injury, 151–152
Paraspinal muscles, strain of, 167
Parastep 1 system, 66–67
Pars screw, C2, for craniocervical injuries, 84
Pavlov/Torg ratio, 165
Pediatric patients
    craniocervical injuries of, **73–90**
    subaxial cervical spine injuries in, **91–102**
    thoracolumbar spine trauma in, **103–114**
Pedicle screw placement, percutaneous, 160–161
Percutaneous kyphoplasty, 159
Percutaneous posterior segmental fixation, 158, 160–161
Percutaneous vertebroplasty, 159
Phenylephrine, for spinal cord injury, 54
Pleural effusion, with spinal cord injury, 149–150
Pluripotent stem cells, transplantation of, 58
Pneumonia, with spinal cord injury, 149–150

Pneumothorax, with spinal cord injury, 149–150
Posterior approach, to cervical spine facet repair, 132–135
Pressure ulcers, with spinal cord injury, 152
Pulmonary complications, with spinal cord injury, 149–150
Pulmonary edema, with spinal cord injury, 152
Pulmonary embolus, with spinal cord injury, 149–150

Q

Quadriplegia, transient, 164–165

R

Radiography
    for central cord syndrome, 43
    for cervical stenosis, 165
    for craniocervical injuries, 77–80
    for odontoid fractures, 116
    for subaxial cervical spine injuries, 92–95
Regeneration, after spinal cord injury, 50
Repulsive guidance molecule, in spinal cord injury, 50
Respiratory failure, with spinal cord injury, 149–150
Return to play, for athletes, **163–171**
RhoA protein, in spinal cord injury, 50
Riluzole, for spinal cord injury, 52, 55–56, 64
Robotic training strategies, for spinal cord injury, 67
ROCK, in spinal cord injury, 50

S

Sacral spine injuries, return to play after, 169
SCIWORA (spinal cord injury without radiographic abnormality)
    of cervical spine, 94
    of thoracolumbar spine, 108–109
Screw fixation
    for craniocervical injuries, 82–86
    for odontoid fractures, 118–120
    for thoracolumbar junction burst fractures, **139–145**
    percutaneous, 160–161
Seat belts
    design of, 104
    thoracolumbar trauma due to, 106–107
Semiphorin, in spinal cord injury, 50
Shock, with spinal cord injury, 152
Skin complications, with spinal cord injury, 151
Skull fractures, with spinal cord injury, 148
Slipped vertebral apophysis injury, 105–106
Slow vehicle crushing injury, of thoracolumbar spine, 107
Spinal cord, monitoring of, intraoperative, 99
Spinal cord injury
    craniocervical, **73–90**

epidemiology of, 147
imaging for, 6–8
incidence of, 49
initial assessment of, 32–33
mechanisms of, 49–51
non-neurologic outcomes and, 35–36
pathophysiology of, 31–32
primary, 49–51
secondary, 49–51
socioeconomic burden of, 31
stages of, 49–51
timing of surgery after, **31–39**
treatment of
    cellular transplantation, 56–58
    combination, 57
    complications of, **147–155**
    historic clinical trials, 51–54
    neuroprotective, 52–56, 63–64
    neuroregenerative, 53
    options for, 51
with central cord syndrome, 34–35
with thoracolumbar junction burst fractures,
    139–145
Spinal cord injury without radiographic abnormality
    (SCIWORA)
of cervical spine, 94
of thoracolumbar spine, 108–109
Spinal trauma
    burst fractures, 24, **103–114, 139–145**
    central cord injury, **41–47**
    cervical spine, facet, **125–137**
    complications of, **147–155**
    craniocervical, **73–90**
    imaging for, **1–21**
    in pediatric patients, **73–114**
    minimally invasive treatment of, **157–162**
    odontoid fractures, **115–123**
    pharmacologic treatment of, **49–62**
    restorative treatment of, **63–71**
    return to play after, **163–171**
    subaxial cervical, **91–102**
    thoracolumbar, **103–114**
        classification of, **23–29**
    timing of surgery after, **31–39**
Spine Trauma Study Group, 93–94
Spondylolisthesis/spondylosis, 107–108, 167–168
STASCIS (Surgical Timing in Acute Spinal Cord Injury
    Study), 33–34, 36
Stem cells, transplantation of, 58, 65–66
Stingers, 164
Stress fractures
    sacral spine, 169
    thoracic spine, 166
Subaxial cervical spine injuries, **91–102**
    anatomy of, 91–92
    biomechanics of, 91–92
    complications of, 99

epidemiology of, 92
evaluation of, 92–95
facet, **125–137**
outcomes of, 99–100
patterns of, 92
treatment of, 95–99
Subaxial Cervical Spine Injury Classification, 93–94,
    126–127
Substance abuse, with spinal cord injury, 153
SUN13817, for spinal cord injury, 56
Supratentorial changes, in spinal cord injury, 16
Susceptibility-weighted imaging, 14
Swann cell transplantation, for spinal cord injury, 64

T

Thoracic spine injuries, return to play after, 166–167
Thoracolumbar Injury Classification Scores, 109–110
Thoracolumbar Injury Classification System, 25–26
Thoracolumbar junction, burst fractures of, **139–145**
Thoracolumbar spine trauma, **103–114**
    classification of, **23–29**, 109–110
        AOSpine Thoracolumbar Spine Injury
            Classification System (2013), 25–28
        historical, 23–24
        Thoracolumbar Injury Classification System,
          25–26
        three-column, 24–25
        two-column, 24–25
    developmental aspects of, 103–104
    epidemiology of, risk 104
    outcomes of, 111–112
    risk factors for, 104
    SCIWORA, 108–109
    treatment of, 109–111
    types of, 104–108
Thorascopy, for thoracolumbar junction burst
    fractures, **139–145**
Three-column classification, of thoracolumbar
    trauma, 24–25
Thrombocytopenia, with spinal cord injury, 150–151
Thyrotropin-releasing hormone, for spinal cord injury,
    51, 53
Traction, for cervical spine facet injuries, 132
Transarticular screw, C1-C2, for craniocervical
    injuries, 83
Translaminar screw, C2, for craniocervical injuries, 84
Translational atlantoaxial subluxation, 75
Transplantation, cellular, 56–58, 64–66
Trilazad mesylate, for spinal cord injury, 54–55
Two-column classification, of thoracolumbar trauma,
    24–25

U

Ulcers, pressure, with spinal cord injury, 152
Unilateral cervical spine facet injuries, 131

Urinary incontinence, with spinal cord injury, 153
Urinary tract infections, with spinal cord injury, 153

V

Vaccaro classification, of thoracolumbar trauma, 25–26
Vascular injury
    imaging for, 10
    with spinal cord injury, 148
Vasoactive agents, for spinal cord injury, 54
Vasopressors, for spinal cord injury, 52

Vasospasm, in spinal cord injury, 50
Ventral fixation, for odontoid fractures, 118–119
Vertebral apophysis fractures, of thoracolumbar spine, 105–106
Vertebroplasty, 158–159

W

Watson-Jones classification, of thoracolumbar trauma, 23
Wire fixation, for craniocervical injuries, 86

Printed and bound by CPI Group (UK) Ltd, Croydon, CR0 4YY

08/05/2025

01864696-0013